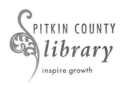

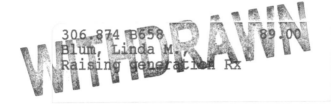

RAISING GENERATION RX

Raising Generation Rx

*Mothering Kids with Invisible Disabilities
in an Age of Inequality*

Linda M. Blum

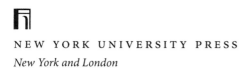

NEW YORK UNIVERSITY PRESS
New York and London

NEW YORK UNIVERSITY PRESS
New York and London
www.nyupress.org

References to Internet websites (URLs) were accurate at the time of writing.
Neither the author nor New York University Press is responsible for URLs that
may have expired or changed since the manuscript was prepared.

Library of Congress Cataloging-in-Publication Data
Blum, Linda M.
Raising generation Rx : mothering kids with invisible disabilities in an age of inequality /
Linda M. Blum.
pages cm
Includes bibliographical references and index.
ISBN 978-1-4798-9187-0 (cl : alk. paper) — ISBN 978-1-4798-7154-4 (pb : alk. paper)
1. Mothers of children with disabilities—United States. 2. Parents of attention-deficit-dis-
ordered children—United States. 3. Parents of children with disabilities—United States. 4.
Mother and child—United States. I. Title.
HQ759.913.B58   2015
306.874'3—dc23   2014040533

New York University Press books are printed on acid-free paper,
and their binding materials are chosen for strength and durability.
We strive to use environmentally responsible suppliers and materials
to the greatest extent possible in publishing our books.

Manufactured in the United States of America

10 9 8 7 6 5 4 3 2 1

Also available as an ebook

CONTENTS

LIST OF TABLES

ACKNOWLEDGMENTS

This project has been with me over a long stretch, from my own years of active mothering to finding myself a middle-aged, menopausal empty-nester. There have been many important sources of support and inspiration along the way, particularly my family and my son Saul Tobin; and though much too late for their help, my beloved graduate-school mentors Michael Burawoy and Arlie Hochschild. I am thankful beyond words for the women who so generously shared their experiences of stigma and isolation. I hope my rendering does justice to their stories and I apologize for taking so long. I also thank the many fictive kin, dear friends, colleagues, and students who encouraged me to keep moving forward, especially Winn Wheeler.

Nena Stracuzzi, when a graduate student at the University of New Hampshire, first started me thinking about the ubiquity of invisible disorders and psychiatric medications and the need to put gender at the center of this story—and the Center for the Humanities at the University of New Hampshire provided the fellowship which made much of the fieldwork and initial analysis possible. UNH graduate students Jennifer Esala, Carol Linsted, and Jennifer Vanderminden provided much-needed research assistance and collegiality; and UNH fellow faculty members Jeany Elson, Rebecca Glauber, Sharyn Potter, and Julia Rodriguez were wonderful all-around sounding boards.

New colleagues at Northeastern University as well as members of the body/embodiment working groups at NEU and at the Centre for Gender Research at Uppsala University, Sweden, offered just the right combination of enthusiasm, probing questions, and e-mailed citations—and the best advice for finishing came from my women colleagues, "We *like* short conclusions!" NEU graduate research assistant Estye Fenton went above and beyond; our numerous conversations honed my thinking about dense statistical relationships and contemporary advice literature. Katrina Uhly also deserves thanks for organizing the bibliography in record time, as does Constance Smith for offering insights on cover design. The interest of audiences at San Diego State University, Texas A&M, the University of Virginia, and the Race and Gender, Capital and State symposium at University of California, Irvine, was more than heartening—as are the friendship of far-flung colleagues Susan Markens, Andrea Press, Jennifer Reich, Victoria Gonzalez-Rivera, and many others from the extended family of Berkeley sociology. Anonymous reviewers as well as editors of earlier pieces that appeared in *Gender & Society*, *Signs*, and the edited collection *Vulnerable Bodies/Embodied Boundaries* improved my arguments in many ways, as did, in the final innings, anonymous reviewers for NYU Press and the editorial savvy of Ilene Kalish. But I am forever indebted to Vicki Smith, Roger Tobin, and Joan Wolf for slogging through drafts of each of these chapters—often more than once—in heroic acts of care, intelligence, and patience.

1

Mother-Child Troubles, Past and Present

In the kid world, too nice equals way nerdy; in the grown-up world, too naughty translates to, well, Ritalin. Below are the holiday season's best ways to keep pint-size characters stylish and happy, whether they're strolling the primrose path, walking on the wild side—or caroming back and forth.
—Ellen Tien, "Don't Make Santa Guess, Dress the Part,"
Sunday Styles, *New York Times*, November 25, 2007

The breakfast buffet at Camp Echo starts at a picnic table covered in gingham-patterned oil cloth. Here, children jostle for their morning medications: Zoloft for depression, Abilify for bipolar disorder . . . and a host of medications for attention deficit disorder. . . . The dispensing of pills and pancakes is over in minutes, all part of a typical day at a typical sleep-away camp in the Catskills.
—Jane Gross, "Checklist for Camp: Bug Spray. Sunscreen. Pills," *New York Times*, July 16, 2006

Every book has a moment of conception, even if the period of gestation, as in this case, is a very long one. This book began as a tiny embryonic idea in 1996 when, like so many mothers of children struggling to navigate their social worlds and perhaps "caroming" between "naughty" and "nice," I scurried to pick up my second-grade son from the after-school program at our quiet suburban elementary school. Once home, he hesitated, but then burst out with his half-secret question, as if he'd learned some new "swear word" on the playground: "Mom? Sean was going, 'Your mother has ADD. *Your mother* has ADD.' *Do* you have it? What *is* it?"

Wow: *your mother has ADD.* My colleagues at work thought this was simply hilarious, the new "yo mama" of the nice white 'burbs. My own initial reaction was also to laugh, to hear it like the recurring references to ADD (or attention deficit disorder) and "pills and pancakes" among the high-status parenting fads often featured in the pages of the *New York Times* Fashion & Style section. To reassure my lanky seven-year-old, my gifted boy with his ill-defined vulnerabilities, almost without thinking I fell on the authority of neuroscience. I explained blandly that doctors think attention deficit disorder affects the brain's chemical balance and that the imbalance makes a person too jumpy and distracted to work. But I ended on an upbeat note; the imbalance can be corrected with medicine. And I tried to reassure: *if* I did have ADD, it was news to me! And it certainly hadn't posed any problems for my work. Since he was all too aware of the hours I spent holed up in my study, he seemed satisfied. Yet as I mulled it over later, I thought how simplistic my response about brain chemistry had been, when the playground chant carried layers of dense cultural meaning. The inversion of race and class disadvantage that my colleagues heard intrigued me,[1] but I also heard with this (elite?) attempt to impugn our family's respectability, a twist on boyhood rituals of shaming and taunting. Rather than explicitly targeting a peer—like the boys incessantly calling one another "retard" when I was growing up, or those decades later captured in C. J. Pascoe's ethnography incessantly calling one another "fag"[2]—"your mother has ADD" seemed to displace stigmatized difference from a boy's body to a mother's brain. This thought was, of course, troubling personally, but what did it signal about our culture if seven year-old boys hurled such labels for invisible brain imbalances and hard-wiring flaws at mothers and sons?

This book begins from the several very clearest factors signaled: the growing prevalence of diagnoses like ADD among U.S. kids, the growing cultural preoccupation with such invisible disabilities and the medications used to treat them, and the pressures and stigma mothers face in dealing with these new diagnoses and treatments. But there are also several larger factors, just behind the scenes, I believe are signaled which figure importantly in this book. First, this is a book about persistence and change in twenty-first-century U.S. families and gender arrangements. Such arrangements have been changed by the wholesale entry of mothers into the labor force and, as I will come to below, the declining opportunities for men's breadwinning. Yet this is, nonetheless, a book about how we persist in assigning mothers primary responsibility for children and the major share of blame when things go wrong. Second, this is also a book about the New Economy and the postindustrial workers it now requires, with sharp divides between its winners and losers. And third, this book is about the neoliberal ideology or belief system which undergirds this high-stakes New Economy, a belief system valuing individual over public responsibility or government protection, beliefs that have created a more challenging context for family life and childrearing in the United States today. In the chapters to follow, I continue to unravel the influence of these three interrelated social factors while moving squarely to the major project of this book: examining how mothers differently situated in this reconfigured social world navigate its institutional arenas on behalf of vulnerable children, taking personal responsibility for their entrance into a yet more perilous future.

But Why Study Mothers?

Historians instruct that mothers have consistently been thought of as the sources or carriers of their children's troubles, though how transmission has been understood has varied. Shifts in past centuries from religious to scientific worldviews relocated the source of mother-harm from the mother's tainted soul to her disordered body, and then to various conceptions of her disordered mind, some more embodied and biological than others. The valorous mother of the modern scientific era has been defined in polar opposition to such disordered, disreputable mothers. With her own fit body, mind, and moral character, she devotes herself to the promotion of her children's and thus the nation's health. She is, therefore, the source of our next generation of productive, well-adjusted citizens.

The stark normative divide between immorality and ill health on the one hand and order, fitness, and productivity on the other, serves to discipline all mothers as we perform boundary work to distance ourselves from any hint that we or our children might ever tax or pollute the community. White middle- and upper-middle-class families like my own have a distinct advantage in this boundary work, as we have the resources to promote our children's demonstrable virtue, attractiveness, and achievement; and to be blunt, our skin color distances us from the long history associating deficiency, degeneracy, and ill health with racialized others. Yet disability, at least in part, signals similar disreputable traits: the unruly and impaired child burdens the community's resources, threatens to disrupt its sense of order and safety, and raises questions about the mother's physical, mental, and moral respectability. Strikingly, we count more of the nation's children as disabled, and in forms more invisible or nebulous than in past eras, raising questions about maternal fitness in our New Economy era of global competitiveness and volatility. Simply put, can the many mothers caught up in this medicalization, many of whom administer psychoactive medications to their kids and seek added services from over-burdened schools and healthcare systems, still be considered good, respectable mothers who secure the nation's future?

I begin to answer this question by considering how a group of forty-eight mothers, widely varied in their social backgrounds and present social locations, wrestled to make sense of their children's troubles, the extent of their own responsibility, and the confusing array of treatments, services, and interventions they might pursue through the educational and medical systems to protect their children's future odds for productive citizenship. While I also observed at special-education parents meetings in several districts, conversed with many other parents, and analyzed professional and popular texts, my major argument rests on the words of the mothers with whom I spoke in greatest depth. My argument about their differences will be multilayered: nearly all the mothers attempted on their own to expertly negotiate the many maze-like obstacles of the educational and medical systems governing invisible disability, defining a mother's responsibility to be relentless in efforts to mitigate her child's issues and the stigmatized difference surrounding them. But at the same time, mothers' options for managing a high-need child were shaped by distinct yet interrelated dimensions of social privilege: their class resources,[3] whether single or married, their ethnoracial location, and the gender and race of their unruly children. Institutional and cultural sorting processes frame the perception and handling of mother-child troubles, I discovered, along these complex lines of advantage and disadvantage, sometimes in paradoxical or counterintuitive ways. With such divergent understandings of mother-child troubles, I argue that we risk masking rising inequality and our collective responsibility for New Economy divides behind newly revised forms of mother-blame.[4]

In my own swirl of emotion and intellect as a mother and feminist sociologist, I had already spent a good deal of time reading about historical understandings of causality, guilt, and children's troubles and how each new science claims to better capture how things go wrong. I discovered that older discourses about not-normal children may fade but are not quite forgotten in the face of new knowledge. In recent decades, for example, neuroscience and biological psychiatry have made important discoveries about the brain's structure and electrical-chemical processes through new drugs and imaging technologies. And several scholars have asked what happens to mother-blame with this neuroscientific turn to innate brain-based explanations for children's troubles. Each found mothers only partially absolved of the blame so predominant during the mid-twentieth-century heyday of Freudian psychiatry.[5] Freudian psychodynamic theories had centered child troubles wholly on mothers' lack of emotional fitness, most famously in Bruno Bettelheim's psychogenic, frigid or "refrigerator" mothers directly blamed for causing their children's autism.[6] And while I take this up in subsequent chapters, I discovered that lack of fitness is now more expansively, if indirectly, defined. Among those I interviewed, mothers emphasized new forms of proximate, secondary blame and self blame, not so much for causing children's troubles as for falling short of the standard of relentless expert management of a child's innate brain issues, whether differences, flaws, or imbalances.[7]

I refer to this way of thinking about children, or really each of us, as "em-brained," a useful term from sociologist Victoria Pitts-Taylor.[8] Much as I had when unthinkingly explaining ADD to my young son, it signals the neoliberal belief that the brain is an embodied object to be individually managed, manipulated, and optimized for improved productivity rather than the site of a potentially deep, self-reflective, unmanageable mind. In the case of normal and not-normal children, each mother must take on this responsibility. But to approximate this neoliberal mission, I discovered that mothers of not-normal children were compelled to master more than the new brain science, but also the highly technical domains of special-education policies and disability law, child psychiatry, an array of related professional fields, and the psychopharmacology that specializes in psychoactive medications.

In the past, mothers who lacked race or class privilege, or the protection of heterosexual marriage, had been believed most at risk for raising degenerate, unfit children. In the chapters to follow, I explore the extent to which fears of those whose offspring would pollute and burden the country are still pushed on to such other-ed women. The category of "disability" itself was originally constructed on the back of such social differences, although primarily to sort adult men into those few deserving public assistance from the larger number of the undeserving. In our era, aspects of sorting still occur in schools and for limited and increasingly stingy forms of public assistance (such as Medicaid or Supplemental Security Income), and I examine these closely in a later chapter. However, the very meaning of disability is transformed, perhaps into several meanings, with increasing numbers of children labeled with terms like ADD and ADHD (attention deficit hyperactivity disorder), other learning disorders, disorders on the autism spectrum, or with any of a host of emotional disorders now crossing all divides of privilege and advantage. In fact, the most prevalent of the invisible disabilities, ADD and ADHD, as well as the autism disorders, seem to have become more evenly distributed across levels of income over time[9]—though I will suggest that meanings and experiences vary significantly and are more stigmatizing for single mothers and those raising children of color. In the course of this research, I also learned how complicated it is to simply count, with all the invisible disabilities said to be "high in comorbidity," meaning that many kids will be diagnosed with more than one such disorder. And I learned that all invisible disabilities are subject to much clinical or diagnostic uncertainty, with neuroscience yet to find clear biomarkers even through brain imaging.[10] The frustration with uncertainty was a major theme sounded by the forty-eight mothers who shared their stories with me, widely shared across gulfs of economic and cultural resources, as will be seen in chapter 2. Even the affluent, whom I examine in chapter 3, told of shifting or conflicting diagnoses typically beginning with ADD or ADHD but then encompassing combined or different labels.[11]

In this book I examine the distinct meanings of these invisible disabilities from mothers' perspectives through a feminist sociological lens. This means, simply put, that I treat women as important, knowing subjects, allowing them as far as possible to construct their own narratives, in their own language and with their own ways of drawing from or challenging dominant discourses.[12] Moreover, rather than taking a strictly constructionist view of invisible disability that pits itself against the biomedical or neuroscientific lens, I attempt to treat invisible disabilities as both real, embodied, *and* as cultural inventions specific to our time and place. Cultural theorist Majia Nadesan similarly attributes the rise in invisible disabilities to a "dialectic of biology and culture" in which subtle differences come to matter, to be made different, only at a particular historical moment—but they are nonetheless real.[13] I am deeply indebted to those who consider burgeoning medical and neuroscientific labels less real than this, but my feminist approach cautions that we should balance such perspectives against attention to those with intensely real lived experiences.

In lengthy interviews, mothers I spoke with revealed that they were neither overreacting to the normal vicissitudes of child development nor being duped by Big Pharma,[14] evil professionals, or a high-stakes culture into blithely labeling and medicating their kids; rather, they were attending to children, not severely impaired, but only quite "precariously normal" and "liable to slip into inappropriate or problem behavior without constant vigilance."[15] At the same time, as this quote suggests, the medicalization of such "precarious normal[ity]" happens within a larger social landscape—a landscape I sketch out in this chapter—fueling the anxieties many of us have for our children's futures. If there is a cultural story I would emphasize in the fast increase of kids' invisible disabilities, it is one of these anxieties about an uncertain world in which boundaries of privilege within and outside the United States are being redrawn and perhaps only the most vigorous-brained will succeed. We might also call this confluence of factors "the age of neuroscience" for, according to cultural theorist Davi Johnson Thornton, "brain-based healthism" and "popular neuroscience [are] changing . . . ultimately, how we understand and live our lives" at a time when "having a normal brain" may no longer be enough.[16] But before I turn to this present context with its pervasive emphasis on medicalization, brain issues, and mothers' personal responsibility, I turn to an obvious question about why I have not mentioned fathers.

What about Fathers?

It may seem wrongheaded to many readers that I have not included fathers in the subtitle or core research focus of a book on families and children. I can perhaps assure some by clarifying that fathers do figure importantly in most narrative accounts of the mothers I interviewed and will not be absent in the chapters to follow. Still, I did not choose to formally interview fathers, though I met several when visiting their homes, and I observed others, if always a minority, during fieldwork at parent meetings. I do not question that fathers care deeply about their struggling children. At the same time, I rely on extensive scholarship which finds that "parenting" remains highly gendered in both material or practical and discursive dimensions.[17] From the practical responsibilities for organizing day-to-day caregiving and engaging with schools and healthcare providers, to, according to sociologist Annette Lareau, "the additional labor of getting children to protect fathers' time and space," women still carry the much larger share. In an influential study including separate in-depth interviews of fathers and mothers, combined with lengthy ethnographic observation in a subset of homes, Lareau bluntly argued that interviewing fathers posed serious methodological problems for understanding the day-to-day lives of diverse families with children. While fathers matter a great deal to their children and partners and may be contributing somewhat more caregiving than in past generations, only those "rare" single fathers or men truly sharing joint custody arrangements (or perhaps in same-sex partnerships) are even "viable sources of information on family life."[18] And much research finds that having a disabled child, whether with visible or invisible impairments, only exacerbates this gender division of labor and responsibility.[19] In any case, as Lareau acknowledged, the numbers of less involved, divorced, or never-married fathers have also increased, trends reflected among those I interviewed, with about half the mothers single parents solely responsible for managing daily life and for coordinating any help and support from fathers (see chapter 4).

Just as important, cultural representations, norms, and values still assign responsibility for children's health and well-being almost exclusively to women and mothers. Feminist scholar Joan Wolf also argues that our current neoliberal political culture only heightens mothers' privatized responsibility for children's health.[20] As I briefly explained, neoliberalism is a political culture celebrating our nation's mythic origins in virtuous entrepreneurial citizens, all of whom pulled themselves up by their own proverbial bootstraps in an unfettered free market. In this milieu, ideas of public protection and social provision come under attack for, among other ills, encouraging dependence and weakening "personal responsibility" for family life. In turn, and with skyrocketing healthcare costs, it is mothers who are exhorted to become expert in exploding sources of health information and to do all they can to minimize their children's risks for obesity, diabetes, and a range of other ills.[21] Burgeoning rates of children's invisible disabilities have led to proliferating sources of narrow expertise on these "ills" alone. And growing numbers of cultural representations of invisible disability—in films, memoirs, television shows, media accounts, and novels—center on the healing presence or tragic absence of the mother with sufficient "love, energy, effort and commitment" to redeem a family shattered by a child's disorder.[22] Put bluntly then, it is still mothers who are the primary parents and accountable for children's troubles. As such, they are my focus.

Framing Mother-Child Troubles in the Twentieth Century: Sorting Brains and Minds

As I've suggested above, troubling behavior among children is not new to our age of neuroscience, yet its contours, causes, and forms of maternal accountability have been differently understood over time, with differing complex interactions with shifting class, gender, and ethnoracial inequalities.[23] Ideas about good and bad children—just as of their reputable and disreputable mothers—often expressed both specific aspirations and fears of an era. Yet the tendency to think in binary terms—good/bad, ruly/unruly, typically developing/disordered—itself represents more continuity than change. Such stark judgments emerged from both genuine desires to help those deemed troubled and desires to protect the (seemingly) moral or natural boundaries surrounding the advantaged conditions producing those "normal" children against whom they were defined. A century ago, more specific social fears were provoked in the United States by the rise of the corporate economy and the erosion of the skilled trades, family farms, and small businesses of the past. From the mothers of the aspiring classes, the United States wanted children to be the future managers and white-collar bureaucrats to work within large organizations and expanding job hierarchies. This well-adjusted child carried forward older notions of self-control and diligence, but emphasized a new need for an outgoing, sociable personality, a shift in "character and society" sociologist David Riesman, in the classic *The Lonely Crowd*, described as the move from "inner" to "other-direction."[24] This model twentieth-century child, successful with peers as well as adults, was valued for being genial and conforming, without today's hyper-cognitive fixation on maximized brain-power.

Along with the rise of the corporate economy, aspiring classes a century ago were also threatened by rising immigration and urbanization. Cultural anxieties fixed on creating social distance or boundaries between normal children and the antisocial children deemed "lawless," delinquent, or truant. Early twentieth-century physicians initiated a medicalization of childhood, first positing that such "badness" might be illness, a biological rather than moral or religious failing with taxonomies of "congenital mental deficiency" or "encephalitis lethargica." Some labels like "moral imbecility" attempted to sort those troubled children with selective or canny intelligence from those with simple "imbecility," "idiocy," "feeble-mindedness," or "retardation"—the latter terms conveying inherently limited cognitive potential, marking a boundary still struggled over today. Enlightened and humanist in many respects, this early shift to biology was also contradictory and imbued with the eugenic and social Darwinist discourse of the era. Even liberal professionals fixated on discovering which lower-income ethnoracial groups were lower in evolutionary "fitness"—and this led to the first widespread testing of schoolchildren. Unsurprisingly, greater rates of heritable deficiency were found through new ostensibly scientific measures among children of color and immigrants.[25]

Enlightened physicians and researchers continued seeking better organic classification of troubled children throughout the century; but the biological perspective lost its stature when all it could offer was dangerous, highly experimental brain surgeries and electroshocks which few wanted to try on children or youths. By mid-century, favored taxonomies nonetheless included the "minimal brain dysfunction" or "hyperkinesis," which later became the hyperactivity now included within

ADHD. Yet it was little treated with drugs until much later. Instead, early- and mid-century reformers and emerging mental health specialists in social work, psychology, and psychiatry formed an expanding "psy sector" of the medical system, moving away from the brain as physical organ toward treating the developing subjectivity of the mind as capable of healing through better nurturance.[26] The child guidance movement, for example, with over two hundred clinics, emphasized countering the effects of bad social-emotional environments when treating juvenile delinquents and other defiant and truant youths understood through "an eclectic interpretation of causation." New mental health specialists also bolstered their professional standing by offering a new kind of treatment from Freudian psychoanalysis targeting the mind's capacity for (at least partially) conscious self-reflection; with the clinical, psychodynamic approach, women social workers tended to provide guidance and education to lower-income mothers. Those more affluent sought the men with PhDs and MDs to become the better mothers their children needed. The psy sector added additional layers to the ways that unfit mothers were understood to produce problem children; and, according to French scholar Jacques Donzelot, these captured more middle-class mothers by distinguishing children "in danger" from the "dangerous children" of the lower classes.[27] Yet, for all its mid-century influence, the psychoanalytic frame never completely supplanted the organic model and the wish for simple, effective, and inexpensive medical treatments for mental disorders.

Historian Andrea Tone has argued compellingly that this desire for simpler treatments for mental troubles drove the early market for patent medicines. And in the second half of the twentieth century after the establishment of greater medical control of such markets, it led to the rise of physician-prescribed psychoactive drugs that were strikingly gendered. First, some number of fathers striving to be the ideal corporate managers and family providers turned to Miltown, followed by a larger number of mothers struggling with suburban isolation turning to Valium, the infamous "mother's little helper" of the 1960s.[28] These unprecedented pharmaceutical success stories, each product a "wonder drug" and somewhat safer than the last, no doubt paved the way for the resurgent, more pervasive medicalization of childhood which this book seeks to explore. If it was inconceivable to treat children with brain surgery or electroshock, it became somewhat easier to conceive of administering pills to circumvent the slow, frustrating, and expensive approaches to changing the mind.

At the start of another new century, we confront mother-child troubles and another shift in "character and society" without the clarity of historical hindsight. It is hard to see what distinguishes norms for the good mother and ideal child from those of the past in this rapidly emerging age of neuroscience with its proliferating psychoactive drugs, categories for those "precariously normal," and vivid brain imagery—all three on display in a number of arresting *Time* magazine cover stories.[29] Mothers themselves never simply conform or react passively to changing ideals and normative discourses. Rather, they selectively draw from old and new cultural vocabularies as they negotiate educational and medical systems on behalf of less typical children. But we can enlarge on the social factors already enumerated that shape the range of available choices. First, to add a layer to gender and family changes mentioned earlier: we now rear children across a greater diversity of household types, in what have been termed postmodern family forms:[30] post-divorce, blended families; families depending on dual earners; small numbers of single custodial fathers, but large numbers of single- and never-married breadwinning mothers; and families of same-sex partners or LGBTQ single parents. Second, as I examine in the next chapter, neoliberal attacks on public provisioning leave mothers negotiating two systems, medical and educational, each in the grips of belt-tightening. As for the latter, though schools no longer sort on the explicit eugenic basis of a century ago, they continue to serve as gatekeepers to future opportunities while organizing children's daily lives. Moreover, as feminist scholars Allison Griffith and Dorothy Smith demonstrate, schools rely on the routine, daily labor of mothers to function,[31] and this may only increase as budgets contract. As for the medical system, managed care and other cost-containment strategies restrict the available choices for those rearing precariously normal children. Insurers, for example, prefer to cover brief, infrequent appointments to monitor medications rather than expensive long-term psychotherapy. According to the American Psychological Association, between 1997 and 2008, the number of patients receiving psychotherapy decreased by 30 percent, and in 2008 nearly 60 percent of children treated received medication alone.[32]

Finally, economic changes also reshape our ideals, fears, and social character as much as they did a century ago. Sociologists are beginning to ask how the rise of the New Economy—the decline of America's twentieth-century industrial base, replaced by technology-, information-, and service-based industries amid increased global competition—may ramp up uncertainty for our children. Some family scholars lament that, as a result, we now have more over-anxious, intrusive "helicopter parents" and "over-scheduled," over-controlled kids than ever before.[33] I would go less far in blaming individual parents. I suggest instead that if there have always been real variations in children's organic vulnerabilities and embodied temperaments, more may be pushed over the threshold into disorder by an overwrought social environment. Our use of language itself points to such an interaction, as we speak of the brain and our neuroscientific understandings through ubiquitous New Economy, new technology metaphors. Brains, like global capital markets, are said to suffer from "misfiring" synapses, "disregulated" circuitry and networks, and "quirks" in "neuronal hard-wiring."[34] And as I will show, the diffusion of such metaphors and ways of thinking about the brain definitely influence notions of valorous motherhood, putting mothers of diagnosed children at once in the vanguard and yet, at the same time, threatening that very status with a child's stigmatized, burdensome difference.

All-or-Nothing Framings of Childhood Medicalization

In subsequent chapters, I will demonstrate that most mothers I spoke with relied on multicausal explanations for their children's troubles, drawing from both neuroscientific and psychodynamic frames or discourses; some fewer number also referred to the kinds of sociocultural or economic factors I've just outlined. However, most explanations for the burgeoning of invisible disabilities circulating in popular culture pay either too much or too little attention to sociocultural context and have a similar all-or-nothing take on biomedical progress. For example, some seizing the voice of reason portray all as straightforward neuroscientific progress: due to breakthroughs, we only now begin to capture the full range and prevalence of organic imbalance that was likely always there.[35] But on the sociocultural side, I was startled by the negative portrayals of mothers, the pervasive assumptions of social privilege, and of parents' seeming willingness to reproduce it "by any means necessary." Psycho-active medications appear to be like performance-enhancing drugs for athletes, a nearly accepted method to ensure that struggling kids receive all the enrichment and cultural capital their families have to offer—from fashions to summer camps.[36] Just as in the sports world, the drugs seem to be met less with outrage than with knowing winks and clever, allitera-tive phrases like the "the dispensing of pills and pancakes." In another such instance linking child to mother, the story line for one of the main characters, Lynette, on the first season of TV megahit *Desperate House-wives* had her taking the Ritalin prescribed for her hyperactive twin boys to spoof escalated norms for stay-at-home mothers (and underscore Lynette's struggle with leaving a successful career). Whether clever or campy, the associations with social advantage are striking—as in the TV "dramedy" *Parenthood* featuring a high-functioning autistic son with over-earnest parents—with gleaming suburban homes, Botoxed, white faces, slim blonde moms, and smart, if smart-alecky kids.

Another popular variation emphasizes the increased numbers of high-powered career mothers—some include fathers, if very secondarily—selfishly medicating their kids rather than questioning the effects of this lifestyle, as in writings of conservative pundit Mary Eberstadt.[37] Left-wing media can be little different. Arianna Huffing-ton once reprimanded mothers who shuttle kids to the dermatologist, podiatrist, and orthodontist, and yet casually administer Prozac with-out full psychiatric evaluation: "Substituting the quick fix of a drug for the often frustrating reality of parenting can be a subtle form of child abuse." Pointing to social privilege, Huffington likened this "Camp Pro-zac" to the boarding schools of earlier "upper classes," each the pre-ferred way for the elite of its era to handle challenging youth. But, at the same time, Huffington worried that "forty percent of American chil-dren live without a father in the house": "how tempting" the thought of medicating kids "will seem to those overwhelmed mothers."[38] Here Huffington chided in one essay both the most and least advantaged of mothers. Distancing herself from the latter with the third-person "those overwhelmed mothers," she tapped new fears of postmodern families and older suspicions of single mothers while also accusing privileged mothers of "subtle" child abuse.

Within sociology important voices such as Peter Conrad have also rejected the biomedical account and seen children's invisible disabilities instead as part of larger trends of medicalizing many forms of deviance and ordinary troubles. Medicalization is thus all about context and cultural invention.[39] The theory of medicalization finds little unique in childhood medicalization, driven by a similar convergence of interests redefining other moral-religious issues such as alcoholism, ordinary sadness, and even short stature into treatable biomedical conditions— initially this was the province of turf-seeking medical specialists, followed by profit-driven pharmaceutical and insurance companies. The corporate interests of Big Pharma have ramped up in recent decades, with psychoactive treatments relentlessly promoted in the United States through direct-to-consumer drug advertising.[40] While this makes an anti-corporate critique very apt, the research of Conrad and related scholars focuses primarily on medical discourse and its institutional forms rather than on lived experiences at home with vulnerable children. Medicalization as an explanatory framework can therefore imply some indictment of mothers for "buying into" such cultural invention.[41] Conrad himself, in his early work observing a diagnostic clinic, had cast mothers as largely overreacting to normal, if annoying, behavior.[42] In contrast, few have actually considered through in-depth study how mothers themselves understand, actively manage, and selectively draw from or challenge the authoritative professional discourses defining their children's invisible troubles.

An insightful group of feminist scholars have begun such investigations. Jacqueline Litt, Claudia Malacrida, and Ilina Singh each studied mothers raising kids with ADHD through in-depth, qualitative interviewing, to reassert mothers' agency in the face of pervasive mother-blame. As I mentioned earlier, Singh discovered that mother blame was ubiquitous, if "reconstituted" by "brain-blame," studying thirty-nine primarily white, middle-class New England mothers.[43] Litt came to a similar conclusion, if in a very different context, studying fifteen low-income midwestern mothers.[44] Similarly Malacrida, who self-reflexively drew from her own experience, found that the thirty-four Canadian and British mothers she interviewed were confronted with "limitless culpability" by the authoritative professionals with whom they had to engage.[45] I aim to extend their work in two directions. First, I intended to capture the full scope of neuroscience and its impact by including other mild to moderate social-emotional-behavioral disorders beyond ADHD and its recommended stimulant treatment. Studying just one diagnosis, while admittedly a much clearer research design, misses the proliferation of diagnostic categories, psychopharmaceutical choices, and neuroscientific discourse itself. And my interviews suggest that for many families, ADHD and its treatment may be the starting point in a longer story of diagnostic uncertainty and varied wonder drugs. Second, none of the three pathbreaking feminist scholars attempted to disentangle the divergent meanings and experiences of medicalization across the classed, gendered, and racialized contexts in which such mothers and children live.[46]

While few take such an intersectional perspective, other public voices allow that mothers might be acting wisely when acquiescing to labels and pills—yet they return us to the flat biomedical account. Journalist Judith Warner, for example, acknowledged setting out to condemn "parents" who turned to psychopharmaceutical treatments for "'fashionable maladies' of questionable reality." Yet, after investigating the professional debates and meeting many affected mothers, she concluded that the children's issues were devastatingly real.[47] (Intriguingly, she also admitted that her previous work, *Perfect Madness: Motherhood in the Age of Anxiety*, may have been insensitive in its indictment of hypercompetitive, "winner-take-all" parenting.)[48] Similarly, the authoritative Harvard University Press tome *Medicating Children*, whose academic authors translated volumes of psychiatric research for a lay audience, struck a reassuring note, instructing as I had done with my young son, that brain disorders are no different from other chronic illnesses: we should not deny needs for psychoactive medications any more than we would deny the needs of diabetics for insulin or of asthmatics for steroid inhalers. Yet both avoid trickier ground: Warner acknowledges that mothers and families now confront an array of drugs, but she ignores the problems of diagnostic uncertainty amid aggressive marketing, which emerged as major themes in the narratives of mothers I interviewed. And Mayes, Bagwell, and Erkulwater in *Medicating Children* look no further than the stimulants like Ritalin with long safety records.[49]

In fact, this narrow focus seems a throwback. The use of Ritalin has skyrocketed since the 1990s, but so too has the use of the antidepressants like Prozac. And these two types, considered the safer first-line approaches to children's disorders, are increasingly augmented by second-line, "big-gun" approaches.[50] The latter, less familiar medications include anticonvulsant or antiseizure drugs like Depakote, Tegretol, Lamictal, and Neurontin initially developed for epilepsy; the "atypical" antipsychotics like Risperdal, Zyprexa, Seroquel, Abilify, and Geodon, developed to improve treatment of schizophrenia; and antihypertensive drugs like Clonidine, nominally for high blood pressure. Concerned specialists increasingly offer such drugs to worried parents as "mood stabilizers" for their vulnerable kids.[51]

To add to the din of competing voices confronting families, there are also those of "the non-neurotypical" who tend to sharply reject such medications and argue instead for the appreciation of neurodiversity. They are alone in embracing the reality of invisible brain differences and the neuroscientific paradigm while at the same time rejecting the core assumption that organic difference is disease. This call for a multicultural-like appreciation of brain difference can be exploited for clever, niche marketing, like the New Age websites promoting merchandise for the "Indigo Children" who are "the next step in human evolution."[52] The more sincere protests, however, have emerged from young adults reclaiming their stigmatized identities through identity-based movement discourse. Although most may identify as high functioning on the autism spectrum with Asperger syndrome, they argue, somewhat as I do, on behalf of a more inclusive umbrella for those whose differences should be honored. Their Internet-based activism could signal a new embodied social movement challenge to biomedicine like those that have arisen from survivors of HIV/AIDS, breast cancer, environmental hazards, and other toxins.[53] Yet rather than engage with psychiatry or the psy sector as other such health movements have engaged with biomedicine, the disability rights' frame of the neurodiverse repudiates the search for a cure.[54] In this sense it bears stronger resemblance to deaf community activists and scholars arguing for the autonomous culture of American Sign Language speakers.[55] The neurodiversity argument for appreciation clearly absolves mothers of blame, but sadly, it appears to be dividing those who come across it. Some mothers, particularly those with children with severe forms of autism, have responded in social media vigorously objecting to the multicultural argument. Such mothers, who are well beyond my focus on mild to moderate disorders, protest any slowing of the urgency in the search for a biomedical cure for autism, thereby provoking important philosophical or bioethical debates.[56]

Invisibility, Visibility, and Stigma

In addition to the varied theories and mother-absolving or blaming attitudes surrounding burgeoning childhood medicalization, mothers like those I interviewed also wrestled with the distinct *invisibility* of their children's troubles. This distinction between the invisibility or visibility of difference and deviance has been under-theorized in current discussions, yet it was crucial to the prominent twentieth-century sociologist Erving Goffman. In his classic *Stigma: Notes on the Management of Spoiled Identity*, Goffman argued that the routine "perceptibility" or "evidentness" of difference lay behind the original Greek concept of stigma as a way to easily convey negative social information: "The signs were cut or burnt into the body and advertised that the bearer was . . . a blemished person . . . to be avoided, especially in public places."[57] Much of his work mulls over types of invisibility, passing, and the heightened tensions in social interaction when "differentness is not immediately apparent."[58] If those with clearly visible stigma faced a lack of privacy and "displeasure in being exposed" in public, they might also more readily find "sympathetic others" than those faced with continuous, anxious decisions about the "management of undisclosed discrediting information" and "invisible failings."[59] I will demonstrate in the next chapter that, as Goffman might have predicted, the "perceptibility" or "evidentness" of traditional disability was envied by many of the mothers I came to know, who drew pained comparisons to the disregard which they and their children received and to their responsibilities for concealing, revealing, or managing discrediting information.

Most Americans, in fact, likely envision disabled children as those with visible, physical impairments like the cerebral palsy, muscular dystrophy, Down syndrome, deafness, or blindness depicted by charitable fund-raising drives. Critical disability studies, as well, has overwhelmingly focused on the visible.[60] From feminist theory and the notion of the objectifying male gaze, critical disability studies has emphasized a politics of appearance to combat "the stare" that pathologizes physical impairment.[61] Disability rights activism has similarly emphasized physical impairment and a social-antidiscrimination model that led to important legal victories and changes to built environments and public spaces.[62] Both theory and activism, however, miss much of the illusive complexity of burgeoning em-brained disorders and the experience and meaning of disability without wheelchairs, leg braces, canes, cochlear implants, signing, computer-assisted speech or prosthetic limbs. Most recently, disability studies collections have paid greater attention to autism and have highlighted issues of passing—though studies of passing still emphasize those with "visible physical impairments" coping with or deflecting "the stare."[63] During the fieldwork portion of my research, I was continually reminded of the tendency to count or consider the large number with invisible em-brained disabilities under the mantle of traditional disability (though see Leiter's treatment of "hidden disabilities" for an exception).[64] I realized, for example, that in the dozen sessions of special-education parent groups I observed, useful referrals or reference materials for psychoactive medications were *never* discussed or made scheduled topics for the monthly gatherings, though meetings often featured outside specialists on other topics. And psychoactive medication, despite its ubiquity, was almost *never* mentioned.[65] In contrast, meetings were specifically held on assistive technologies and assistive sports of less relevance for many in the groups who, as discussion often revealed, had children with invisible disorders.

Just how many children and youths might be ignored by this grouping with traditional, physical disability? I found this apparently simple question hard to answer because rates of diagnosis have been increasing faster than the generation and analysis of nationally representative surveys can keep up with—and on top of that, measures of disability vary. Demographer Dennis Hogan and his research group provide important analysis of families with disabled children, but it is drawn from a data set—the National Longitudinal Survey of Youth, 1997—with too few impaired children to disaggregate by type of disability.[66] The more focused 2005–6 National Survey of Children with Special Health Care Needs included invisible and traditional disabilities with chronic illnesses, reckoning that some 22 percent of U.S. children from birth to age eighteen were, broadly speaking, "disabled."[67] In the largest categories of invisible disabilities, the survey found 4 percent of all children diagnosed with ADD or ADHD and less than 1 percent with autism spectrum disorders, and the two together including some 3.5 million kids.[68] But the Centers for Disease Control, which updates prevalence reports more often, estimated that autism spectrum disorder diagnoses are increasing 10 to 17 percent per year, and ADHD about 5.5 percent per year. For the autism spectrum, this yielded a 2008 prevalence estimate of one in eighty-eight children (just over 1 percent),[69] and for ADHD an estimate of nearly 10 percent of those school-aged.[70] By one particularly intriguing measure, the National Institute of Mental Health estimated lifetime odds of nearly 25 percent for experiencing an "impulse-control" disorder, a term used to include ADD/ADHD as well as conduct- and oppositional-defiant disorders, but excluding autism spectrum disorders, many mood and emotional disorders, and other learning disabilities.[71] But following the CDC, perhaps the "ballpark" for school-aged kids might be somewhere around 12 percent counted with invisible disabilities.

This is, of course, a messy estimate because the educational system's categories do not completely square with biomedical diagnostic categories.[72] For example, some who might qualify for special-education programs may not be enrolled due to budgetary constraints or poor-quality services, others with mild impairments might not require educational services but be counted as medically diagnosed, and some with learning differences that require services might not have medical diagnoses (or perhaps, in this age of neuroscience, I should say such differences are not *yet medicalized*). And the high level of diagnostic uncertainty itself leads to questions of both over- *and* underdiagnoses.[73] That is, there are no blood tests for the invisible disabilities, none which capture hypothesized imbalances in neurotransmitting chemicals the way that diabetics can test for blood sugar or asthmatics for blood oxygen. There is no known genetic marker, as with Down syndrome. And to date, even the most advanced brain-imaging technologies have failed to capture hypothesized differences in brain development and activation. Most invisible disabilities are diagnosed through observation of kids from the outside and fairly subjective assessment against traits listed in the American Psychiatric Association's *Diagnostic and Statistical Manual of Mental Disorders* (*DSM*); while in its fourth edition during the time of this research, the revised fifth edition has been an object of contention, particularly because it retains such descriptive criteria for diagnosing the em-brained disorders.[74] The best assessments of the most prevalent attentional disorders, ADD and ADHD, still rely on questionnaires from parents and teachers with items from the psychiatry manual querying how fidgety and distracted a child is, how often he jumps out of his seat at school, and how often she leaves tasks unfinished.[75]

Without observable biological evidence, drug treatment itself has become a major route of diagnosis; that is, worried parents have no better, objective way to know if a drug might be suitable or called for than to test its effectiveness for post hoc confirmation. The stimulant Ritalin was approved to treat kids back in 1961, but its use was fairly limited until the 1990s, increasing in that decade by some 700 percent. In that decade the United States produced and consumed nearly 90 percent of the world's supply of the drug,[76] but trends indicate that at least Canada and Australia may be following our lead.[77] Prozac, the first of the selective serotonin reuptake inhibitor antidepressants (SSRIs), hit the U.S. market at the end of 1987, and its instant popularity among adults (mainly women) has been credited for Ritalin's surge. SSRI use for kids, in combination with stimulants like Ritalin or separately, increased between 200 to 400 percent in the 1990s. The decade also saw less steep but definite increases in the use of the "big gun" mood stabilizers—and by the end of the twentieth century, more than 6 percent of American kids were estimated to be on some form of psychotropic drug treatment, an increase from about 2.5 percent in 1987. A significant minority were on at least two such medications simultaneously.[78] No wonder that a decade into the new century, with rates still escalating, pundits began to dub this cohort of youths "Generation Rx."[79]

The 48 mothers who shared their experiences in great depth, though not randomly selected, still reflect and illuminate much of this aggregate picture.[80] Through the subsequent chapters, I will share their stories with pieces of my fieldwork observations in an effort to understand the complex processes hidden in any composite snapshot. For example, about two-thirds of the mothers had children whose diagnoses at some point had included ADD or ADHD, but as mentioned earlier, for many the attentional disorder diagnosis was only a starting point. And while about five had as yet avoided psychiatric medications, nearly all faced regular questions about whether to try, change, or add drugs, or adjust dosages. Most had developed a range of expertise across medical and educational fields; and all from the most affluent to those few in "hard-living" low-income families wrestled with questions of self-blame about whether they might still be good mothers.[81] But their ability to draw boundaries and distance themselves from truly bad mothers with hopelessly burdensome children depended in large part on the familial economic and cultural resources they could marshal.

How are the truly bad, the most stigmatized portrayed in the age of neuroscience? Although I began from an observation of the pervasive social advantage in much popular discussion of mothers and invisibly disabled kids, I should add that we also find very stark contrasts, cautionary tales from the other extreme of the economic spectrum. Affluent mothers may pack their kids off to "Camp Prozac," but the few stories of hard-living low-income mothers who drug their kids instruct us of deeper moral wrong, ominously recapitulating the demonization of other mothers. Beginning at Christmastime in 2006, the New England media followed such a morality tale in the tragic death of four-year-old Rebecca Riley. The young girl had been diagnosed with ADHD and then bipolar disorder by specialists at a leading research university, a diagnosis she shared with two school-aged siblings. Her parents, graduates of a local area high school, were charged with murder for knowingly administering lethal doses of the Clonidine, Depakote, and Seroquel prescribed to calm Rebecca's tantrums.[82] Though white and married, Carolyn Riley in other ways conformed to stereotype: unemployed, living in subsidized housing, she allegedly had her children diagnosed and medicated only to qualify for more SSI, the Supplemental Security Income for the indigent disabled on which she and her husband survived.[83] At trial she was convicted of second-degree murder, after being portrayed as routinely putting the needs of a violent, child-abusing husband above those of her own children.[84] While her husband was convicted of first-degree murder, this did little to counter the horrific image of a parasitic mother who would heavily drug her babies only to increase the size of her government checks.

In contrast, the portrayal of the professional-managerial class might make mothers out to be too anxious about their kids' achievement or too caught up with competitive display and their own careers—but the consequences for medicated kids are hardly portrayed as life-threatening or as a drain on society. Even in accounts of the thriving black markets in ADHD drugs like Ritalin, or "Vitamin R" as it is called in the nation's high schools and colleges, the privileged subtext speaks loudly: these kids are in affluent high schools in Advanced Placement courses or are excelling at selective colleges and universities. Such "straight-arrow" kids may use psychoactive drugs illegally, but only to comply with class-specific demands for high achievement and productivity. And their mothers are neither indicted nor condemned.[85]

Gendering Disorder and Disability

While I have spoken at length about the gender binary still dividing parenting in both its practical and cultural aspects, I have neglected until now the obvious point that norms and ideals for successful, well-adjusted children—and the bad children they are defined against—are also deeply gendered, if in historically shaped ways. A century ago with manhood unquestionably based on breadwinning, ideals for well-adjusted, "outer-directed" children primarily addressed boys to steer them toward future productive citizenship within large bureaucratic organizations.[86] Boys were, as a result, also more vulnerable to contrasting charges of unruliness than girls, whose "badness" and "goodness" were defined in terms of the private sphere and sexual respectability. The child guidance clinics, for example, overwhelmingly treated the boys or young men whose delinquency rates threatened law and order and the docility of the next blue-collar labor force.[87] In our era, boys' troubles are far more likely to be medicalized than are those of girls. And the current binary en-gendering of disorder recapitulates that of a century ago, though ramped up at significantly higher prevalence and reconstituted around traits desired in the New Economy. Today boys are over twice as likely as girls to receive diagnoses of ADHD and three times more likely to be on stimulant medications.[88] Boys are also four to five times more likely to be labeled with an autism spectrum disorder.[89] Girls begin to converge in rates of medication in the high school years but still remain lower, and their diagnoses and drugs are primarily for depression and eating disorders.[90] The drugs themselves take on a gendered character, like the earlier generation of psychoactives. Countless ads and occasional cartoons depict Ritalin and the stimulants for boys and the Prozac-type SSRIs for girls, each pill bringing youths closer to newly desired forms of productive citizenship still divided in binary terms.

The category of disability itself was originally, a century ago, a gendered category, defined through norms of honorable manhood, masculine embodiment, and the reliance of an industrial nation on manly breadwinning labor. As such, the first federal government programs to assist disabled men were Veterans Benefits and Workmen's Compensation; together with the first forms of welfare, these programs also assisted the widows of the honorable soldiers and workers who had not survived. Both forms of public assistance were stingy and intent on helping only the truly deserving—for widows this meant proving they were chaste and keeping a "suitable home"; for men this meant proving they were neither feigning impairment nor shirking their own responsibility for injuries. Unions and veterans organizations won some concessions over time, but claims of men of color tended to be dismissed, their injuries blamed on either "congenital weakness" or "willful misconduct."[91] Moreover, early confusion in defining and measuring impairment in some ways prefigured today's diagnostic uncertainty with invisible disability. The original Veterans Benefits and Workmen's Compensation policies were written for starkly evident, embodied impairments, for the amputee or cripple, the blind or tubercular.[92] But the standard Goffman termed "perceptibility" was quickly modified to recognize at least the worst of those with trauma and shell shock among World War I veterans.[93] This recognition of honorable soldiers was still on a small scale compared to our current era; disability now seems a nearly ubiquitous label, though still with meanings influenced by race, class, and gender.

Today's threats to manhood and manly wholeness stem less from war than from economic restructuring[94]—and these threats are enormous, with one major magazine cover story and the attention-grabbing book which followed simply declaring, "The End of Men."[95] Decades of industrial decline, followed by the "Great Recession" and the burst of the housing bubble in 2008, have gutted the numbers of manly breadwinning jobs at the core of the U.S. economy. And journalist and author of "The End of Men" Hanna Rosin readily employed the neuroscience paradigm and computer-brain metaphors to describe this transformation of gender and economy. She noted, for example, that men might have been evolutionarily "hardwired" for "the drive to win on Wall Street" while women were similarly "programmed" to "more-nurturing and more-flexible behavior," with postindustrial jobs demanding much more of the latter. Also alluding to young men's lack of em-brained fitness for our age, Rosin further argued "the attributes that are most valuable today—social intelligence, open communication, the ability to sit still and focus—are, at minimum, *not* predominantly male."[96]

Sociologist Michael Kimmel, who specializes in understanding masculinity and changing norms for men, has also linked "massive" economic restructuring and the rise of millions of dead-end service-sector jobs to new forms of vulnerability among young men who had expected middle-class opportunities.[97] Kimmel's analysis, like Rosin's, reminds us that the transformation was well underway before the 2008 recession, exemplified by the several decades since the nation's largest private employer had shifted from General Motors to Walmart. Many jobs moved offshore to Latin America, Asia, and India, and by one estimate, the ability of the New Economy to generate jobs any better than those at Walmart had declined by 25 to 30 percent in the quarter century before the 2008 crisis. In short, young men raised to be manly providers and productive citizens instead face uncertainty, more and more contingent jobs, and the entrepreneurial pressures of neoliberalism to get out and create their own opportunities. With the increasingly rapid circulation of global capital and embrace of market volatility, some innovations and start-ups have and will continue to pay off—but on the whole, economic gains, as the Occupy Wall Street activists emphasized, tend to benefit the "One Percent."[98] The young college-aged and twenty-something men in Kimmel's study are either adrift in the extended adolescence of "Guyland" or scrambling for increasingly rare spots in finance, high-tech, and elite professions.[99] If we were to do a new "character and society" study in the same vein as the 1948 classic *The Lonely Crowd*, we would notice New Economy neoliberalism and its mantra of personal responsibility everywhere, with incessant advice to be flexible and creative, to market yourself, embrace change, and (my personal favorite) educate yourself for the jobs that don't yet exist.[100]

In fact, several child psychiatrists have written that the degree of economic uncertainty and neoliberal pressure surrounding all of us—if they do not precisely use such sociological jargon—produce a specifically toxic "ADD-ogenic" culture. Working parents pressured by "high stress, long hours, and a perform-or-else mentality" cannot help but carry this volatility home; and if their patience is further tried by a sensitive, highly reactive child, a child with temperamental or genetic vulnerabilities, this spiraling of stress might well exacerbate the child's issues, also, over time, more negatively influencing brain chemistry.[101] And with the highest rates of childhood medicalization around the globe, we do have a singularly harsh brand of postindustrial capitalism, as no other advanced nation works its parents as much or cushions them less.[102] This lack of public policy support for working families might also influence our higher marriage "metabolism," burning through marital and cohabiting partners faster and exposing kids to more stressful household disruption.[103]

I find such multicausal or interactive frameworks most useful because they do not make neurochemistry our destiny apart from culture and the institutions shaping family life, though sometimes the arguments are a bit overheated or hyperbolic. However, most also ignore the prominence of gendered norms, the great gulf in expectations dividing mothers from fathers, and sons from daughters, at the center of the story—a point obvious to sociologist Kimmel. Though mothers' responsibilities for invisible disabilities were not the topic of his investigation of young men adrift, he sees "guys" lacking clear routes to masculine adulthood, "disconnected" from fathers' guidance and suppressing the feminine emotionality that threaten to make them "mama's boys": "No wonder boys drop out of school and are diagnosed as emotionally disturbed four times as often as girls, get into fights twice as often, and are six times more likely than girls to be diagnosed with Attention Deficit and Hyperactivity Disorder."[104]

To be clear, postindustrial restructuring and its ADD-ogenic culture have not and cannot alone cause children's troubles, as of course is evident in the large majority of children who are resilient in the face of all kinds of family stress. But the line between kids expressing "normal" stress and "pathology" may not be as sharp as those in the flat biomedical camp describe,[105] particularly when most diagnosed kids fall into the mild, moderate, or high-functioning range of impairment which I focus on in this book.[106] If they are exquisitely attuned to their psychosocial environments, and if (as medicalization critics assert) we are primed to interpret their distress as disability, perhaps increasing numbers fall or are pushed over the threshold into special needs. Moreover, as a group of cultural studies scholars studying autism instruct, it is no coincidence that such invisible troubles fuel "an epidemic" of worry about boys just when manly status is so destabilized.[107] In contrast—and back to all-or-nothing frames—some neuropsychologists posit that autism, particularly at the high-functioning end, is caused solely by an "extreme male brain" "hard-wired" in utero by prenatal hormones, a hotly contested, shaky hypothesis even in the biomedical paradigm.[108] But to cultural theorist Majia Holmer Nadesan the debate itself signals our fascination with technical, engineering prowess and the current "'crisis' of masculinity."[109] Nadesan, who coined the term "dialectic of biology and culture," suggests we construct high-functioning autism as "an alien form of intelligence that is simultaneously seductive and threatening." For her, popular speculation that Albert Einstein, Isaac Newton, and Bill Gates might have been afflicted by Asperger syndrome reflects an unspoken assumption that such "men must pay for their inherent technical/analytical superiority."[110]

Nadesan's insights might be extended, at least in part, to the broader category of mild to moderate invisible disability which forms the heart of my analysis. In line with the advocates of neurodiversity, "geeky" or "alien" intelligence may rescue some youths with what Nadesan describes as "an eccentric but *potentially productive* cognitive style, a cognitive style most found in *men*."[111] I add that this may tend to benefit young men, largely those in affluent white families, while redoubling the responsibilities of their mothers to cultivate their potential for this twenty-first-century productive citizenship. If neurodiversity may rescue such young men, however, its ubiquity may also threaten the gender binary and push mothers to intensify their efforts to police boundaries of gender and heterosexuality. As both Kimmel and cultural studies scholar Stuart Murray suggest, boys and young men with invisible disability signal feminine vulnerability and violate norms for tough, manly heterosexuality.[112] And what of the minority of girls diagnosed with invisible disabilities? While the jury is still out on whether the differential rates rest on any neurological or biogenetic foundation, I will argue, extending the arguments of Nadesan and Murray, that these rates may rest on the "neurodiverse" girls' lack of cultural intelligibility at the present moment.[113] Mothers of vulnerable girls—a minority among those I interviewed as well as on the national level—face somewhat different challenges from those of vulnerable boys, particularly in a culture still obsessed with maintaining gender as a binary divide.

Those with wildly different political views may nonetheless share deep anxieties about future gender relations and the boundaries of gender and sexuality called into question by our "epidemic" of vulnerable boys. And many may wish in some deep-seated way that mothers alone might resolve these fears by producing the flexible, hyper-cognitive, yet manly sons who can restore the ailing U.S. opportunity structure and shaky global dominance. Prominent conservatives' alarm that invisible disabilities pathologize "boyhood" and are tied to women's rejection of domesticity may come closest to revealing such wishes. Scholars like Francis Fukuyama and George Will tend to blame feminism for these gendered family changes and argue for a return to industrial-era nuclear families and women's full-time homemaking to heal them. They also claim that Ritalin—which Phyllis Schlafly dubbed "kiddie cocaine"— makes boys behave more like girls, furthering a "feminist conspiracy" and "androgyny agenda."[114] Thomas Sowell wrote similarly that ADHD is an attempt to alter "natural male traits" through "repression, re-education, and Ritalin."[115] Conservative radio pundit Michael Savage extended this to autism spectrum disorders when he argued every "kid" with autism is just "a brat who hasn't been told to cut the act out." His solution? Tell them: "Don't act like a moron. You'll get nowhere in life." And: "Straighten up. Act Like a *Man*."[116]

Motherhood in a Risk Culture: "Personal Responsibility" in the Age of Neuroscience

Though conservatives may lay the blame on a feminist "androgyny agenda" and argue for private solutions to burgeoning childhood disabilities, they are little different on that score from many liberal voices—all in one way or another, from Mary Eberstadt and Rush Limbaugh to Arianna Huffington and Judith Warner, expect mothers to understand, love, nurture, and find a way to control, help, or cure these kids largely on their own. From a sociological perspective, however, additional public factors extend from economic uncertainty to constrain mothers' abilities to offer such care. Notably, squeezed educational and medical systems, on top of ADD-ogenic workplaces, make it unreasonable to see mothers' efforts as simply the result of their good or bad private choices. In the next chapter, I will illustrate one of the main arguments of this book: across widely varied social backgrounds and locations, it was difficult for all the mothers I came to know to navigate such constrained institutions on behalf of highly reactive children. This was particularly the case because each tackled multiple bureaucratic obstacles and expert knowledges so privately. While only a quarter of those I interviewed were full-time homemakers with time for such demanding care work,[117] nearly all were pushed into becoming what I will term vigilantes on lone quests for justice when institutions had largely failed their kids. Vigilante is, I admit, an imperfect metaphor for mothers who were neither reckless nor violent (nor men); but nearly all seized authority and took "the law" into their own hands, engaging with and often challenging multiply credentialed professionals as they stood guard to protect their families.

In fact, cultural theorists might see the reversion to private solutions for invisible disability itself as one of many expressions of pervasive neoliberalism and our "risk culture"—a culture particularly burdensome for mothers and caregivers. Neoliberalism, the nation-state's corollary to New Economy entrepreneurialism, valorizes independence, small government, and the free market, while demanding that each citizen take extensive "personal responsibility" for all life outcomes, from wealth and poverty to health and illness.[118] With assisted reproduction, organ transplantation, imaging technologies, and genetic testing—as well as psychopharmaceuticals, steroids, Viagra, and human growth hormone—"risk culture" promotes the sense that all life down to the cellular level may be manipulated, planned, and controlled much like a consumer should make purchasing decisions. Good citizens should thus make disciplined risk assessments and appropriate health choices for themselves, but maternal citizens must also do this for family members. As feminist scholar Joan Wolf explains, "What is new in risk culture is not the centrality of care to maternal citizenship, but the scope and complexity of that responsibility . . . and the reach and precision of the sciences on which demands of mothers are founded."[119]

Neuroscience is clearly at the center of this neoliberal imperative, with mothers now confronted with a plethora of advice on the fragility

and intricacy of the children's brains, which they are personally responsible to nurture and manage.[120] From *Brain Rules for Babies* (2010), to
The Whole-Brain Child (2012) or *Welcome to Your Child's Brain* (2011),
to *The Science of Parenting: How Today's Brain Research Can Help You
Raise Happy, Emotionally Balanced Children* (2006), mothers read that
their "parenting can dramatically determine whether or not your child's
brain systems and brain chemistries are activated in such a way as to
enable him to enjoy a rich and rewarding life."[121] Even the relatively sedate American Academy of Pediatrics publication *Caring for Your Baby
and Young Child*, a perennial best seller, provides detailed advice in its
fifth edition for stimulating brain growth; its authors advise that all children, those with and without "disabilities and other special healthcare
needs[,] . . . greatly benefit from close monitoring of early brain development."[122] In our risk culture, good mothers simply must be fluent in
the new brain sciences. Infants may come "preloaded with lots of software in their neural hard drives," but it falls to their mothers, each on
her own, to learn to monitor, activate, stimulate, and maximize the potential in her child's very individualized "wiring."[123]

I will also detail how navigating the educational system is experienced as each mother's "personal responsibility," an isolated task on behalf of vulnerable children regardless of social advantage or privilege.
Education remains one of our major, unquestioned public rights, but
neoliberal belt-tightening and the accountability movement have had a
major impact, changing education in ways that even the more affluent
cannot entirely escape. Mothers of vulnerable kids confront educational
authorities with pleas for more at a time of less, for diverse learning
models at a time of standardization, and for buffering from competitive pressures while, increasingly, children too must "perform or else."
Moreover, all the mothers I spoke with, across wide divides of class and
race privilege, faced with their disordered kids some degree of stigma in
schools. As social researchers at Indiana University discovered, over 20
percent of Americans across class lines admit that they would prefer that
invisibly disabled kids' were *not* in the classroom with their children or
making friends with them.[124]

If these difficulties in navigating the education system weren't enough,
mothers whose kids have invisible, ill-defined needs are thrown deeply
into the U.S. healthcare system at a tense moment. Perhaps some years

from now, new generations of parents will no longer confront the maze
of private insurers and HMOs, barely able to decode the extent of their
families' coverage let alone the array of emerging hyper-specialized fields.
But for now we're left with the fact that pills are cheaper, more profitable,
and a relatively quick fix compared to labor-intensive forms of one-on-
one or family therapies, or to the multimodal approaches incorporating
such practices with medications that have been found to be most effective.[125] There are also many less legitimated alternatives to sort through,
such as those from complementary medicine. The *New York Times* estimated, for example, that as many as two-thirds of children with ADHD
have used some form of alternative, nondrug treatment, often in tandem with psychopharmaceuticals and/or psychotherapies. These range
from vitamins, fish oils, herbs, or diet changes to biofeedback, massage,
yoga, and then to numerous interactive software packages, leaving "parents" basically on their own to sort the useful from the fads and outright
fraudulent: "The challenge is to find a doctor who will help explore the
range of options."[126] As I found among the forty-eight mothers I came
to know, each mother is left to research and patch together potentially
helpful therapies, treatments, and wonder drugs on her own, as she is to
research and patch together the insurance or other funds to cover the
many expenses. Such mothers experience most harshly the imperative
that they alone must engage deeply with neuroscience to minimize all
risks and maximize all health outcomes for their children.

In contrast to the near consensus across popular and scholarly discourse on the newness of childhood medicalization and neoliberal risk
culture, researcher Ilina Singh has provocatively asked whether medicating the child is so different from past eras which endorsed medicating the mother. Mothers today may dispense wonder drugs to kids,
but in earlier generations many depended on "mother's little helpers" to
live up to gendered family ideals and to produce normatively gendered
children. Singh intends to underscore that we have yet to hold fathers,
other family caregivers, or communities responsible for child and family
well-being—a contention with which I largely agree.[127] Yet the changes
in wonder drugs governed by authoritative new brain discourses, and
the vastly increased usage among children as well as mothers, express
and contribute to important changes in gender relations and the form of
maternal responsibilities.

Plan of the Book

I begin my analysis of diverse mothers by emphasizing what all or nearly all of those I interviewed shared: the need to negotiate two systems in the grip of economic austerity, with authority over invisible disability divided, at times arbitrarily, between medical and educational systems. Having to take "personal responsibility" for managing a vulnerable, burdensome child propelled mothers to become vigilantes, painstakingly acquiring expertise to locate possible ameliorative services and treatments when many such sources were hidden. Because they do this in a culture surrounded with old and new forms of mother-blame, I scrutinize the difference good or even good-enough social support and marital partners might make to mothers across wide divides of economic and cultural resources. I also explore the extent to which mothers, managing needy kids often on top of paid work and busy households, turned to psychoactive medication themselves, under duress from the stigma and fear of contagion surrounding their kids' less perceptible disabilities.

In the third chapter, I turn to those mothers with the most social class advantage in terms of income, educational backgrounds, and familial economic and cultural capital. I ask how such mothers, protected from the worst of postindustrial volatility, understood their children's troubles amid forms of mother-blame, finding that their resources helped less than I might have guessed to escape the stigma of invisible disorder within schools and neighborhoods. Their resources may have helped to ease the navigation of the medical system, though even those few full-time homemakers with high-earning husbands and supportive kin struggled with diagnostic uncertainty, the fragmentation of expertise, and the side effects of psychoactive medications. I discovered that for affluent mothers the imperative to ensure the transmission of class advantage and cultural capital to their children while also engaging in vigilant management of a child with special needs created several paradoxes, not the least of which was placing considerable strain on marriages. In short, their lives were far from the easy images of "Camp Prozac."

For the many women who are single mothers, as I show in chapter 4, more time at home often comes at a sharp cost to financial security. Nonetheless, it is a sacrifice some with high-need children make, though the chapter will demonstrate that, among those single mothers I interviewed, households and work-family strategies varied and often demonstrated remarkable strengths. I argue that such mothers, on the whole, faced greater stigma and suspicion of their maternal fitness. While free of the burden of a husband's prerogative or demands, they faced the double blow of burdensome children and the lack of public legitimation that a legal husband and father in the home still provides. This was evident in narratives of relentless vigilance navigating educational and medical systems, though having class resources and race privilege mitigated some of the illegitimacy of being outside heterosexual marriage. Institutional sorting on class and ethnoracial lines was most evident for those compelled to engage with the state, either for meager public resources, or because suspicions of maternal unfitness provoked surveillance by child protective services. This process, while most challenging for single mothers of color, was not without irony: meager public support can be an escape from relentless isolation and can sometimes make more services available for managing a high-need child.

In chapter 5 I return to the centrality of gender in understanding and sorting troubled children, developing the line of argument begun in this introductory chapter that, both in statistical prevalence and cultural understandings, invisible disability is about boys, and the threatened or disabled masculinity of our current historical moment. I examine the frustration expressed by mothers as they attempt to strengthen vulnerable young sons' embodied masculinity and physical sense of assurance in the face of stigmatization and bullying. I also take up the distinct vantage point of the much smaller subgroup of mothers raising daughters with invisible disabilities. I argue that they wrestle with greater layers of invisibility negotiating for treatments and services precisely because of the lack of cultural intelligibility of such similarly disordered girls. At the same time, however, I explore whether experiences and understandings of a vulnerable child's stigma, bullying, or harassment differ significantly between mothers of sons and of daughters. And I show that the greater invisibility of troubled daughters may pose a paradoxical benefit in the face of the zero-tolerance policies for school aggression that ensnare many vulnerable boys.

In chapter 6 I hone in on the sixteen mothers among those I interviewed raising children of color. Several raised questions and unprompted concerns about the extent to which their vulnerable children had fared worse because they were "Black"—the term they supplied most often for a range of more specific ethnoracial identities, such as "Black Honduran," "Afro-American/American Indian," biracial, and African American. While their concerns varied, from having sons unnecessarily labeled, to having medications pushed too hard, to being denied much-wanted special-ed services, their stories help us make sense of the larger context of racialization surrounding invisible disabilities. Paradoxically, boys of color are *more* likely than either girls of color or white Euro-American boys to be labeled with invisible disabilities, but they are much *less* likely than white Euro-American boys to be treated with psychiatric medications.[128] I argue that the mothers of vulnerable children of color in my research group demonstrated a complex ambivalence toward such childhood medicalization, sometimes challenging and sometimes reluctantly acquiescing to pressure from schools still engaged in racial sorting. Rather than simply being ill-informed, lacking access to care, or carrying cultural difference—explanations most often posed by aggregated psychiatric studies of the lower medication rates—I found that such mothers were, if anything, more vigilant in managing vulnerable kids. This was particularly true for those with sons of color, sons most likely to be cast as dangerous and truly bad,[129] though I suggest this was partially mitigated if mothers could shrewdly marshal class resources.

The final chapter, "Mothers, Children, and Families in a Precarious Time," will summarize the book's multidimensional argument: while it is difficult for all mothers to manage sons and daughters labeled with invisible disorders, disability itself comes to have multiple meanings inflected by class, race, and gender and is likely to perpetuate inequality based on these dimensions. To be a good neoliberal mother, taking extensive personal responsibility for the health of one's family also means vigilantly monitoring and maximizing children's brain development, working relentlessly to resolve or ameliorate innate flaws and imbalances. This demand is particularly heightened by the emphasis on brain power in an information- and innovation-based economy, and conscious and unconscious fears for boys, for manly status and for preserving the gender binary itself. Mothers of disordered children may thus represent a moral vanguard in the age of neuroscience, with their heightened attentiveness to changed forms of productive citizenship—but those raising children outside of heterosexual marriage or without class and race privilege are still more easily cast as suspect or even monstrous mothers.

2

"Welcome to Your Child's Brain"

Mothers Managing Dense Bureaucracies, Medications, and Stigma

When I first met Charlotte Sperling, a long-married mother whose three invisibly disordered sons were nearly grown, she announced that she was reading books on the adult ADHD brain and had concluded her husband, too, must suffer from the disorder. Charlotte lamented that her oldest son spoke often of his "bad brain"—and she referred to her own position in the family, managing four disordered males, as "brain central": "Like I don't have to be just my brain, I have to be the kids' brains, but I have to be my husband's brain too . . . I am *so* tired of being everybody's brain and not feeling like there's a point at which it's going to stop." During the course of this research, I was continually struck by such images of the brain as a sort of coordinating bodily super-organ, an object for which mothers were directly responsible—though few painted images as vivid as Charlotte's. These images circulated in mothers' talk about their troubled kids and in the popular sources of information they turned to, with the brain now distinct from the mind, the latter the site (or potential, emerging site) of self-reflexive intelligence and the very sense of being a subject. Though certainly not the only way in which mothers spoke about their volatile children, mothers clearly took on the responsibility to know this object. When I spoke with Cassie Mueller, for example, who managed just one volatile young son, she said she was in the midst of reading *A User's Guide to the Brain*.[1] And Lucia Santos was reading about alternatives to medications for her young son: "This teacher, a great, great teacher in the middle school recommended fish oil, it helps the brain he recommended that before we talk about medication. And I agree with him." Indeed, I recognized nearly all the mothers I had come to know and their arduous efforts to understand and manage vulnerable kids in the apt title of a recent best seller, *Welcome to Your Child's Brain*.[2]

In this chapter I emphasize that the forty-eight women I interviewed shared this experience across wide gulfs of economic and cultural resources, work and household situations. Nearly all took to heart being good neoliberal mothers, engaging with neuroscience, trying on their own to make sense of the inner workings of their children's brains and painstakingly educating themselves to negotiate with authoritative professionals on their children's behalf. They did this all with trying, unpredictable daily challenges, with kids prone to excessive impulsiveness, irritability, frustration, and tantrums. If the mothers did not all describe themselves like Charlotte Sperling as their families' "brain central," all were carrying heavy care burdens, compelled to navigate at home as well as in educational and medical systems without maps, compasses, or GPS devices. I discovered that nearly all the mothers reported difficulty identifying and locating the increasingly fragmented specialty fields providing services and treatments within and across these two systems: not only pediatricians, special-ed teachers, and school counselors, but also child psychiatrists, speech and language pathologists, occupational and cognitive behavior therapists, varieties of private tutors and reading specialists, psychologists, family therapists and clinical social workers, neurologists, neuropsychological evaluators, pediatric psychopharmacologists, and more. Because fragmented specializations were so hidden within large impersonal organizations subject to strict cost controls—and each woman was left to search out what she hoped might be most appropriate for her child largely on her own and then to ferret out the necessary referrals, forms, and documentation—I refer to these institutional settings as dense bureaucracies. I will illustrate how these bureaucracies have become dense or more irrational through turf wars concerning who has more professional authority over the invisible brain disabilities—and I will share fieldwork observations at special-ed parent meetings to illuminate these irrationalities, augmenting the insights of the mothers.

This chapter will also detail the stigma shared across wide gulfs of social advantage and disadvantage by mothers and their invisibly disabled children. All reported some degree of taint from a child's disturbing difference. In addition to the social isolation and marital strains created by such stigma, I will also explore the complicated ways in which the lack of visibility or "evidentness" of a child's troubles may create more shame and disgrace for mothers than if their children had been visibly, and thus some felt legitimately, disabled. But before I turn to the dense bureaucracies and mothers' sense of stigma, let me briefly introduce those I interviewed.

The Mothers Themselves

Between 2003 and 2008 I used several strategies to recruit women who might share with me their stories of raising kids with invisible special needs:[3] I was given names by several school contacts who first asked mothers if they might be interested; I placed announcements in several relevant newsletters; I approached some at the parents meetings I observed in three public-school districts and at one parents night at an independent special-needs day school; and I utilized snowball techniques, asking mothers for names of relevant friends or neighbors. Of the final forty-eight women, twenty-one were married, twenty-three were single, and four were in some stage of divorcing.[4] Thirty-three were employed, the majority full time, and fifteen were full-time homemakers. Seventeen women had low household incomes, near or below the poverty level; another twenty-one were roughly middle level, with household incomes between $35,000 and $70,000 per year; and ten had high incomes of $100,000 a year or more. While only twelve among those I interviewed were women of color, four of the thirty-six white Euro-American mothers were raising children of color, three from interracial relationships and one who had adopted an African American son. The interviews themselves ranged from two and a half to five hours and I conducted them all face-to-face, though we had always communicated first by phone and e-mail, sometimes a good deal. Most of the interviews were conducted in women's homes, and the longer narratives over multiple visits; but a few women preferred I take them out for coffee or join them at a restaurant, and one took me to a nearby park where I proceeded to get a nasty sunburn and a record number of bug bites over a long afternoon. I had additional contact with a few mothers over the years by e-mail and phone. And along the way I was informed by numerous shorter conversations with mothers unable to spare the time for lengthy interviews, as well as by conversations with staff at three independent special-needs day schools, and most important, by participant observation at a dozen public-school special-ed parents meetings. The latter were divided among three districts: one affluent and white, two largely working-class and ethnoracially diverse. While subsequent chapters, each looking at only a subgroup of mothers, will hopefully provide readers with some sense of the interviewees as particular individuals—sharing moments of themselves as funny, knowing, tired or upbeat, angry, sarcastic, optimistic or sad—this chapter will in some sense run roughshod in demonstrating what all shared. But I offer a summary of the household circumstances of each of the forty-eight women in tables 2.1 and 2.2.[5]

Caught between Educational and Medical Systems

At the present moment, authority over invisible disabilities is divided somewhat arbitrarily between medical and educational systems. Schools deliver many ameliorative services through special ed—occupational, physical, or speech and language therapy, social pragmatics or social skills groups, math and reading tutors, aides for inclusion in regular-ed classrooms, and work with school counselors or psychologists. Children must often have formal medical diagnoses to be eligible—though this is not always the case for impairments not (or not yet) considered "medical" such as dyslexia and related learning disorders—but this is an increasingly blurry distinction when all such impairments ostensibly involve brain processes and functioning. Mothers, in the meantime, attempt to learn the rules of two systems torn by competing objectives. Both educators and healthcare professionals gain authority from expanding expertise into this burgeoning market, but each system pushes responsibility away when budgets are at issue. Mothers are left to scramble between school meetings and doctors' offices, between calls to health insurance providers, psy-sector mental health professionals,[6] and special-ed directors.

Both the educational and the medical systems are dense bureaucracies, seemingly impenetrable, in which mothers discover layers and layers of impersonal rules, forms to be filled out, signatures or approvals to be obtained, half-hidden offices or phone numbers to be located. Providers are often so specialized or in such newly emerging subfields that treatment for vulnerable children is fragmented within

TABLE 2.1. The Forty-Eight Mothers Who Shared Their Stories with Me: A Glance at Their Diversity by Income, Household, and Ethnoracial Location

Income	Married (21)	Separated/Divorcing (4)	Single (23)
High income	Angie Thompson	Abby Martin	
	Colleen Janeway		
	Elaine Irving		
	Gabriella Ramos-Garza		
	Judith Lowenthal		
	Molly Greer		
	Sandra Barbieri		
	Theresa Kelleher		
	Virginia Caldwell-Starret		
Middle income	Blayne Gregorson	Jenny Tedeschi	Brooke Donnelly
	Charlotte Sperling	Kelly Caruthers	*Cara Withers*
	Faith Prenniker		Donna Simon
	Hermalina Riega		*Dory Buchanan*
	Lucy Nguyen		Kay Raso
	Meg O'Toole		Lenore Savage
	Renee Riverton		*Marika Booth*
	Rosemary Hardesty		*May Royce*
			Nora Jorgenson
			Shauna Lapine
			Susan Atkinson
Low income	Heather Dunn	Louise Richardson	Barbara Donato
	Lucia Santos		Beverly (Bev) Peterson
	Marilyn Chester		*Caron Ross*
	Rosa Branca		Cassie Mueller
			Greta Roigerson
			Jerri Dougherty
			Joann McGinnis
			Leesha Baker
			Mildred Andujar
			Patricia Gwarten
			Rhonda Salter
			Vivian Kotler

Note: **Women of color raising children of color** (12); **white women raising children of color** (4); white women raising white children (32).

TABLE 2.2. The Forty-Eight Mothers Who Shared Their Stories with Me: Detailed Information

Mothers	# Kids	Focal Child (FC)	FC Age	$$$	Educ.	Hshld.	Race	Emply.	How Contacted
Abby Martin	Two	Jessica	12	High	Post-grad.	Divorcing	White	Full	Snowball
Angie Thompson	Two	Spencer	14	High	2 yr. coll.	Married	White	Prt.	Private school 2
Barbara Donato	Four	Craig	12	Low	H.s.	Single	White	Prt.	Snowball
Bev Peterson	Two	Natalie	16	Low	H.s.	Single	White	Hmmk.	NH high-risk prgrm.
Blayne Gregorson	Two	Brandon	13	Mid	2 yr. coll.	Married	White	Full	Private school 3
Brooke Donnelly	One	Taylor	5	Mid	Post-grad.	Single	White	Full	Newsletter
Cara Withers	Two	Michael	12	Mid	4 yr. coll. +	Single	**Af. Carr.**	Full	Private school 3
Caron Ross	Two	Rashaun	18	Low	1 yr. coll.	Single	**Af. Carr.**	Hmmk.	Private school 1
Cassie Mueller	One	Ned	9	Low	Post-grad.	Single	White	Prt.	Snowball
Charlotte Sperling	Three	Timothy Daniel Isaac	22 20 18	Mid	4 yr. coll. +	Married	White	Prt.	Snowball
Colleen Janeway	Four	James	12	High	4 yr. coll.	Married	White	Hmmk.	Private school 2
Donna Simon	Three	Lynn Ann	20 18	Mid	2 yr. coll.	Single	White	Full	Private school 1
Dory Buchanan	Two	Khari	4.5	Mid	Post-grad.	Single	White/ FC **Af. Amer.**	Full	Public school 1
Elaine Irving	Two	Micah	11	High	Post-grad.	Married	White	Prt.	Private school 2
Faith Prenniker	One	Miller	12	Mid	2 yr. coll.	Married	White	Full	Snowball
Gabriella Ramos-Garza	Two	Diego	4	High	Post-grad.	Married	**Latina**	Full	Snowball
Greta Roigerson	Three	Paul	18	Low	H.s.	Single	White	Prt.	Private School 1
Heather Dunn	Two	Jared, Terry	11 9	Low	H.s.	Married	White	Hmmk.	Public school 1

Mothers	# Kids	Focal Child (FC)	FC Age	$$$	Educ.	Hshld.	Race	Emply.	How Contacted
Hermalina Riega	Three	Mateo	6	Mid	2 yr. coll.	Married	**Black/ Latina Centrl. Amer.**	Full	Latino org.
Jenny Tedeschi	One	Will	13	Mid	4 yr. coll.	Divorcing	White	Prt.	Private school 1
Jerri Dougherty	Three	Carl	18	Low	H.s.	Single	White	Prt.	NH high-risk prgrm.
Joann McGinnis	One	Thomas	15	Low	H.s.	Single	White/ FC **Black**	Hm./DS	NH high-risk prgrm.
Judith Lowenthal	Four	Allan	12	High	4 yr. coll.	Married	White	Hmmk.	Snowball
Kay Raso	One	David	13	Mid	4 yr. coll.	Single	White	Full	Private school 2
Kelly Caruthers	One	Stacey	13	Mid	1 yr. coll.	Divorcing	White	Full	Private school 1
Leesha Baker	Three	Dion	11	Low	H.s.	Single	**Af. Amer.**	Hm./DS	Private school 1
Lenore Savage	Two	Noah	17	Mid	Post-grad.	Single	White	Full	Private school 1
Louise Richardson	Five	Eric	16	Low	H.s.	Divorcing	White	Full	Private school 1
Lucia Santos*	Three	Grace Carlos Eduardo	18 14 13	Low	H.s.	Married	**Latina/ Puerto Rican**	Prt.	Latino org.
Lucy Nguyen	Two	Ken	17	Mid	H.s.	Married	Wh/FC biracial **Viet./ white**	Hmmk.	Private school 1
Marika Booth	One	Geneva	15	Mid	H.s.	Single	**Af. Amer./ Amer. Indian**	Full	Public school 2
Marilyn Chester	Three	Drake	15	Low	H.s.	Married	White	Hm./DS	NH high-risk prgrm.
May Royce	One	Robert	8	Mid	Post-grad.	Single	**Cape Verdean**	Full	Public school 3
Meg O'Toole	Four	Ryan	17	Mid	3 yr. coll.	Married	White	Full	Public school 1

TABLE 2.2. (*Continued*)

TABLE 2.2. (Continued)

Mothers	# Kids	Focal Child (FC)	FC Age	$$$	Educ.	Hshld.	Race	Emply.	How Contacted
Mildred Andujar*	Two	Gil	7	Low	1 yr. coll.	Single	**Latina/ Domini-can**	Prt.	Latino org.
Molly Greer	Two	Andrea	12	High	2 yr. coll.	Married	White	Prt.	Public school 1
Nora Jorgenson	Two	Stephen	11	Mid	Post-grad.	Single	White	Prt	Snowball
Patricia Gwarten	One	Jacob	6	Low	1 yr. coll.	Single	**Af. Amer.**	Prt.	Public school 1
Renee Riverton	Two	Bobby	21	Mid	2 yr. coll.	Married	White	Prt.	Snowball
Rhonda Salter	Four	Rachael	15	Low	H.s.	Single	White	Hm./DS	NH high-risk prgrm.
Rosa Branca	Four plus two step.	Frank Justin	20, 19	Low	H.s.	Married	**Black/ Hondu-ran**	Hmmk.	Snowball
Rosemary Hardesty	Three	Josh	16	Mid	2 yr. coll.	Married	White	Full	Private school 1
Sandra Barbieri	Three	Chris	10	High	2 yr. coll.	Married	White	Full	Private school 2
Shauna Lapine	Three	Leo	12	Mid	Post-grad	Single	White	Prt.	Snowball
Susan Atkinson	Two	Mary	12	Mid	4 yr. coll.	Single	White	Hmmk.	Private school 2
Theresa Kelleher	Two	Colin	10	High	Post-grad.	Married	White	Hmmk.	Private school 3
Virginia Caldwell-Starret	One	Henry	6	High	Post-grad.	Married	**Af. Amer.**	Full	Snowball
Vivian Kotler	One	Isabel	12	Low	4 yr. coll.	Single	White/ FC biracial **Af. Amer./ white**	Hmmk.	Private school 1

Note: In a few instances I modified details to protect interviewees' confidentiality. All names are pseudonyms except in two cases (*) in which participants requested their names be used. Interviews occurred between 2003 and 2008, averaging two and a half to four hours, most in women's homes, with some over more than one visit. Nonwhite racial identification is indicated by boldface, using the identifications mothers supplied. Employment is indicated as fulltime, parttime, (fulltime) homemaker, or at home and on disability (DS). The three public school special-ed parent meetings at which I met many of the mothers are coded as: 1 = a diverse urban district, 2 = a diverse suburban district, 3 = a white affluent district. All private schools were special-needs day schools with some whose tuition was paid by public districts.

and across organizations, with only mothers to research and coordinate each potentially helpful piece of expertise. In his qualitative study of how family caregivers cope with mental illness, sociologist David Karp described such exhausting dealings as "bureaucratic gymnastics," explaining that he, "an intelligent enough person," would find his "eyes glaz[ing] over" each time conversations turned to the complexities of gaining private insurance, public coverage, or access to treatment. "Caregivers," he poignantly emphasized, "become ensnared in a bewildering and endless maze of paper, policies, [and] unanswered telephone calls."[7]

Many I interviewed explained that just to start seeking eligibility for assistance in school required weeks, even months of phone calls to coordinate an initial evaluation from a psy specialist who might be located on either the ed or med side—months in which a "normal-looking" child was left to struggle with peers, schoolwork, and frustrated or overwhelmed teachers. Theresa Kelleher, whose son in the second grade was barely interacting with other kids, explained that she was on wait lists for months for a child psychiatrist on the med side, finally seeing someone "two weeks before school got out." Because Theresa and her husband had chosen to purchase a home in a wealthy school district, she had been taken aback by foot-dragging on the ed side as well: "I'd requested a core [evaluation] in October . . . they sent the forms in December, and we didn't get the results until March. Pretty much the whole school year had gone by!" Other married women reported the same frustration. Sandra Barbieri, who resided in a solidly middle-class town, described hounding her son's school for eight months before they conducted his core evaluation. Blayne Gregorson exemplified the frustration and extra care burden which this medical-educational divide creates:

> Brandon [who frustrated easily and was prone to prolonged tantrums], he needed an evaluation. But pursuing that through normal [school] channels, there was a six- to eight-month wait. So I went ahead and just booked it at St. Joseph's [Hospital]. So who was going to pay? It's from three to five thousand dollars . . . Call the HMO for the "medical reasons," the town for the "learning" piece. I had to call the pediatrician to get a referral, but I could not say "educational," no, no, no. I have to say the problem is "medical" or we're back to square one!

Blayne did have one key source of support, a woman psychotherapist, to coach her through these confusing impersonal channels: "The psychologist became my advocate. She said to use certain words, you could get further." But Blayne had gone through an arduous effort just to gain access to this sympathetic expert by wresting information out of her pediatrician's practice. Moreover, cultivating the psychotherapist's sympathy represented, at least in part, a commodified, instrumental transaction involving significant insurance payments and copayments as opposed to any reciprocal relation of shared support or any larger collective or community responsibility for children's troubles.

While Blayne, with two years of college, had been successful in this instance, Dory Buchanan was having less success despite a master's degree in education. Like Blayne, she could not wait months for the school to evaluate her four-year-old son while the prekindergarten teachers complained about his loud, disruptive behavior and the school district denied more therapeutic services. Dory explained that she acted on her own, as Khari, adopted out of foster care, could be "fast-tracked at Children's [Hospital]" with the Department of Social Services picking up the bill. But then Dory was caught unprepared when the school system rejected the evaluation, an obviously medical account calling for a costly full-day inclusion program for Khari. "How could they reject it?" I asked naively. "None of those doctor reports counted because they're from doctors, not *educators*," Dory mimicked sarcastically.

Just so no reader will think it is only the educational system trying to shirk costly responsibilities, I can also supply tales in which the medical system was as difficult to manage. Gabriella Ramos-Garza, for example, was seeking a diagnosis through the medical system for her younger child, a bright boy with subtle speech delays given to irritability and tantrums. With high earnings and excellent benefits, Gabriella had consulted numerous specialists, neurologists, psychologists, geneticists, even allergists—yet none was able to definitively explain why, "for some reason, his brain just works differently." And then her medical insurance denied coverage for a $900 autism evaluation: "They had a *fit* with the autism evaluation. They didn't want to pay for it. They were like, 'Oh, that's *not medical.*'"[8]

I heard a most astute assessment of the medical-educational turf war from a mother at one of the special-education parents meetings I observed.[9] It was a particularly frustrating meeting in which the town's special-ed director was addressing the school system's shrinking budgets. The two dozen parents in attendance, primarily mothers, inquired about paraprofessionals and discussed relative costs for more occupational, speech, and language therapy for their kids. The special-ed director vigorously responded, "Why come to us? Those are *medical* needs. Why should the schools have to provide for *medical* needs?" Finally, an astute mother spoke up: "Look, we know the schools are stretched. We don't like it; we have typically developing kids too. But in the U.S. today we don't have the *right* to medical care. We *do* still have the right to a public education." She was correct that privatized medical care combined with public education has been the "American way" for over a century; and even if political contention over President Obama's healthcare reform leaves it more or less intact, we will still be left with a largely privatized, competitive system of care providers rather than the universal access of European or Canadian national healthcare.[10] In the United States, however, the right of universal access to publicly provided primary and secondary education has not eroded and in fact was enhanced by late twentieth-century disability rights legislation: Section 504 of the Vocational Rehabilitation Act (1973) prohibited discrimination against disabled children in public education; and more recently, the Individuals with Disabilities Education Act (1990) positively mandated that children with certified disabilities, if not making "effective" academic progress, must receive "appropriate" services in the "least restrictive" environment possible.

Special-ed parent advisory councils (PACs) such as those I observed were often mandated by state disability rights legislation and would seem to provide a "natural," already-existing location for stigmatized mothers to find genuine non-commodified community and support in navigating educational and medical systems. But my fieldwork in New England suggests that such community may be unusual. I found it surprisingly difficult to locate groups and their monthly drop-in, informational meetings. It seemed I was not alone as I overheard comments like this from a young mother who had traveled over an hour on a cold, snowy night: "There's no PAC in my town—or I can't find it. I thought there was, but I can't find it." (Similarly, several of my interviewees reported that PAC groups were helpful, but that they had been years into dealing with special ed before learning such groups even existed.) On another night I drove for an hour, after a string of phone calls and e-mails, to find a desultory group of five at an urban PAC meeting; the mother-volunteer who led the group explained that she had simply not had time to circulate an announcement (she had dragooned instead a co-leader and a few stalwarts to come out to meet me).[11] I discovered from such mothers that confidentiality rules prohibit systematic outreach to eligible families, that sole reliance on mother-volunteers to run PACs leaves some districts un- or underserved, and that public notices buried within regular-ed announcements assume some insider knowledge. For example, I had at first embarked on this research assuming that "advisory councils" were elected bodies with closed monthly evening meetings. I only subsequently stumbled into finding that PACs are open to all on a drop-in basis.

In addition, because PACs were originally mandated before the burgeoning of invisible disabilities, based on a traditional model of disabilities as unambiguous and often severe, mothers of children with mild to moderate invisible disabilities might wonder if they are included or welcomed. Strikingly, the two or three mother-volunteers leading each of the three public-school PACs I observed (each in a different district) had children either physically disabled or with full-spectrum autism rather than a mild to moderate disorder. One of my interviewees who lived in another district (Lucy Nguyen) raised precisely this issue, unprompted, observing that she felt bad to speak of her son's ADHD when the PAC leader was dealing with a severely impaired child. Once, however, when I attempted to ask the co-leaders in an affluent town if they saw a distinction or could speak to the needs of other, less visible disabilities, they seemed quick to understand, with one nodding to the others sympathetically, "oh, she means if a kid can pass." And often in the meetings I observed, either a cursory sweep around the room for introductions or later questions revealed at least some number whose kids were diagnosed with more moderate social-emotional and learning disorders.

"Raise the Bar on Being a Parent Professional": Into the Ed System

Nearly all the monthly PAC meetings I observed were structured for rapid-fire delivery of information by a guest expert. I felt that we parents, again primarily mothers, were there to be schooled to comply with the bureaucratic demands of special ed rather than to find support or community: we each sat hurriedly taking notes, scanning multiple handouts and PowerPoint slides, with little time to engage one another. Not surprisingly, many I attempted to speak with as the meetings broke up admitted they had attended only once or twice and weren't likely to return.

A few mothers, like Blayne Gregorson, spoke quite positively of their weekly parent support groups; but these, I learned, were within independent special-needs day schools and were organized just for those families with children attending, largely for noninstrumental or therapeutic purposes. Ironically, such already existing, institutionally provided locations of support were only for those who had *already* gained entry to a more supportive setting. In contrast, the overwhelming majority of families with struggling kids will remain in a public-school setting simply because special-needs independent day schools can cost as much as private colleges. And those few who fight successfully to have an "out of district" placement funded by the local district,[12] as Blayne Gregorson had, are likely to have experienced their most distressing years prior to gaining entry. Blayne, in fact, had described years of painful isolation.

For the mothers of disordered children remaining in public school, as for most of those I met, contestation over needs occurs in writing the Individual Education Plan (IEP). This is the contract for specific services and accommodations for each eligible child required by disability legislation to be drawn up by a "team" including school personnel and parents. I discovered that the entire IEP process was arduous, more obscure and ongoing than I might have guessed.[13] Though parents are promised a voice, most mothers I spoke with were angered by the "team" rhetoric and described their meetings as surprisingly adversarial. Most found it hard to get full commitments for services in writing or to get regular follow-up to ensure services were implemented. Even a privileged mother like Theresa Kelleher, who had been an elite finance professional before resigning to deal with son Colin's needs, was intimidated facing some half-dozen school personnel:

> I did not really know what to ask for. . . . I have no idea about [child] development . . . I'm not a psychologist. I wasn't a, you know, physician, and I wasn't a teacher of special ed, or any of this. . . . I thought all these

people are taking care of my child, that's *their job*. . . . [But] I was so naive and idealistic . . . I never thought people would put cost over children's needs.

A local journalist explained why even mothers like Theresa in wealthier districts are not made more aware of available special-ed options: when schools are "stretched" and educational funds embattled, communities tend to resent legal entitlements for "budget-buster" kids in special ed.[14] (A PAC co-leader in another area once offered me her own sarcastic explanation: within such dense bureaucracies, district administrators don't even know themselves what's available from one school to the next.) Moreover, the if-not-making "effective [academic] progress" standard for services leaves much room for interpretation and, as several mothers told me, lowered expectations. I heard more about this from Rhonda Salter, in night school to complete her high school equivalency degree and trying to secure more help for a dyslexic daughter:

> They always say "Parents are a valued member of the IEP team"—but as a parent, if you argue, then OK, you're the Uncooperative Parent. I've actually had that written on reports . . . For them to develop a plan is really easy. Getting them to carry out the plan, *all* of the plan, is the hardest part. They want you to read the IEP, ask a few nice questions, and then go away.

Molly Greer, another with a bright daughter frustrated by dyslexia and ADD, had considerably more economic resources to call upon and eventually hired an attorney to gain full compliance from the local school district. At a later PAC meeting, I learned that this can easily run between $20,000 to $30,000, with an initial $3,000 to $5,000 just for an attorney to look over the records (perhaps as a very partial substitute, both PACs in the less affluent districts I visited had invited educational attorneys in to field questions). Molly confirmed Rhonda's assessment of dealing with the school without such commodified expert support: "You're at a complete disadvantage at that team meeting, completely."

What was required of mothers in team meetings, and how easily their expectations for a child might be manipulated or lowered, was vividly displayed in one of the monthly special-ed parent meetings I observed, this one in a diverse, largely working-class district with some creeping gentrification. An informational session on effective communication within the IEP process, it was offered fairly routinely in the region by a local nonprofit, the Federation for Children with Special Needs, and was part of its training for educational advocates. Such advocates—who charge much less than attorneys, but can still ask for several thousand dollars to prepare and attend team meetings—add to the fragmentation of expertise which mothers negotiate, and at the same time further commodify and privatize social support. At the effective communication meeting I observed, an advocate regaled us while seemingly unaware of the irony:

> I strongly recommend that you bring someone to the meeting with you. I had someone calling me the other day, "I want to hire you to come with me. Can you do it?" I'm like, "I really don't want to overbook. Do you have someone [else]?" . . . But she's new to the state, no relatives here, no friends yet. I said, "Do you have a dog?" She laughingly turned to us and announced, "If all else fails, bring your dog!"

At this same meeting, the advocate barraged us with advice seemingly impossible to follow without paid professional help. She chastised us never to go into an IEP meeting without the latest information on our child's specific disability, written objectives for the following year in the classroom with appropriate assessment measures for each, a five-year vision statement, and a grasp of what was covered under both state and federal disability law. There was also a distinct message that this gathering of extensive expert information was every good mother's personal responsibility: "If there's something you don't understand in a report, have it explained *before* the meeting. Go to a reliable source. Call the clinician, the OT, the PT, the speech and language therapist. I have a friend who's an OT, another who's a PT. I'll still call them." She went so far as to suggest that each of us become a legal expert:[15] "I'm the type of person, I bring the federal legislation to the beach with me to read. So know your laws. Peruse the laws you expect to be coming up at the meeting. . . . Raise the bar on being a parent professional. They'll listen to you more effectively if you know the relevant legislation." In several role-play exercises, we were further instructed never to agree to inadequate services through "power plays" by school officials. Yet we had been emphatically advised to avoid being confrontational, to "take the olive branch, acknowledge we're part of the problem."

Several in attendance resisted this last message that "we're part of the problem." For example, subsequently when asked, "What as a parent makes it difficult to communicate?" two women and one of the few men in the room shifted the responsibility decidedly to school officials: "When they're not returning my calls"; when they use "the technical terms"; and "when they won't tell you what [services] are available." Our presenter ignored these comments and marched ahead, prodding us to take back our responsibility, to "raise the bar" on ourselves, by writing "EMOTIONS" with a felt-tip marker up on a large pad of white paper. She next asked a young, eager-looking mother, "Katie," to share her feelings: "Do you mind, since you're about to have your first team meeting?" What followed was a striking interaction in which Katie sounded as if she was well informed rather than "part of the problem." This is the exchange as recorded in my fieldnotes:

Katie: OK, no, I don't mind. Well . . . it turns out the early intervention person can't be there. I thought she'd be there, that there'd be someone on my side.

Advocate: So you're ANGRY? [Writing ANGER up next to EMOTIONS.] So what else?

Katie: Well, I took the course [a related PAC workshop] on basic rights. I read on the Internet. I've talked to other parents. We have the diagnosis autism. I'm worried, will it be appropriate services?

Advocate: Confusion?

Katie: Yeah, what are the services available? They won't tell me. I want [my daughter] to have full-time appropriate placement. We want a year-round ABA [Applied Behavior Analysis] program. She's not ready for an integrated program yet, but she turns three this summer, so starting then.

Advocate: Oh, it's often difficult. We don't really know what our child needs. We can't be experts on every disability . . . but sometimes anger, anger at having a disabled child, shifts to a sense of entitlement, to a demand to fix it. And it can't be fixed.

Despite the advocate's repeated misreading of her comments, Katie evidenced little confusion. While she may have been angry on some level at having a disabled child, the decision to request Applied Behavior Analysis was quite clear and legitimate—ABA is not uncontroversial and may not be every family's choice, but the intensive behavior modification program is widely recommended. And rather than raising unreasonable demands, Katie acknowledged that her toddler was "not ready for an integrated program yet" (such intervention programs are small preschool classes with highly trained teachers integrating three- and four-year-olds with special needs with a small number who are typically developing). The young mother's desire for a "full-time" or "year-round" program demonstrated further clarity and reasonableness; in fact, research finds that two years of "year-round" ABA at preschool age improves odds for success in a regular-ed classroom later on.[16] The advocate's comment, "We can't be experts on *every* disability," while hitting a sympathetic note, was oddly dissonant with a mother who seemed to be very well informed about her daughter's autism. It also seemed to contradict her own (the advocate's) emphasis throughout the evening, that you must become an expert and "raise the bar on being a parent professional."[17] And sadly, throughout the interaction the educational consultant failed to hear anything of the educational system's irrationality, its lack of support, its withholding of crucial information.

Individual mothers at the present moment might have little choice but to "raise the bar" on their individual efforts to ameliorate a child's issues. To mobilize greater political support for much-maligned special-ed budgets seems at best a long-run project. While a few valiant mothers I met at the urban PAC meetings were attempting to challenge city leaders, this only increased their already heavy care burden (and evidently had cut into their ability to sustain the PAC itself). Moreover, mothers must attend to their high-need children in the present and cannot put off seeking possible help for longer range institutional or cultural change. Most had a sense of urgency that, as one (Susan Atkinson) explained to me, each additional humiliation at school or explosive episode and "meltdown" at home only added more painful "scar tissue" to the original brain differences. Even those lucky few who find their way to PAC meetings may find only mixed messages of support, with the formal presentations reiterating the need for strictly individual, nearly overwhelming forms of maternal accountability.

I did observe moments that seemed like genuinely mutual support at the PAC meetings—for example, on the secrecy of special-ed services— but these were almost in spite of the meeting's planned program. When Katie had complained that she could not find what services were available in her outlying district, recounting that "they *won't* tell me," I overheard another knowingly nod and whisper out of range of the speaker, "Our town has great services, *if* you can find them." At another PAC, I observed two mothers sharing similar complaints of secrecy about what one might request for a child; one was caustic as her companion nodded in agreement about district personnel: "They just lie!" Yet the predominant takeaway message was clear: any worthy mother can overcome this on her own (and without being so confrontational). A handout I picked up offering "Eight Rules of Advocacy" for parents distilled this neoliberal wisdom in the eighth and final rule: "Do it yourself."[18]

Two of the dozen PAC meetings I observed were geared directly to mothers (and the few fathers, partners, or other caregivers who attended) of kids with invisible disabilities, organized to introduce neuroscientific terms and new specialty fields with the very latest thinking about brain disorders. These two monthly sessions were also the best attended. At the first a "psychoeducational diagnostician" in private practice, according to a handout, would "unravel the mysteries of cognitive/ psychological, neuropsychological, and academic tests." The handout also noted her master's degree in education. She initially informed us as she began her presentation:

> Neuropsychological assessment is hot. Everybody wants it. It includes the WISC [Wechsler Intelligence Scale for Children, one of several commonly used IQ tests] *but* it's a way of *thinking* about the tests. *Why* are they performing as they do? It's a way of thinking about behavior with the brain in mind.

Next she drew on a white board, diagramming four regions of the brain with intersecting circles: the "planning, organizing" and "self-correcting" "Executive Function" was on top, "Language" and "Visual-Spatial" were to each side, with "Memory" on the bottom. She also introduced the term "cortical" with an arrow down to the "subcortical" region. In a vigorous question-and-answer session among some twenty-five women and perhaps three men crowding the room, many of the questions had to do with brain functions, "word retrieval," "motor planning," "auditory processing." The main gist of each was, as one mother queried bluntly, "Can you fix that?" The specialist's mixed responses— for example, "brain function is *hard* to change though the nice thing about brains is they do develop"—seemed to reflect both the many unanswered questions about the brain's plasticity and the wish to protect parents from unrealistic expectations.[19] Several questions then took a different tack, concerned with managing the arbitrary divide between educational and medical systems and understanding the jurisdiction of our speaker's narrow specialization. For example, one mother asked, "But if you want a diagnosis, do you have to see *someone else* with an MD degree?" This seemed to be getting at the limits of our guest's authority and to challenge the value of seeking out her private practice. Our "psychoeducational diagnostician" responded again with somewhat unclear logic, seeming to say that parents ought to know beforehand whether they sought a medical or an educational diagnosis: "Well, it depends on the diagnosis. Schools won't do ADHD, it's medical. But they might do dyslexia."

The second PAC meeting geared to those managing kids with invisible disabilities honed in on the executive function introduced in the earlier meeting. It was attended by a larger number of parents, mostly mothers, and the first ten or fifteen minutes were actually spent reassembling in a larger room. With our guest speaker this time a speech and language pathologist with master's degree, certification, and a private practice, we were told she specialized in "cognition and attention" and would offer "strategies [parents] can use at home to help children get organized from homework to chores." I did learn more about the brain, the subcortical drives, the frontal lobe (home of executive function), and the neuro-integrative ability that lets you add information, "schemas," and past experiences to the brain's "filing cabinet." With advice like "teach to the executive function" or "to stop a tantrum, access the frontal lobe," there was an earnestness to the tone of the evening befitting the difficulties of shepherding a volatile, highly reactive child through day-to-day life. At one point our guest speaker was refreshingly honest and sympathetic: "There are *not* a lot of great strategies out there." But she largely reinforced the notion that mothers must diligently increase their managerial skills if hoping to increase the odds of a child's future success. In addition to purchasing homework planners and teaching "forecasting," we were provocatively asked "Does your child's brain seem to have no CEO on board?" A handout reviewed in the meeting carried this analogy further asking, beside a small drawing of the brain and the frontal lobe which should be the brain's CEO, "What does a CEO do?" and what makes "a good CEO" successful. This was followed by: "Imagine a CEO who had difficulty organizing, reasoning, and problem-solving. What if he could not negotiate? What if she was unaware of what was happening in the company? What if they did not set goals and follow through on them? What if they did not make changes in the company based upon performance evaluations? The company would not run efficiently."

Mothers, I was struck, have yet more fields and more vocabularies to master—from the rigors of special-ed procedures, disability law and diagnostic categories, and the "secret services" to be ferreted out of schools, to all the terms and acronyms associated with new methods of testing, and now this "Welcome to Your Child's Brain" as a corporate board. It became clearer and clearer to me that simply to locate the increasingly narrow specialists, to figure out what they might have to offer, and then to negotiate for services within recalcitrant, belt-tightening institutions compelled mothers to become something like the lone vigilante heroes of so many films, like Clint Eastwood in the *Dirty Harry* series, or in Westerns like the Lone Ranger, Zorro, or the cult classic *Walking Tall*, seeking justice when institutions fail one's family. That is, like an extreme of neoliberal citizenship, each mother was to heroically take the "law" into her own hands, seize authoritative knowledge, and attempt to get tough with multiply credentialed professionals. Sociologist Jacqueline Litt, in a qualitative study of low-income mothers whose kids had ADHD, argued more literally that so much of this bureaucratic "advocacy work" was required that it should be distinguished from daily care work and interaction with children.[20] The image of the vigilante, an imperfect metaphor because of its associations with excessive violence (and at times with racist hate crimes), kept coming to my mind in its more positive version to better capture the lone adversarial positions and the illicit feel of scrounging for hidden information that so many of the mothers I interviewed described.[21] The term's original meaning also captures the sense of unrelenting watchfulness, of standing guard over vulnerable children.[22] Amy Sousa, studying memoirs by mothers of autistic children, similarly suggests that mothers draw on or "reinvent" the masculine "warrior-hero" cultural archetype, invoking acts of bravery, determination, and the "isolation of the hero."[23] Dory Buchanan, for one, expressed many of these aspects, wondering how she, a "white middle-class parent," had ended up so "incredibly frustrated" in her battle for more therapeutic intervention for her young son Khari. Dory observed the irony that as a parent with an advanced degree in education "who works in the school system," she had nonetheless been pushed into a confrontational position, with her concerns treated as illegitimate, "I feel really stupid. I feel humiliated. I have an advocate, we went to mediation, and it's just like, oh my God, *if I* feel this way . . . *Unbelievable!*" Dory laughed ruefully, knowing she would soldier on and try to better master the vocabulary: "You know what? I was overwhelmed by the language. . . . It's your own kid so you're kind of not objective anyway. But you walk in and they all have this big language they're using, and lots of acronyms. And oh my God."

Across a wide expanse of class difference, many mothers similarly complained of the professional jargon they had to penetrate to navigate the educational system. Heather Dunn, only a high-school graduate, nonetheless shared Dory Buchanan's exasperation with acronyms: "The ETF, the um, what do they call them? Aaaaah, what does it stand for? Educational team leader? . . . It's like all these acronyms!" *New York Times* journalist Judith Warner was also struck when she visited a parents meeting for those whose kids had invisible special needs: "It was all acronyms and codes for navigating the public school system."[24]

And Mothers as Vigilantes in the Medical System . . .

In addition to taking the law into their own hands to navigate the educational system, mothers challenged dense bureaucracies and narrowly specialized elite professionals in the medical system. Amid the larger strains in U.S. healthcare touched on above, mothers' accounts often began with struggles to wrest coverage from private health insurance providers. The long story of May Royce, single mother of eight-year-old

Robert, also exemplified a struggle to gain entry along with coverage. But May's detailed narrative highlighted the surprising maze of hurdles and obstacles for someone armed already with her own professional experience. As a physical therapist well versed in such intricacies, May's story of frustration and sense of illicit action parallels educator Dory Buchanan's humiliation at the hands of the educational system. May had been desperate to make sense of her son's volatile moods and found herself paying out of pocket for psychotherapy for two years. On just one good but "womanly" income this was unsustainable, and she described the ensuing "war":

> The therapist suggested testing [to obtain the diagnosis code required by insurers]. So I call [the specialty diagnostic clinic], "Well, you need to get approved from the insurance company." . . . "Well, give me the forms." . . . So they give me this one-page form for justification. I said, "All right, it looks pretty straightforward." So I said, "Who needs to write this?" They said, "Oh your therapist can do this." . . . So [after eight weeks] I'm yelling at the therapist . . . "I understand you're busy . . . [but] I'm paying you $130 an hour out of my pocket!" [Finally] we get it to the insurance company—of course, what happens? They deny it. They deny it because they think my son needs to see a psychiatrist. . . . Wait a minute. "I called and checked with you people. . . . You said my clinical psychotherapist can do it." . . . [After filing a lengthy, stalled appeal] "OK, you know what? I'll take him to a psychiatrist!" Then I started calling all these psychiatrists and no one would call me back . . . you've got to see, here [bringing out a notebook, with information logged by call]. All of these people, look at this: "no new patients," "no new patients," . . . "he's no longer here," "left message," "left message."

I met May some ten months after she had logged these numerous calls, encountering a serious bottleneck in access to the properly credentialed specialists, a feature of dense bureaucratization mentioned by many of the mothers. By our first meeting, May had succeeded in demanding the insurance provider locate a psychiatrist for her. However, she described "cajoling" "the Quack" to approve costly neuropsychological testing rather than just, without a glance at Robert, "whipping out his prescription pad for Prozac." Finally, after additional months, she was armed with a diagnosis of ADD and "mood disorder, possibly bipolar"; and May sighed deeply at the extent of relentless vigilante action this had required: "OK, now I've battled the insurance, I've done that piece. Next is the school, his IEP."

May's story also raises the controversial issue of medicating kids, as she relented to administering both an atypical antipsychotic and an ADD pill after Robert's neuropsychological evaluation had urged such use. Despite the burgeoning rates, large-scale surveys find low approval for the practice among the American public,[25] and a small-scale survey of parents in New England found fully 40 percent agreeing that parents use psychiatric drugs as a "quick fix" for their children's "normal, but annoying behaviors."[26] May was outraged when a talk radio program similarly condemned parents like her and revealed the larger stigma attached to such mother-child troubles: "They are ignorant! We are like any responsible parent. We don't want to medicate our children. They should be open and listen, and give us as much support as if he [Robert] had cancer. What if he had a tumor?"

As is evident in May's story, mothers may paradoxically experience both relief and dread in obtaining a medicalized diagnosis and label for a troubled child. Mothers shared pain or sadness that the seriousness of a child's troubles had been confirmed, and in ways that invited overstatement and the finger-wagging of other parents; however, they also very much wanted language to name chaotic events and to speak of them to others. This helps explain why mothers actively seek medicalization: labels provide access to resources within the ed and med systems, but more than this, a meaningful diagnosis can also be, as working-class mother Kelly Caruthers exclaimed, "a *great relief!*"[27] Influential labeling and antipsychiatry theories of the 1960s and 1970s cast diagnoses of mental disorder as damaging myths, actually producing as well as heavily stigmatizing difference;[28] however, multiple voices, including those of feminist scholars, have since demonstrated that medicalized labels also provide important validation of the reality of distressing experiences.[29] Affluent Theresa Kelleher, who had struggled long months to get school testing and then confronted a wait list to see a child psychiatrist, illuminated the two-sidedness of labels in the reaction she depicted to her son Colin's eventual diagnosis of anxiety disorder and ADHD and subsequent out-of-district school placement:

That [they would pay] for the transportation and the cost to send him to a different school . . . there was no argument there. And that was why I was, on the one hand, happy. And on the other hand, it also was *very sad* because I felt that he was, it must be a terrible thing that he has if he can't, you know, if they're willing to do that.

In fact, Theresa still sought further diagnostic evaluation despite Colin's successful placement in an independent therapeutic school at the time I met her. Like other mothers I spoke with, it was not just a question of resources to be gained, but the need to make better sense of a child's issues, to do all they possibly could to understand or ameliorate those issues, which made diagnosis itself a more ongoing process.[30]

At the same time, however, the interviewed mothers spoke poignantly about stigma and the isolating weight of painful decisions to use, as one mother put it, "a brain-altering medication on a child." I discovered from mothers' narratives, but also from my fieldwork observation at special-ed parents meetings, that indeed there is little social support for such decisions or acknowledgment of how difficult they may be, how shameful to a mother's sense of self. Mothers, for example, spoke a great deal of the disapproval of family members: "My mom . . . she says, 'How can you give him all those meds?'" or, "My sister, she'll say, 'He doesn't need the meds.'" Others tried to keep the administering of meds a secret, perhaps increasing their own sense of shame to save face with kin. When Faith Prenniker discussed her secret, she ruefully acknowledged what many might think: that she had doomed her son to a lifetime of drug abuse: "I felt like I was sending my child to *The Valley of the Dolls*."[31]

At the special-ed PAC meetings, there was much silence on the question of whether to use psychiatric medications, certainly due in large part to the assumption that this would be a purely medical rather than an educational matter. The silences and the uncomfortable, dismissive responses to the few queries from unknowing parents, however, suggested something stronger than a turf war. It felt more like a taboo which made the subject unspeakable, confirming its shamefulness, even as it was omnipresent. Questions about medications were only very briefly raised by parents at three of the twelve meetings which I observed. While I thought each query appropriate in the context of the evening's discussion, this was evidently not the opinion of the speakers and leaders. Eleven of these twelve meetings—spread over three public-school districts—featured guest experts with a range of expertise which extended into the medical realm: if not the advocates or attorneys, then certainly the neuropsychological evaluator and the speech pathologist instructing us about the brain's structure and functions. Guest speakers and volunteer leaders also offered numerous references, handouts, pamphlets, business cards, and URLs for numerous websites, many of which again appeared to span educational and medical realms. Yet no guest or leader pointed to resources to support decision-making about psychoactive medications.[32] In fact, at the year-end planning meeting in the affluent district, volunteer leaders asked us to choose our top ten from the thirty informational topics covered in the previous six years to set the upcoming year's schedule—and none of the thirty dealt with information or resources on medication issues.

At each of two meetings in which medications came up in the affluent district, it was because a parent in attendance raised the question. At the meeting described featuring the "psychoeducational diagnostician," one mother asked if she ought to have her young daughter skip medication on the days of her testing. The question was answered politely but dismissively: "I prefer on it [meds] to do their best, but some do it some scales [tests] on, some off. There's no specific protocol." The speaker then marched abruptly on to change the topic, eliciting no follow-up or related questions from some thirty other adults in the room. I would have guessed, however, that many if not most others who showed up that midweek evening would have been soon facing similar dilemmas. Two months later the larger audience gathered for the speech pathologist presenting on the brain's executive function. One of the few males in attendance asked an entirely impersonal question: "How does medication affect executive function?" Our guest expert replied, "It depends, there's a lot of meds out there. The idea is to reduce overstimulation that leads to overload, to increase capacity. But that *doesn't teach* executive function or information integration." Needless to say, with this hint of a reprimand that we might medicate to shirk our parenting duties or to avoid the heavy lifting of developing a child's brain functions, the well-dressed, well-behaved audience let the topic drop.

Because of troubles locating PAC meetings, and the intermittency of one of the groups, I was able to observe only five meetings in the

two diverse, less affluent districts.[33] But I witnessed only one instance
in which mothers raised medications. This occurred in the dense urban
district at a meeting with quite a different tenor from any other I had
seen, with mothers jesting and speaking back to the pair of attorneys
attending as guest speakers. This could have been due to the attorneys'
youthfulness and the fact that they skipped a formal presentation; or it
might have been because the meeting included a casual potluck supper
with kids wandering in and out, loosely supervised by two older girls (I
did not find food or kids at any other PAC meeting I attended). There
were visible class and ethnoracial differences from the affluent town,
but not from the other diverse district in which I had observed. Yet,
when the talk shifted from contesting school placements to overly harsh
disciplinary practices, a mother angrily demanded to know if the school
could force her to increase her son's ADHD medication. Both attorneys
hesitated uncomfortably and the room filled with tittering as another
woman called out, "We stumped the lawyers!" Embarrassed, the female
attorney replied, "I don't have an answer how to stop that," though indicating between them that they had defended others in similar situations.
At the same time another disgruntled woman interrupted: "My son, they
keep saying he's ADD and to medicate him. I took him to neurologists
and they said no." At this, the woman attorney followed up more sup-
portively, "They can't force you to medicate." However, one of the two
volunteer coordinators quickly inserted a neoliberal message of personal
responsibility (and one that seemed to reflect her sense of relative social
advantage): "No. But a lot of parents don't know any better. They feel the
school will do the right thing. I tell parents all the time, 'Don't take everything [schools tell you] at face value.'" In other words, as in the "Eight
Rules for Advocacy," "Do it yourself."

Mothers and Pills

Many of the mothers I came to know described themselves as "very,
very resistant" to medications. They recounted that decisions to turn to
psychoactive drugs for their troubled kids had been among the most difficult of their lives, hardly something in which they took any suggestion
at "face value." Only six had avoided this turn, though three of those with
children just beginning their school years admitted they could not rule it

out for the future. Indeed, for Patricia Gwarten, a focus on diet, exercise, and several therapies was more about postponing than preventing the turn to medications. With few resources, and her own education having ended after a year at a community college, Patricia's vigilante efforts were impressive. On behalf of six-year-old Jacob, who struggled with learning and attentional issues and motor skill delays, Patricia had cut back to low-paid part-time work, resorting to public Medicaid coverage for his needs. When I came to their home, Patricia was awaiting results from the prior week's dyslexia evaluation, which she had arranged at a local university hospital; she planned to have the specialty ADD clinic at another hospital follow up on their ambiguous test results in one year. She described taking Jacob, through a third university's training clinics, two or three times per week to speech and language therapy and to family counseling. When I asked if Jacob's public school had helped locate or obtain these resources, since at least speech and language therapy and dyslexia tend to be considered *educational* rather than medical, Patricia shook her head vigorously: "It was *my* idea . . . That's something the school said they did not do and they would not know who to contact. And I said, 'Thank you very much, I'll call the hospitals.'"

Another five mothers had allowed only trials of medication, from just one weekend to three months, stopping because of either difficult side effects or a lack of benefit. Meg O'Toole, also with some college courses after high school, finally relented to a trial after her son's school had been suggesting medications for over a year. Meg's son Stephen struggled with dyslexia, as Patricia worried her son did as well. There is currently no known medication for dyslexia, a broad category of problems with the visual processing of language and the written word, though it is also considered to stem from physiological brain differences.[34] School personnel "were trying to claim it was ADD," although "they always said he was well behaved in class." Meg recalled the mother-blaming responses when school authorities disputed the neurologist's evaluation of dyslexia she obtained privately: "They told me I didn't know what I was talking about, that all he needed was discipline at home and with his homework [but] . . . homework that should take a child a half an hour was taking him three hours." Finally, turning to the family's pediatrician for help, "He said to me, 'He could be borderline . . . let's try him on this medication for thirty days, just see what happens.'" Meg laughed recalling that his teacher then noticed nothing different: "We tried it for two weeks, [but the doctor said,] 'There's no reason for him to be on it. You can say to them, we tried the drugs, didn't work, that's it.'"

For the five mothers (including Meg) who managed brief trials and for the thirty-seven who were administering (or had administered) medications to vulnerable children over lengthier periods, I discovered a great deal of vigilantism was required. Across differences of income, education, ethnoracial background, and families' cultural capital, mothers labored to research the commercially driven proliferation of drugs, to monitor effects and side effects in logbooks, charts, and files, to modify dosages and decide when to intervene. Meg, a full-time office worker, had "log[ged] and monitor[ed] everything" during her son's two-week drug trial. Only nine mothers were administering or had administered just Ritalin or a stimulant pill, a practice that the social science research treats as the extent of childhood medicalization,[35] Though a few others administered only an antidepressant, the majority described a turn to multiple medications, sometimes simultaneously. While this is a higher proportion than aggregate estimates for concomitant psychopharmaceutical use—and my volunteer sample may be unusual—it is nonetheless in line with trends showing steady increases. By 2005, for example, some 28 percent of those on a medication for ADHD were taking this in combination with another psychoactive.[36] Moreover, nearly half of the mothers, twenty-two out of forty-eight, found themselves over time in the world of proliferating, second-line psychoactive medications used for "mood stabilization"—the antihypertensives, atypical antipsychotics, and anticonvulsants described in the first chapter—many used "off-label" or without specific approval to treat kids' social-emotional disorders.[37] Managing medications, like diagnosis itself, thus represents a more ongoing process—much tougher than the often-assumed one-time decisions regarding stimulant or antidepressant use. In earlier decades, these first-line medications may have themselves seemed frightening, but I discovered that mothers found the stimulants and antidepressants less scary than the mood stabilizers some termed the "heavy hitters" or the "extreme medications."

Rosemary Hardesty's story exemplified the work of managing medications over time. Rosemary's oldest child, Josh, was in high school when we met. He had received several diagnoses, the earliest ADHD, then the addition of the less familiar oppositional defiant disorder, and finally the more controversial suggestion of possible bipolar disorder.[38] Rosemary, a licensed practical nurse who routinely administered drug cocktails for geriatric patients at her workplace, had concluded that psychopharmaceuticals offered no panacea, no magic resolution. But typical of many I came to know, Rosemary continued to closely monitor and dispense a drug combination for the partial help it provided Josh, on track to graduate high school, holding down a part-time job, and responsibly driving her old car. Rosemary reported that Josh had been a very challenging child who had been rejected by preschools, asked to leave catechism class in their Catholic parish, and spent many grade-school days in detention. He had been diagnosed first in kindergarten and initially put on Ritalin:

> Miracle drug! Miracle. Oh yeah, immediate, what a different child. Alert, attentive. The teacher called up the very next day and said, "I couldn't believe it was the same kid." Didn't last. Did *not* last. He maxed out the Ritalin . . . Then they switched him, I believe to the extended release. Which in the beginning worked wonderfully until he maxed out the dose on that too . . . He's been on every single medication for ADHD . . . every stimulant on the market . . . now he's on lithium and Prozac and Strattera, that brand-new [non-stimulant] drug for ADHD.[39]

Rosemary tried to sound matter-of-fact and make light of her discomfort, but she worried terribly with this mix on top of asthma medications: "At one point I think he was on like seven drugs!" Yet Rosemary had also worked diligently on family therapy and behavior modification, had consulted many specialists, and had listened painfully to her son's emerging self-knowledge: "He knew he wasn't normal and he was begging Dr. G. and Dr. W. at [a regional psychiatric clinic], he wanted an EEG done, he demanded an EEG, an MRI. Why? 'Because there's something in my brain. Maybe I have a tumor. And they can take it out and I'll be normal.'"

It may be less surprising that highly educated, affluent mothers do well handling medications. Judith Lowenthal, for example, kept detailed logbooks like office-worker Meg O'Toole in the months when her son was on multiple psychoactive drugs; yet Judith, graduate of a prestigious university, also culled articles on "pediatric psychopharmacology" from the Internet, discussed these in chat rooms, and took decisions about stopping particular drugs out of specialists' hands. I discovered, however, that others with far less in the way of research skills still intervened knowledgeably. Marika Booth, a high-school graduate, acted independently when her daughter's increased dose of antipsychotic Seroquel caused excessive fatigue. Similarly, Hermalina Riega, with a junior college certificate, had acted when her son's school behavior and irritability worsened. Together with his classroom teacher, an important source of support for several mothers, Hermalina challenged the psychiatrist's prescription of Clonidine: "I knew Clonidine was a blood pressure med with a lot of side effects. So we compared the research. I did America Online WebMD, and she did Google. She printed out like twenty-five pages, and I gave her eight or nine, and we both read it all. We kept in touch on a daily basis. So then I took him off it. And he has been fine ever since. I mean, not fine, but you know, not lashing out. A plus for me!"

Stigma, Invisibility, and Fear of Disorder

I found that experiences of social disgrace and mother-blame were to a surprising extent shared even among those most affluent and multiply privileged. Similar to mothers of kids with traditional disabilities, the mothers of invisibly disabled kids perceived themselves to share the stigma assigned to their sons and daughters. Kay Raso, a single mother with decent earnings, sadly ruminated on her loss of friends: "Everybody gradually, you know, got rid of me because they couldn't deal with [my son] David." Another single mother, but one living in poverty—Vivian Kotler—put it just as bluntly: "You don't have much support because nobody really wants to be your friend. Nobody wanted to be my daughter's friend. But nobody wanted to be my friend either." But Blayne Gregorson, who was long married to a blue-collar husband, similarly recounted that even with her son's out-of-district placement and its weekly parent-support group, "I'm very, very isolated." And this differed little from the report of loneliness and sadness of Theresa Kelleher, living in a wealthy community with her high-earning husband.

Historically, many believed that illness or handicap reflected a curse on the family, particularly transmitted by the mother.[40] In this way, as sociologist Erving Goffman maintained, the mark of stigma was literal; as with the early religious stigmata, the body was a reflection of a tainted soul.[41] Meg O'Toole reminded me of this not-altogether-lost cultural history; like her youngest son, Stephen, she had endured a lifelong struggle with dyslexia. Although her three older children were typically developing, she still recalled being admonished as a child in an observant Irish Catholic household, "Don't tell *anyone*. It's a curse." Several other mothers indicated that such views persist even in our high-tech, postmodern era. Patricia Gwarten observed more abstractly, "It seems like when you have a disability of some sort, it's still taboo, you know? [People think,] 'I don't want to catch it. I don't want to be around you.'" And Heather Dunn was emphatic: "You know, I think there's also always an element of, 'Is my kid gonna catch this?' . . . I really get that off of people. It's like, OK, [my son] Jared's *not* gonna give it to them. You know, this is [just] Jared." Researchers studying stigma lend weight to such insights about possible contagion: it bears repeating from the last chapter that in surveys at least 20 percent of Americans were willing to admit that they did not want kids with ADHD or depression in their children's classes or to have their families as neighbors, with somewhat higher percentages reporting that they prefer their children not befriend such kids. And these estimates may *understate* the extent of prejudice, with respondents unlikely to acknowledge more deep-seated, "virulent" beliefs.[42]

The precariousness of opportunities in an innovation- and information-based economy, and the fear of some sort of contagion from growing brain disorders, may make the stigma of invisible disorder particularly acute in U.S. culture today. Indeed at this historical juncture, in which the daily news refers to the successful as "the knowledge-class,"[43] brains are particularly at stake—and the experience of stigma compared to that of families whose children have immediately perceptible physical impairments may be more distinct than in other eras. I discovered, for example, that fully thirteen out of the forty-eight mothers (or 27 percent) emphasized (rightly or wrongly) that they perceived a *greater* stigma to the invisible disability they shared with a relatively unmarked child than that of mothers with visibly marked ill or disabled children.

Several, for example, compared their invisibly disordered child to one in a wheelchair, claiming the latter received far more sympathy. After all, the symbol of the child in a wheelchair is often evoked in popular culture as a sentimental trope, particularly for charitable fund-raising purposes but often in other contexts as well.[44] May Royce, who had complained that son Robert's disorders were not taken as seriously as if he had had cancer, later remarked of unsympathetic school personnel, "What about a wheelchair, an obvious disability? They wouldn't think twice about being extra nice." Angie Thompson specifically pointed to the paradox of looking "normal" as a factor *increasing* son Spencer's stigmatized identity:

> My brother has four *perfect kids*. I think about, what if my son was handicapped, in a wheelchair, with a bib. What would they think? Would they accept it? I want them to know he [her son Spencer, diagnosed with Asperger syndrome and depression] has a list of disabilities a mile long. I know what they're thinking "Why is he so weird?" Because he looks normal.

What is behind this resentment? Some mothers' comments suggested they may envy medical certainty itself, the legitimacy and the sympathy it offers. For example, across the economic divide from well-off Angie Thompson, working-class Heather Dunn complained that the inclusion program at the local school found her son Jared's disabilities nearly incomprehensible,[45] making daily life "very hard" for her and her otherwise gifted young boy:

> The coordinator [for inclusion] said to me, "You know, we've never dealt with a child with the kind of special needs that Jared has. We have *no idea* what we're doing because a lot of it's social-emotional for him." And they don't have a clue . . . [they have] kids with Down syndrome . . . [and] kids with physical handicaps [like] cerebral palsy.

Other mothers also pointed to the paradox of children who looked normal and appealing, with claims of impairment incomprehensible to those who might have been expected to provide the most support. Divorced mother Susan Atkinson, who clung to a middle-class life only with the financial help of her own parents, lamented that they and the extended family network refused to understand the disabilities of her attractive and highly verbal young daughter: "It's very, very difficult for parents and for family members, aunts, uncles, grandparents, to understand LD [learning disabled] kids who don't have *a physical* handicap. *They don't see it!* . . . It's very, very difficult for them to recognize that there's an issue in a child who . . . has tremendous verbal skills. . . . And they start isolating you."

Similarly, Brooke Donnelly, a white single mother, envied her own mother the kin and community admiration she received for rearing a son (Brooke's brother) with immediately evident, severe mental retardation. In contrast, Brooke, though a social worker, maintained some secrecy around her own "good-looking" son's occasionally crippling emotional turmoil. And from those very few close kin to whom she confided Brooke received added shame, such as from an "adoring" nearby sister: "She thinks he does *not* need to be on medication; she *really* questions it." Patricia Gwarten, an African American single mother, recounted frustration with her own mother's similar criticism: "'Stop trying to find things wrong with Jacob!' But something *is* still wrong. I just can't say what it is. It's *invisible*."

In short, to these women, if the devoted mother of a traditionally disabled child can simply accept the clear diagnosis, she may be relieved of a good amount of stigma and mother-blame, if not of an arduous care burden. That is, as in Brooke Donnelly's estimation, her own mother's devotion was evident and admired—although she and her perceptibly impaired son were still sometimes treated to the objectifying stares so worrisome to disability scholars and activists.[46] In contrast, in the face of medical uncertainty and a largely unmarked child, mothers I spoke with expressed a sense of both being held to and holding themselves to an impossibly high standard: they had to keep up relentless lone heroic efforts to resolve their child's issues all the while managing the degree to which their child might pass as normal. As sociologist Erving Goffman suggested a half century ago, passing to avoid stigma is fraught with continuous decisions about which "discrediting information" to conceal, which to disclose, when, and to whom—and Goffman, decades before burgeoning childhood medicalization, was speaking only of adults managing their own presentation of self when he pondered "the great rewards in being considered normal."[47] For mothers managing disordered kids, attempts to pass are yet more complex, fraught and inviting, with possibilities to fuel mother-blame at every turn. On the one hand, even with a diagnostic label, disclosures of a "good-looking" child's invisible issues often invite incredulity, a mother trying to shirk responsibility or deflect blame, as in many of the incidents offered by my interviewees. On the other hand, normalcy and "ruliness" in daily life, if much wanted, were always potentially disrupted by the unpredictable episodes of children's emotional outbursts, moodiness, or impulsive behavior—in which case a mother can be blamed for failing to disclose, especially by school personnel and other concerned parents.

Certainly in this sense, when medications work well enough, they can ease public life and increase the odds of successful, consistent social and peer interactions as well as school performance. Yet, at the same time and almost tragically, medications ramp up the amount of discrediting, disgraceful information mothers must manage. Although Goffman's framework can hardly envision the fraught presentation of interdependent *selves* involved for mothers of the Rx generation—with children who often elude the best laid plans—his analysis of invisibility provides a most helpful corrective to disability studies scholarship and any singular focus on the immediately, predictably evident. But because his analysis centers so much on the taint of mental illness, I turn now to ask how the mothers categorized invisible brain disorder and its very confused relation with the term "mental illness."

Is This Mental Illness?

I heard few mothers use this arguably most stigmatizing term to describe a child's invisible disability. Just five white Euro-American mothers used this term: affluent Judith Lowenthal, Colleen Janeway, and Abby Martin; Brooke Donnelly, the social worker whom we just met; and working-class Jenny Tedeschi. As a sociologist, I might say I avoided the term to remain neutral, to allow mothers to draw on their own language and categorization. Yet I was also confused about the relation between these categories, stumbling for terms to signal the burgeoning mild to moderate range in my research design and to politely exclude those with children in the severe range. In the end, I offered only the terms invisible "special needs" or sometimes "in special education" when introducing myself and my project, thinking that their ubiquity in the educational system normalized these terms. (I discovered later in the research that the latter terms may be more pejorative than I had suspected, at least among kids.) Mothers commonly supplied the terms "disorder" or "disability," which I use in this writing fairly interchangeably, perhaps the medical system's most normalized equivalents to the educational system's "special needs." Other terms were often added: Lenore Savage, also a social worker, at one point employed the more specific "neurobiological disorder." May Royce, the physical therapist who battled for insurance coverage, at one point observed, "The psychiatric illnesses have really gotten a bad rap," yet she repeatedly referred to her son Robert as "emotionally disordered." To me these terms sounded serious, but still less loaded than "mental illness," perhaps because only the latter connotes losing one's mind, one's reasoned self-awareness, or one's contact with reality. Other terms seemed to invoke the centuries-old mind/body dichotomy, but to signal that the mind was intact and illness resided only in the embodied brain.

Did mothers employ more serious terms when diagnoses became more serious, as, for example, when bipolar disorder was suggested? Bipolar—in the past labeled "manic depression" due to the volatile cycling from terribly high to desperately low moods—is more serious than most learning disorders or ADHD. It carries a higher risk of suicide than other disorders, is harder to treat, and more often leads to recommendations for the "heavy hitting" mood stabilizing medications. Yet fully fourteen of the forty-eight mothers I interviewed—about 30 percent—had children whose diagnoses had shifted to include bipolar or possible bipolar after initially less serious labels. And while some child psychiatrists maintain that bipolar cannot truly be manifest or diagnosed in children, others stand by early treatment, fueling an estimated forty-fold expansion in such diagnoses over the past decade.[48] Indeed, in 2013, well after I completed these interviews, the American Psychiatric Association added a new category, "Disruptive Mood Dysregulation Disorder," to its fifth revised edition of the *DSM* to help stem this rise. It remains to be seen whether such change under the depressive disorders—along with changes in the autism spectrum disorders, like folding in Asperger syndrome rather than naming it separately—will have a meaningful impact on burgeoning childhood medicalization. It may be that new labels will just become synonymous with the past, much as manic depression became bipolar. In either case, the appearance of such technical changes, amid highly specialized biomedical debates in the first major, controversy-plagued revision of the *DSM* since 1994, only amplifies my larger argument concerning the relentless work across multiple institutional-professional domains that mothers must engage in to manage vulnerable children.[49]

While my small sample precludes drawing any conclusions about whether families in general consider invisible disabilities, in categories of *DSM*-4 or *DSM*-5, to be "mental illnesses," the varied responses among the fourteen mothers who encountered the serious bipolar disorder diagnosis suggest little cultural agreement. Only three (Judith L., Brooke D., and Jenny T.) mentioned the term "mental illness," with others employing only more normalized terms. Vivian Kotler, for example, had just received a suggestion that this diagnosis might fit her daughter, previously diagnosed with ADHD. But Vivian only described twelve-year-old Isabel as "special needs." She also challenged the bipolar label, questioning whether Isabel's escalating oppositional behavior and aggression could be due to the hormonal surges of puberty. A few others shared such skepticism with me, aware, despite a varied range of class and cultural resources, that bipolar diagnoses were the latest trend in child psychiatry. Blayne Gregorson, with a community college degree, rejected any suggestion of this label for her challenging son: "Bipolar with kids is [just] the newest thing going on." And like Vivian, who had a four-year college degree, Blayne never employed the term "mental illness." But Heather Dunn, whose education ended with a high-school degree, explicitly contested this term when it was applied to her son Jared: "I took offense to the fact that the [school personnel] kept saying, 'Jared's mental illness,' you know, 'his mental illness,' 'his mental illness.' OK, listen to me: '*it's not* a mental illness!' [Jared] is perfectly normal, but he has these things to deal with."

Experts themselves debate where the lines should be drawn delineating mental health from illness, and in terms of *DSM* categories, at what level of severity disorders become something qualitatively more distressing or pathological.[50] The National Institute of Mental Health employs a wide umbrella in large-scale decennial surveys of "mental illness," in the past including mood disorders like bipolar, but also ADHD and mild to moderate depression. The 2005 report suggested that, counted this broadly, 55 percent of Americans would experience episodes of mental illness in their lifetime.[51] Other authorities in the field, however, contest the expansive definition, arguing that it trivializes serious issues and is too vague to guide families and practitioners to appropriate treatments. I noticed, more in line with this latter view, that the Massachusetts Association of Approved Special-Needs Private Schools retained more narrow delineations, with "mental illness" just one of several categories and a seemingly small one; it delineated conditions such as psychosis and schizophrenia with severe symptomatology and a loss of touch with reality.[52] Most schools in the association do not include this category, only serving the larger market of special needs: ADHD, autism spectrum disorders, learning and language disabilities, and somewhat less often, the mood and conduct disorders grouped in 2002 as "emotionally disturbed" or "behaviorally disordered." Bipolar disorder, which was categorized with the latter in the 2002 catalog, by 2008 had received its own delineation on the organization's website, but still not grouped with "mental illness."[53]

The Indiana University research group whose large-scale surveys of stigma and children's invisible disorders I have cited repeatedly also acknowledged that "mental illness" is a matter of "scientific debate and public controversy."[54] Their methodology therefore asked respondents, a random sample of American adults, to categorize unlabeled symptoms typical of ADHD and of depression as mental illness, physical illness, or as part of the "normal ups and downs" of life. Not surprisingly, results varied, but found that attributing such symptoms to mental illness did not alone explain the stigma of invisible disorder (although when assigned, it significantly worsened the stigmatizing effect). I would hazard a guess that the sheer amount of childhood medicalization, the proliferation of relevant specialists and service providers, and the pervasiveness of neuroscientific discourse in everyday life might together make a collapsing of em-brained disorder into mental illness unlikely. Moreover, if advocates of neurodiversity gain in influence, they will certainly argue for an even greater distinction between the non-neurotypical and the pathological.

Popular Advice, Brain Talk, and Twenty-First-Century Mother-Blame

Amid the present swirl of mainly negative attitudes and associations, however, what do mothers find if they look to the most popular parenting advice? Would the mothers I spoke with find support for neurodiverse children or any counter to the stigma and isolation they experience? Instead they might more readily discover fear of invisible disability and more reinforcement of their singular responsibility to manage it. Popular works repeatedly on the Amazon list of top parenting books in 2011, for example, revealed the rising authority of neuroscience but also a plethora of messages of twenty-first-century mother-blame.[55] About 40 percent of titles on the list were devoted, in whole or substantial part, to explaining the intricacy of children's brains and all that can easily go wrong with them if not properly managed. A parent's responsibility stretches from "conception to college," according to the subtitle of *Welcome to Your Child's Brain*.[56] In addition to newer titles like *The Whole-Brain Child*[57] and *Brain Rules for Baby*,[58] discussion of brain issues increased in updated editions of long-standing best sellers like *What to Expect When You're Expecting* and *Caring for Your Baby and Young Child: Birth to Age 5*, the latter published by the American Academy of Pediatrics. With sometimes striking visual imagery from the high-tech wonders of functional magnetic resonance imaging (fMRI) or positron emission tomography, readers "see" into the fragile ordering of genetic, chemical and hard-wired neuroanatomy in their hands. As the American Pediatric Association instructs, "the new science" demonstrates "exactly *how significant our role is* in the development of the child's brain" as all children, those *with and without* "disabilities and other special healthcare needs[,] . . . greatly benefit from *close monitoring* of early brain development."[59] The Amazon description for another best seller (*Parenting from the Inside Out*) also signaled the weighty responsibilities: "Drawing upon stunning new findings in neurobiology and attachment research, [the authors] explain how *interpersonal relationships* directly impact the development of the brain."[60]

Beneath the hyperbole, much of today's advice is really not new: it recapitulates the century-old discourse of scientific motherhood in which good mothers were to be guided by the latest in biomedicine;[61] and it recycles a half century of the "intensive motherhood" ideal holding maximized child development as a moral-political imperative.[62] Some tomes specifically echo the hyper-intensive "attachment parenting,"[63] exhorting "parents" (i.e., mothers) to practice the extended breastfeeding and co-sleeping claimed to enhance psychological bonding—but now to "promote brain development by feeding the brain the right kind of information."[64] But for fear-mongering about bad mothers, we now read of brain damage rather than just of fears of abandonment: low attachment brings high "cortisol and stress hormones," and "low dopamine and norepinephrine levels make it more difficult for a child to focus and concentrate[and] low serotonin levels are a key component in many forms of depression and violent behavior."[65] Or in this somewhat more benign comment mixing old and new conceptions of harm, the cost of less intensive mothering is "IQ points, emotional well-being, ADHD, and obesity."[66]

In a more general sense and for all citizens, sociologist Victoria Pitts-Taylor has argued that the popular diffusion of neuroscientific discourse *is* new—and a crucial part of the neoliberal nation's push toward dismantling public programs and individualizing responsibility for health, risk reduction, and the "welfare" of the nation's population. Pitts-Taylor suggests that much falls to mothers because they bear responsibility for the nation's future, now in need of vigorous brains for its global competitiveness. Sociologist Glenda Wall has also demonstrated that intensive mothering in Canadian advice literature is now linked, as I found in the United States, to brain development and neoliberal privatization of all child outcomes.[67] But neither Wall nor Pitts-Taylor note the growth in diagnoses of em-brained child disorders and the consequent fears, hopes, and needs that may drive mothers of both more and less vulnerable kids to consume such advice or to draw from its brain-talk vocabulary. I had not initially set out to include such popular advice literature in this project. In the course of the research, however, as mothers brought up the works they turned to, made insistent recommendations to me, or employed metaphors from the popular literature, the evidence that it mattered became impossible to ignore.

Charlotte Sperling, who reported that she felt like her family's "brain central," might best exemplify this. Charlotte had turned to a great deal of parenting advice to sort out contrasting images of the brain, whether plastic or predetermined by inheritance. What were the possibilities and limits for privatized maternal intervention?

> Well, there's a great book . . . on developing a high IQ in your child. . . . It takes you right from birth. I mean it's incredible, three months, how they should be responding at three months. And not to panic. But if they're not, you know, these are the kinds of things that will help . . . I thought, "Well that's great." But you know it's really contingent on the parents having a high IQ . . . So that was the flaw.

Later, however, Charlotte backtracked, returning to a more neoliberal sense of unrelenting maternal responsibility and brain plasticity: "You still *have to manage the genetics*. I mean, you have to say, 'OK, this is what we're facing, we need some compensatory skills developed.'" An overwhelming majority, some thirty-six of the forty-eight mothers I spoke with, drew specifically from neuroscientific vocabularies and brain talk, while nearly all drew complex multicausal models to explain their children's invisible disorders.

May Royce also spoke eloquently about the solace she took from advice books and brain talk as she sought to make sense of her son Robert's troubles at home and school: "OK, I'd gotten a lot of books on attention deficit. My brother, for my birthday, gave me two books on attention deficit. I mean I was living and breathing this." When she realized Robert's volatility might be beyond the ADHD profile, May navigated the arduous process to obtain a formal diagnosis, but she also sought out much more specialized advice to grapple with the question of medications. In the level of detail and repetition in her remarks, May revealed discomfort and the understandable defensiveness that, in turning to psychoactive drugs, she might seem a very bad mother:

> I got some books about some holistic natural ways [to treat my son]. I was against medication, I was actually against it. But back to the library I went, and I got some books on bipolar disease, and I got another book called *It's Nobody's Fault* [subtitled *New Hope and Help for Difficult Children and Their Parents*].[68] And these books stand out, and I read this book, and this book helped me come to terms . . . And it's biological. It's not emotional, it's *not* some crock. It's legitimate. There are different

chemical receptors that are just not right and need medication to correct. It's like diabetes. And so the book made me feel better that . . . I was going to *have to* medicate [my son], that it was going to be OK. And that I was doing it to help him, because he needed it. And that I had sought out the best, and I was questioning, and I was educated. And you know, I wasn't just doing this because *I* wanted to sleep at night!

Colleen Janeway, an affluent mother, was less explicit about which books she had consulted. But she nonetheless took on a teaching role with me, sharing what she had learned about the brain from books and from the "pediatric neuro-psychopharmacologist" she relied on to treat a young son diagnosed on the high-functioning end of the autism spectrum and with a mood disorder:

It's actually a wire, it's described as a wiring. And it's also described as like a right brain dysfunction. So there are various theories . . . I think that the brain is a very, very complicated thing, we all know that. And there is no one model brain. There just isn't. So along with this nonverbal learning disorder [that he] has . . . his intelligence level is very high . . . But the problem is he has what doctors call a dysregulation anxiety disorder.

This depiction of a son's brain as "a very, very complicated thing," employing the computer metaphors of "wiring" and "dysregulation" (along with at other points discussion of chemistry and chemical "receptors"), might seem the purview of only highly educated mothers. But less educated mothers also aptly described complexity, for example, Marika Booth, a Black single mother with a high-school education. After mentioning heredity and computer-like information processing in the brain, she offered this description of the newest connectivity hypothesis to explain a daughter's learning and emotional disorders: "She was a very bright child . . . but to sit and arrange something the way it's supposed to be arranged, she has that problem. Why is that? . . . I'm really trying to read a lot on that . . . because . . . there are certain cells or nerves on the brain that, if one doesn't connect to the other one for some reason, they're not going to learn how to do that function."[69]

Quite unusual was Lucy Nguyen, a married homemaker with two biracial children. With her oldest, a son, diagnosed with ADHD and language-based learning disabilities, Lucy was the only mother among the forty-eight I spoke with who engaged with neuroscience primarily to reject it. Lucy, who had quit high school without graduating, had just begun recovery from drug and alcohol addiction when she became pregnant with her son, who was seventeen when I met her. She judged her own early mothering harshly and questioned so much focus on brain-blame theories, explaining, "I read a lot. I read that *Driven to Distraction*,[70] all those books on ADD," but clearly laying out her objections:

> There are so many mothers who don't want to admit they screwed up. But *I* admit it: I screwed up. My old therapist, she said she had a son just like mine. She had this poster, "ADD, it's in the brain." It showed like the brain and the blood, and it not going into different parts of the brain or something. She said, "No, it's in the brain." OK, but I thought to myself, "You are in denial." I believe, well, that *nurture* affects nature.

Of course, the latest neuroscientific thinking about brain plasticity is in line with Lucy's belief that *nurture*, at least to some extent, affects nature; however, Lucy complicated her thinking about causality when she questioned her own troubled youth and the possibility of heritable disabilities: "Was that why I was a high-school drop out? . . . I found drugs. [But] which came first, was it the drugs that got in the way of school? Or was I self-medicating my ADD?" And Lucy was not all harsh self-criticism—she expressed pride in her long sobriety and brought out file boxes, carefully organized, testifying to years of vigilante efforts on her son's behalf, displaying for me multiple evaluations and IEPs, with reports from therapists, tutors, teachers, and an educational advocate.

With the standard for good neoliberal mothers to be absolutely unrelenting in efforts to optimize development of their children's brains—and to "Do it yourself"—every mother I met in some way blamed herself for falling short. Patricia Gwarten, with few resources, seemed to have located every possible reduced-fee service or relevant public clinic for her son Jacob since he had been a two-year-old—as well as working on his diet and exercise directly. Nonetheless, Patricia blamed herself for not beginning early intervention in his infancy. "Maybe I should have read more books," she confessed. As an always-suspect single mother and a mother of color, Patricia's experiences point to the much needed but largely missing intersectional analysis of invisible disability, stigma, and twenty-first-century mother-blame. But I turn first to two final experiences shared by the mothers across divides of resources and ethnoracial locations: a mixed bag of marital strain and support and the question of whether to take psychoactive medications themselves.

Marriage and Invisible Disorder

Lucy Nguyen, critical of many aspects of her own mothering and regretful of her lack of education, counted herself nonetheless very lucky in her happy marriage. Though the couple did not marry until Lucy's second pregnancy when she was four years into her sobriety, her partner had remained a constant source of support throughout: "He stayed in my life . . . My husband always, he is so great, the nicest person. He always accepted me." In contrast, lacking such support, single mom Patricia Gwarten recounted turning to a family counselor, a nonreciprocal, partly commodified support, to quell her continuous worries that she was not doing enough for her son: "I had to have someone else [the counselor] tell me . . . 'OK, you *are* doing enough. You are doing what you are supposed to do and more.'" Yet marriage, I discovered, did not always bring the contentment and mutual support that Lucy enjoyed. Many of the married women spoke of strained relationships and of husbands who offered little emotional or practical support for their vigilante efforts. Some reported husbands who contributed to the mother-blame and stigma surrounding them on all sides—or who questioned their credibility as much as other kin or bureaucratized professionals. And of the twenty-five who had told me originally that they were married, four revealed, either at the end of our long meetings or in later phone conversations, that they were actually in the midst of separation or divorce proceedings and did not foresee ever reconciling.

The marital satisfaction Lucy Nguyen described—with just a few others like affluent Judith Lowenthal—also stands out in light of research on families with disabled children. Many studies have found that having a disabled child is associated with higher rates of marital strain, divorce, and single-mother households. A well-controlled, longitudinal study, for example, comparing parents raising kids with ADHD to those with only typically developing children found a significantly higher divorce rate among the ADHD group, as well as significant evidence of a causal relation, with ADHD kids increasing the odds of divorce. Specifically, researchers concluded that it was the severity of children's oppositional behaviors which strained marriages to the breaking point: "Disruptive child behavior likely interacts over time with additional family stressors to spark marital conflict and, ultimately, divorce."[71] This causal ordering is debated, however, with some contending that it is parental discord and divorce which induce children's issues. Another large-scale survey (but one without longitudinal data) provocatively found children of divorce twice as likely to be on Ritalin. While Lisa Strohschein, Canadian sociologist and the study's author, was more cautious,[72] at least one media pundit could not resist observing, "And now we have Strohschein's study, not the first to arrive at the same conclusions, which suggests that divorce appears to be some sort of carrier for this disorder. Could there be some sort of virus that thrives in law offices? Or will we be forced to concede a significant place for parenting in the development of the ADHD child's symptoms?"[73]

Other interpretations are also possible of what exactly links divorce and kids' disorder, including one that emphasizes heritability and genetic transmission. According to the Wymbs longitudinal survey, for example, fathers' disorder could be another significant predictor (or perhaps an antecedent cause) of divorce, along with children's challenging behavior.[74] However, Strohschein mentioned other intervening factors that might plausibly explain higher rates of medication, such as simply kids' increased contact with health professionals after divorce.[75]

What's interesting is that neither the clear causal data of Wymbs nor these alternative explanations garner anywhere near as much public attention as interpretations which lend themselves to mother-blame. This was evident in Arianna Huffington's concern that overwhelmed single mothers would be the most prone to medicate children for normal troubles. Popular advice books steeped in neuroscience also circulate such notions of causality, with mothers to blame for failed marriages and thus for kids' em-brained harm, *as if* these causal linkages (rather than just correlations) were well established in the research: one of the top ten rules in *Brain Rules for Babies* states emphatically that parents *must stay married* because a young child "will *rewire* his developing nervous system depending upon the turbulence he perceives" with stress hormones that may "lower your baby's IQ," "inhibit your baby's future motor skills, attentional states, and ability to concentrate," and may even "shrink the size of your baby's brain."[76] And *Brain Rules* makes mothers who do not preserve their marriages and their children's brain development responsible for far more, including their child's chances for upward mobility: "Children from divorced households are 25 percent more likely to abuse drugs by the time they are 14. They are more likely to get pregnant out of wedlock . . . In school, they get worse grades than children in stable households. . . . So much for Harvard."[77] (These last linkages are highly contentious, with *Brain Rules* overlooking the significant intervening factors—economic and residential insecurity—which account for most, if not all, of the harm of divorce itself.)[78]

Going beyond the focus on ADHD alone, other studies indicate that marital strain and divorce may vary by the type of invisible disorder. Studies of parents with autistic children have reported little increased odds of divorce.[79] Several, however, found negative outcomes short of divorce, including high likelihood of marital strain and mothers' depression, particularly following the common reversion to nuclear-family gender specialization, mothers' reduced labor force participation and disproportionate responsibility for care work.[80] The larger family-disabilities literature, though it primarily emphasizes traditional, perceptible disabilities like Down syndrome or cerebral palsy, also finds an overwhelming tendency for reversion to nuclear-family gender arrangements with at-home mothers, and resulting high maternal stress and depression among those raising such children.[81]

In my research some of those who were (already) divorced spoke of the conflict, blame, guilt, and denial that can accompany rearing a troubled child as a major reason for their marital breakup; others attributed their divorce to multiple strains, with their child as one among several major stressors. Never-married and financially struggling Vivian Kotler thus saw marital support aptly as something of a paradox. On the one hand, she recounted at length, and unprompted, how stressful and isolating it was raising a high-need child alone and how much she could use a husband's practical and emotional support. On the other hand, she suggested that husbands impose their own needs and often, in couples she knew, had trouble prioritizing high-need children, which would only increase a mothers' stress and her care burden. When I eventually responded to Vivian's pointed remarks by asking, "What do you imagine it would be like if you weren't a single parent?" she immediately blurted out, "If I had a special-needs kid *and* I had a husband? That would just cause a divorce!"

While fully happy marriages may be anomalous among those raising disordered kids, I discovered a suggestive pattern for something like a good-enough marriage based on shared acknowledgment and acceptance of a child's issues. I believe finding such shared acknowledgment may explain why some of the women I interviewed remained in relatively strained relationships—and why others left. I do *not* mean to say, like *Brain Rules for Babies*, that women *should* stay. But the threat of more isolation poses a steep additional cost to divorce for mothers already alone with a stigmatized and stigmatizing child amid a culture of mother-blame. Most married women described accepting relationships with what sociologist Arlie Hochschild might agree was a fairly stingy "economy of gratitude,"[82] with the appreciation each offered the other, to my mind, strained. Most performed the lion's share of household work, yet the need for that core, shared acknowledgment seemed to override substantial inequities in caregiving as well as persisting conflict. Put differently, I discovered that a somewhat impoverished marriage became unbearable only if a husband persisted in denying a child's invisible issues.

I learned a great deal from two heartfelt accounts in which a husband's long denial gave way perhaps just in time to save a marriage. Both Rosemary Hardesty and Blayne Gregorson were raising struggling sons and typically developing daughters at modest income levels with blue-collar husbands. Each graciously invited me into her well-kept, smaller suburban home and introduced me to her family members before we went off into other rooms. Stan Hardesty, Rosemary's husband, asked very quietly if he could speak with me after I had turned off the tape recorder on the long evening I spent listening to and speaking with Rosemary. During much of the evening, while Rosemary and I were in an adjoining dining area, Stan supervised the couple's two young daughters' bedtime activities, while high-school-aged Josh (as mentioned earlier, diagnosed with multiple disorders) came in and out. In a sad, confessional tone—as I recorded later that night in my fieldnotes, respecting his wishes not to be taped—Stan asked if I'd met other fathers, if any had been as bad as him, denying a child's troubles as long as he had. I found this very touching; he seemed shy and remorseful and I offered, perhaps too sympathetically, that many parents found it hard to accept, only truly wanting the best for their children.

In both accounts of surviving marriages the larger societal factors— New Economy restructuring, the "end of men," and the destabilization of manly provider status—lurked in the background. Both Stan Hardesty and Louis Gregorson had long been their families' breadwinners, with wives Rosemary and Blayne each employed part-time in and around the needs of their households and challenging sons. But each couple experienced a gender shift when providers Stan and Louis were pushed out of the labor force on disability, unable to find decent alternatives after long years of physically taxing work.[83] Only after this gender shift had each father accepted his child's issues and validated his wife's experience. Certainly more time at home played a part, but with wives taking on more breadwinning perhaps a shift in marital power also accounted for the husbands' remorse. Extensive research on household labor indicates that when husbands face job loss, couples are more likely to revert to a conventional division of the household to shore up men's shaken masculinity.[84] Indeed, while Stan Hardesty and Lou Gregorson spent lots more time at home with their kids, neither took on anything close to equal caregiving or housework. Nonetheless, they seemed to finally appreciate their sons' struggles and to begin to understand all their wives had endured.

When I met Rosemary Hardesty she was working fifty hours a week as a licensed practical nurse, though for most of their married years (prior to Stan's injuries) she had been employed only part-time. Despite this change in breadwinning—and the accompanying move of Stan's mother into the rental unit beneath their home to assist with childcare— Rosemary was still the one who set up son Josh's medical and therapy appointments and dispensed his medications. Yet she chuckled with pleasure explaining that these tasks were easy while her husband now had to ensure that Josh was actually taking his daily pills and showing up to weekly appointments. In the three hours I spent at the Hardesty's home over a long evening, after getting the two younger daughters to bed, Stan occasionally added supportive, knowing details, following Rosemary's lead, about Josh's issues, the lack of communication from his school, and some troubling dealings with neighborhood kids. Although this respectful dynamic may have been influenced by my presence and obvious prioritizing of Rosemary's perspective, Stan did not disagree or attempt to explain when Rosemary described their long-strained marital relationship: "As Josh was getting older [in middle school], things were getting worse in the battles with the school. And then I turned to my mother more and more. [Be]cause, then, my husband was NO help. He just wouldn't admit—or he couldn't come to terms with his son. [That he] was not a whole, his son was not 'normal' per se."

Louis Gregorson, the other changed blue-collar husband, had been out of the labor force for some two years when I met him briefly during my long visit with his wife, Blayne. Blayne had taken over breadwinning, if not as capably as Rosemary Hardesty, but she worked as many hours as she could get in a local retail establishment. And just as in the Hardesty household, husband Louis was finally gaining firsthand experience of day-to-day life with their troubled son Brandon (also diagnosed with multiple disorders): "For the past two years, Louis has been out on a medical disability, injured at work. But up until then [over twelve years], he worked sixty or more hours a week [with two jobs in maintenance services] . . . Louis didn't really see a lot of what was happening. He wasn't around . . . he has had a harder time admitting Brandon's issues." Blayne explained her relief that Louis was finally changing; in treatment for anger management and on antidepressant medication, he had become enthusiastic about the weekly family support group at Brandon's special-needs day school: "We never miss a meeting." With an older daughter already on her own and just teenaged Brandon at home, Louis did less caregiving than Stan Hardesty and it was clear, as in the exchange below about a dentist appointment, that Blayne still fulfilled the "executive function" in their home. Nonetheless, Blayne—like Rosemary—reported happily that, "since Louis has been home on disability, he does more with Brandon. 'Oh, OK, Brandon has a dentist appointment. Guess you'll have to take him.' . . . He also does go to the support group. And at one point he went to a dads group. That was *some* distance, too, but he went!"

The example of another middle-income couple, the lower-white-collar Prennikers, adds to the suggestion that the key to marital survival in such families lies in mutual acknowledgment of a child's troubles.

That is, if mothers shoulder an inequitable work-family burden like Rosemary and Blayne, rough equity in the economy of gratitude can nonetheless emerge from acknowledgment of her difficult experience, and this can be sufficient to maintain marital bonds. In the Prennikers' case, both accepted their only child's, a boy's, diagnosis of ADHD and nonverbal learning disorder. Faith and husband Brian shared breadwinning, with Faith employed as an accounting assistant and Brian in a feminized position as a public-school teaching aide. Neither had finished college, though Brian was attempting to through online and extension courses.

Faith praised her husband's shared parenting and explained that her job usually allowed a flexible schedule so that they could easily stagger their hours, with Faith covering mornings before school and Brian, after school. Yet she confided, just like her friend Charlotte Sperling, that she was "tired, always tired" from being the family "brain." Much like Blayne and Rosemary, Faith scheduled and kept track of multiple medical and therapy appointments, school conferences, household tasks, and even her son's daily homework assignments. "Every day, I'm at work and they're at home . . . they get home about the same time. But I call every day and say, 'What's the homework story?' . . . My husband's wonderful but he just doesn't pay attention the same way that I do." Despite her desire to be home, the family relied on Faith's stable year-round job; so a less attentive father employed only for school terms and school hours was home with a son unable to manage extended day or summer camp settings. Faith nonetheless described a stable marriage. Intriguingly, her words switched from the "we" of parenting with Brian to the "I" of maternal exclusivity as she concluded with the worries that plagued her. From: "The fear is of time going by, if there's something *we're* missing that *we* should be doing, something *we* don't know is even out there that would help him." To: "Sometimes *I* just will get this fear, like there's something else. And *nobody else* is going to find it, and *I* don't know what it is."

"What Kind of Family *Is* This *If Mom* Is on Meds?"

Between the daily stress of managing highly reactive kids while surrounded by stigma and the pressure to live up to a standard of relentless vigilantism, it was unsurprising that mothers navigating childhood medicalization themselves turned to psychoactive medications in nearly half the families I studied. Twenty-one of the forty-eight reported that they had used medication during some parenting years or were currently using such medication; another two were in counseling and actively considering a trial. To be sure, several attributed their need for psychoactive medication to troubles or serious trauma long predating their children's, as with Heather Dunn, who had been sexually abused as a child. Others recounted interacting stressors: troubled kids and busy households, the loss of elderly parents, financial worries and workplace demands, marital strains and separations. But with unknown causal mechanisms, variable individual reactions, uncertain long-term effects, and an array of side effects like suppressed sexual responsiveness, medications were not simply embraced as wonder drugs. Rosa Branca, at her doctor's urging, turned to an antidepressant, but for just a year after being "overwhelmed" by "problem after problem" with her kids, her extended family, and her own health. Similarly, Shauna Lapine had tried anti-anxiety medications for just the months following her divorce and the death of her father, months in which she had also relocated with her children to a new city—but she was never sure they had really helped. And Bev Peterson recounted limiting the months she used antidepressants over difficult years after leaving an abusive early marriage and struggling to pay the bills while caring for two young kids. Situational factors on top of demanding children may have accounted for somewhat greater use of psychopharmaceuticals by the single mothers I interviewed. Fewer married mothers reported relying on such medications, perhaps evidence that even a good-enough marriage offers important protection—though there are likely many factors at play. But some mothers, both married and single, also claimed their turn to medication was solely due to the stress of life with an invisibly disabled child.

Both single middle-income May Royce and married high-earning Virginia Caldwell-Starret, for example, described turning to antidepressants. May observed, "It's helped take the edge off and it's helped me be a little more patient with Robert. Because he needs the patience despite the fact that he's throwing his breakfast around the house. He needs . . . me not [to] get so worked up about that . . . So it's, it's really helped." Virginia, in contrast, had originally turned to antidepressants for postpartum depression, but had continued for six years: "My sister was teasing me, 'I think he's a little old for that now, so you can drop the *postpartum.*' But, yeah, I still take medication . . . I was taking just Celexa, then Wellbutrin and Celexa, and now just Wellbutrin."

The use of psychoactive medications, predominantly antidepressants,[85] by mothers I interviewed must, of course, be seen in the context of high rates of use among *all* American women. The CDC reports that over 15 percent of American girls (older than twelve) and women are taking an antidepressant, and 23 percent of women aged forty to fifty-nine, figures which are two and half times greater than those for men and have grown by 400 percent since Prozac entered the market in 1987.[86] A half century ago, women, in lesser but still large numbers, had turned instead to the Valium made famous in the 1966 Rolling Stones song "Mother's Little Helper." But Valium, a diazepam tranquilizer, induced a sleepy, slightly euphoric, "ambition-thwarting" mood appropriate to an era when nearly all white, middle-class mothers—and many of the white, working class as well—were full-time, married homemakers. In current generations, diverse families depend on mothers' agility, energy, and earnings to adapt to a volatile, high-stakes economy (mothers who are also busy maximizing their kids' brain development). Not surprisingly, the most popular psychoactive medications, far surpassing Valium in its heyday, are the SSRI, Prozac-type antidepressants. Although surrounded by concerns about Big Pharma's unscrupulous promotion, many experts claim that SSRIs safely induce precisely the feelings of ambition and energized optimism that Valium sedated. Influential psychiatrist Peter Kramer described Prozac as the "drug for our time" which "helps produce" a nation of efficient, "extrovert go-getters." He elaborated, writing that SSRIs are "the corporate equivalent of steroids," producing a "muscular assertiveness" so that we are "taut," "lean," and able to "juggle competing priorities" "gracefully," "with a more buoyant personality"—though he acknowledged the ethical quandaries and potential for overuse. Psychiatrist and feminist cultural theorist Jonathan Metzl argued similarly that though gendered feminine, "Prozac . . . is a productivity narrative." And journalists have noted that, in today's globally competitive economy, it's hard to be a "super mom" without "a little chemical help."[87] Earlier I noted that several experts connect Prozac's rapid popularity to the upsurge in Ritalin use for kids in the 1990s.[88]

And feminist researcher Ilina Singh, who went so far as to contend that there was little difference between mothers drugging themselves or their children to conform to dominant gendered family norms,[89] may have been at least partially correct. I found that for many women the thought of medicating children became, if never an easy decision, more thinkable when they themselves, or their friends, coworkers, or kin, had at some time done so as well. As Cassie Mueller, who was reading *A User's Guide to the Brain*,[90] quipped to me, "It seemed like every woman I knew was on Prozac"—though Cassie herself actually had never been.

With this ubiquity, I found it fascinating that four mothers, two married and two single, offered that they could not allow themselves to turn to psychoactive help. Each had administered medications to a struggling child and engaged in valiant efforts to resolve or improve his or her issues. Blayne Gregorson had administered medications to son Brandon since grade school. She revealed in discussion of her almost-broken but good-enough marriage that her husband had been on and off SSRIs as part of treatment for anger management. Her next words surprised me with what seemed a husband's spiteful provocation and a wife's self-abnegating response: "My husband said, 'You should take them, too.' But my God, what kind of family *is* this *if Mom* is on meds?"

Angie Thompson expressed a similar sense of needing to be the member of the household to literally embody family order, strength, and keeping it together. With her son Spencer diagnosed with Asperger syndrome and depression, Angie revealed that she sometimes became overwhelmed and "weepy" facing the additional chronic health issues of her daughter (with diabetes) and her husband. Both their family counselor and her son's psychopharmacologist had recommended she consider taking something, but she rejected any such suggestion:

Really I was like, "Oh no!" Will, my husband, has Crohn's,[91] so I've got [laughs] three out of four of us on medication [which she supervised]. I wouldn't be able to remember to take it. It was when I was really weepy and crying, you know? She [our family counselor] says, "Do you want to talk to Dr. C. who Spencer sees?" And I did . . . and he says, "If you do feel like you need it, something, just call me." But I keep myself busy. I walk, I go to the gym as soon as they got on the bus I would go over to the gym. . . . And then I would go to work. And then come home and start dinner.

While sticking to her gym routine was doubtless a positive coping mechanism for Angie, who worked only part-time supplementing a husband's high earnings, it was one unavailable to single mothers living on low incomes like Vivian Kotler or Jerri Doherty. Vivian also preferred "natural ways" to combat her stress and explained that "aerobic activity" would have been best, but it was not something she could afford in either time or extra expenses. Vivian also emphasized the need for mothers to literally embody strength, much like the two married mothers:

> Oh my gosh! If I medicated myself, where will my daughter be if I medicated for stress? I just feel like oh, you know, I want to be strong for my daughter. And I want to show, I want to model strength and I don't want to rely upon pills. Yeah . . . but I've once thought about it for depression.

Following this, Vivian described waking at 5:00 a.m. to exercise with some small free weights a neighbor had discarded.

Jerri Doherty, another low-income single mother on Medicaid since her divorce, found any healthcare for herself an unaffordable luxury. One of four mothers who smoked, perhaps as a form of self-medication, Jerri surprisingly burst out with the wish that she could afford treatment when recounting how her son had been helped by his medications: "Oh yeah, I think it would be a great idea if I was on something. Like Paxil. Yeah."

Conclusion: Lone Bureaucratic Rangers

It may well be that to a broad swath of the American public the idea of twenty-first-century mothers administering brain-altering medications to their kids appears not just as sending children to the tragic 1960s *Valley of the Dolls* of drug abuse—but additionally, as an affront to core neoliberal values, a shirking of the most vital responsibilities of women citizens to selflessly devote themselves to maximizing their children's health and odds for future success.[92] Only bad mothers seek a quick fix from drugs, or as one *New York Times* pundit asserted baldly, "With Ritalin, the parent [read "mother"] stupefies the child for the parent's good."[93] I learned a great deal about the extent of mothers' individual responsibilities at the PAC meetings for special-ed parents, where medicating kids was all but unspeakable. But from the mothers I spoke with I learned that navigating the medical system and medicating a struggling child was nothing like the quick fix so widely imagined. Locating specialists, gaining insurance coverage, obtaining diagnoses and researching medications seemed arduous and involved wrestling with decisions about whether and how long to medicate, whether to seek additional diagnoses, adjust dosages, or change drugs. In fact, most mothers I spoke with turned to multiple means of treatment and did not see medications as a "panacea" but at best as offering partial help.

In this chapter I have emphasized two major experiences which mothers seemed to share across divides of social advantage and disadvantage as they raised vulnerable kids: first, all had to navigate through the clouded institutional waters of the educational and medical systems, seeking sources of increasingly fragmented, narrowly specialized expertise on behalf of struggling kids. In both large, impersonal, rule-bound systems mothers, across disparate levels of education, income, and cultural capital, were largely on their own whether facing a school's IEP team, an insurance firm's appeals process, or a child psychiatrist's voice-mail system.

Such mothers, I argue, resemble vigilantes taking the law into their own hands, pursuing an ideal of lone relentless action to resolve their children's issues—though mainly they do this by working within existing institutions and with their own detailed records, logbooks, and files. Many showed me these artifacts of their efforts: Faith Prenniker tried to enlist my view of whether to reorganize her files chronologically or by specialist; Lucy Nguyen pulled out samples of her son's report cards and IEPs, reading some choice snippets aloud; and several quipped about better uses for all that paper, like wallpapering a family room. And yet, even the hostile *New York Times* pundit conceded that it is the pressure from the shrinking U.S. opportunity structure that ramps up expectations for kids in ways "cruel" to those more temperamentally vulnerable: "As we as a society become desperate financially, and more regulated and conformist, our ideals of competence become misleading and cruel."[94] (Or as two New England mothers raising invisibly disabled kids who started their own web business announce hilariously, "Shut Up about Your Perfect Kids!")[95]

The second major experience I found that the mothers shared across divergent life circumstances and ethnoracial identities was the painful stigma and disgrace surrounding a child's invisible disorder. A substantial number also resented the greater generosity or sympathy offered those whose children have traditional, visible impairments. This distinct stigma expressed by the mothers I spoke with may be under-theorized in disability studies with its focus on traditional disabilities and the objectifying stare.[96] A model of biology and culture together shaping what counts as disability in particular historical moments is useful,[97] but I suggest we add two insights gleaned from mothers' accounts. The tool kit of twentieth-century sociologist Erving Goffman of individually managing a soiled identity is inadequate to capture the interdependent presentation of selves involved in family life and childrearing; and to the core concept of the stare of disability studies, we must add the fear, the anxious distancing, or the disbelief with which invisible em-brained disability is received in our present historical context.

3

"The Multimillion-Dollar Child"

Raising Kids with Invisible Disabilities in the Context of Privilege

My husband's closest friends have three children, each with a
separate behavioral diagnosis (ADHD, Asperger's, dyslexia).
The mother spends a tremendous amount of time researching and navigating this world. Unfortunately, it's all she talks
about . . . How should I deal with this?
—Stephanie, Boston, from the *New York Times* Sunday
Styles "Social Qs" column, October 23, 2011

My son Jack, 7, and the neighbors' kids play together all the
time. Recently, the neighbors had a party for their boy and
didn't invite Jack. Jack is autistic . . . I am angry. What should
I do?
—Name withheld, from the *Parade Magazine* "Manner Up!"
column, October 30, 2011

I first met Judith Lowenthal on a gray fall weekday, a month into the
school year for her four children. With one each in high school and
middle school, and two in elementary school, Judith had asked me to
come to her home late in the morning after she'd finished her regular
hour-long run. We had scheduled weeks ahead, in and around the Jewish New Year holidays and the studio art and photography courses she
attended. Driving through the Lowenthals' neighborhood of generous,
landscaped yards and spacious three-story homes, I smiled thinking of
Judith's directions over the phone when she had teasingly insisted that
her house was just a "stucco box."

A slim, youthful woman greeted me at the door, and we strode into
a high-ceilinged living room where Judith pointed out a few of her finished collages on the walls. I was charmed, as I had been over the phone,

with her casual, self-deprecating humor. We settled down to talk in a large kitchen displaying neat rows of teas, health-food cereals, environmentally correct soaps, and under the counter, the family's rain clogs. Judith, in dark slacks, red fleece sweater-jacket, unadorned wedding band, and simple bead necklace, certainly dressed like the mother of this gracious home, even if she at times did not quite sound like it. When I complimented her home, for example, she snorted, "The cleaning people come Tuesday, so Wednesdays it looks great. Then it's like a bomb hit later in the week." While I set up my tape recorder, she checked her phone messages, chuckling, "I did my cell message over and over and over, and I still hate it."

This youthful playfulness alternated with another side of Judith, serious, discerning, even a bit condescending when our conversation focused on her middle-school child, Allan, then nearly twelve. Always more needy than his older sister or younger brothers, Judith described her second child as very gifted, with incredible focus for hands-on projects like building with his programmable Lego toys. Yet, she recounted, such focus could veer into fixation, as during the hot summer when, at age five or six, he refused to remove the winter coat that served his play-acting of imagined army battles. As a baby, Allan would sometimes become "a little ball of rage" and the continuing outbursts and "major tantrums" had long troubled Judith. She and her husband, Rick, had first seen a therapist when Allan was three, shortly after the birth of the third of their four children: "[Allan] was a very bright, charming, good-looking little boy. He went to preschool, he was somebody the teachers loved." But at home, "Why was he so difficult?" "It always came back to, 'Well, he's acting out at home, it must be something that we're doing. Or I'm doing.'"

By the time of our meeting, Judith had experienced several "cycles," each with its own diagnoses and specialists, and Allan was perhaps making gains, if unevenly, with the diagnosis of bipolar disorder during his fifth-grade year together with the dyslexia diagnosed the year before. In the multiple hours I spent with Judith, I heard of ongoing stresses, but mainly of the years of concerted efforts to obtain each diagnosis. Judith's three other children were typically developing, but she had wrestled deeply with Allan's issues, seeking out many specialists and treatment approaches. Judith's narrative of mother-child troubles overlaid the subtext of a privileged life, one in which a mother was more careful to whom she disclosed potentially discrediting, stigmatizing information as she managed the presentation of *selves* and the display of family order. Judith's story exemplifies a key paradox I discovered facing affluent, married mothers raising kids with invisible disabilities: Raising a troubled child with generous economic, cultural, and social resources to call upon is of course somewhat easier; however, at the same time, it may be more difficult precisely because so much class transmission is at stake. Tensions surrounding stigma and visibility seemed to become more freighted within the elite neighborhoods, schools, and communities affluent mothers described, and within their marriages themselves. With each family having significant forms of social privilege to protect and pass on, the presence of a challenging, needy child may heighten tensions in gendered processes already assigning much of this care and organizing of daily lives to mothers. Moreover, if it was Judith's primary responsibility to maintain family order and handle social slights, she was one of the exceptional few whose marriage withstood such blows. This chapter will suggest that the challenge to maintain class and community standing in the face of a struggling child can be formidable, as stigma affects even highly resourced families and exacerbates the strain that difficult children may place on a marriage.

In this chapter I also scrutinize the plausibility of mother-blaming theories for the burgeoning medicalization of childhood. To briefly recap, these arguments hold harried working mothers largely responsible for rising diagnoses and psychoactive drug use among kids. And yet, Judith and several of the affluent mothers featured here who remain outside or only part-time in the labor force represent a privileged exception at a time when few men earn enough to (so amply) support women's homemaking. Macro-economic restructuring across the last several decades has led to a decline in good, breadwinning jobs, intensifying 24/7 competitive pressures and families' reliance on mothers' earnings. This trend is particularly sharpened with the increase in households headed by single mothers. Yet American workplaces remain nearly as inflexible to family needs as in the heyday of the gender-divided nuclear family and the manly industrial economy.[1] I begin with Judith Lowenthal because she was one of only three among the ten affluent women living that twentieth-century ideal of manly breadwinning, womanly homemaking (each of the ten affluent mothers lived in households with income at or over $100,000 annually; all had at least two years of college, seven had four-year degrees or more).[2] Four other affluent mothers, in contrast, were employed on a part-time basis, with three employed full-time in elite professional positions.[3] I was not surprised to find so few fully at-home mothers when nationally nearly 80 percent of women with school-aged children and some 65 percent with children under five are employed.[4] But Judith also captures the chapter's central focus because she so readily embraced full-time domesticity and primary responsibility for managing a disabled child. And yet Allan's issues remained unresolved and were described by Judith in terms no less distressing than those whose mothers had greater involvement in the labor force.

Judith, because she had spent all but a few months at home full-time since having her first child, described herself as a "highly attuned mother," particularly with regard to her vulnerable son Allan; and her account was filled with relentless advocacy on Allan's behalf. She exemplified my notion of the vigilante mother who seized authority, without masculine recklessness, despite a lack of specialized training or relevant professional credentials. Enlarging an argument suggested by Claudia Malacrida in her study of Canadian and British mothers raising kids with ADHD, I suggest that even mothers with a large class advantage could call on little authority of their own to confront authoritative discourses and specialists in the educational and medical systems.[5] In the current neoliberal U.S. context, each had to rely on painstaking individual efforts to research the two densely bureaucratized systems, acquiring expertise in special-education policies and disability rights law; the current state of the relevant psy-sector mental health fields and neuroscientific diagnostic categories and assessments; and perhaps the most charged realm, psychiatric medications. I argue that a major reason why mothers of vulnerable children must act so strenuously as vigilantes is the need for such extensive engagement with technical information and the advanced sciences. Because of this, as Colin Ong-Dean has argued for the United States and Malacrida suggests for the Canadian and British context,[6] class *does* matter. Mothers who can activate economic and cultural resources on behalf of vulnerable children are likely to fare better, whether in paying for private services, more easily researching technical questions, negotiating with specialists with a sense of entitlement, or deploying a presentation of self more likely to garner respect. These researchers, however, miss the key paradox suggested by my highly resourced respondents: mothers with class privilege face an extra burden in the imperative to maintain class transmission despite a child's struggles.

I also look more closely at the peculiarity of neoliberal conditions under which even the most advantaged mothers had to locate and patch together their own sources of emotional and expert support with little help from existing institutions (paradoxically, if there was support to be had from existing institutions, it tended to be through state social services, available to only less resourced mothers, and carrying its own heightened stigma and dangers). Consequently, many with resources found support through the purchase of services in commodified, client-provider transactions. In one sense such support is fundamentally social as it is simply between people. In another sense, however, if locating all forms of needed assistance for managing difficult children and mitigating their issues becomes each mother's "personal responsibility"— with little public or collective imperative to even gather and proffer information—then perhaps such an impoverished notion should not be considered truly "social."

Maternal Devotion, Cultural Capital, and the Transmission of Class Privilege

Judith Lowenthal herself was admirably aware that she mothered a troubled child under the best possible material circumstances. But sociological tools allow us to enlarge on her reflections, particularly those developed by Pierre Bourdieu, and in his footsteps Annette Lareau, to scrutinize the dynamics of class privilege and its reproduction in postmodern, postindustrial families. For Bourdieu, class privilege is disguised and legitimated by "cultural capital," a range of educational advantages, adeptness with language and vocabulary, and "soft" skills such as the easy ability to build and activate networks of "social capital," all of which provide one with a "self-assured relation to the world" and make class dominance appear to be justly and individually deserved.[7] Cultural capital thus includes deeply internalized codes for the cultivation of "superior tastes" in the arts, food, and politics, but also intangible aspects of presentation of self, including nuances of dress and bodily comportment or "body capital." Bourdieu wrote of such "good manners, good taste or physical charm" as the "cultural capital most directly transmitted by the family."[8] Indeed, without the accumulated financial assets of corporate wealth—the stocks, bonds, and trust funds concentrated among a tiny fraction of Americans—cultural capital represents the major inherited advantage of middle- and upper-middle-class children and is particularly valuable in the context of shrinking opportunities. Elite professionals—for example, the doctors, lawyers, scientists, engineers, and affiliated specialists with whom Judith was raised and continued to surround herself—may still receive a fairly high return on education and thus fare better with economic restructuring. Although to Bourdieu such professionals represented *dominated* fractions, these were nonetheless fractions of the *dominant* class.[9]

With Bourdieu in mind, the Lowenthals' home and its artful display of "superior tastes" represents parents determined to pass on the same intangible assets they had received. According to Lareau, because families raise kids in a time of economic transformation and uncertainty, middle- and upper-middle-class parenting requires more "concerted" or deliberate action for such transmission than in the past, action to "cultivate" children's every possible avenue for maximizing cultural capital.[10] To both Bourdieu and Lareau, maternal responsibility far overrides fatherly involvement in this process, even among dual-earner couples. Bourdieu, in fact, wrote, "[In] the dominated fractions of the dominant class . . . women, whose labour has a high market value (and who, perhaps as a result, have a higher sense of their own value) tend to devote their spare time rather to child care and the transmission of cultural capital" than to any other household tasks.[11] Lareau similarly found that affluent mothers rather than fathers engage in an intensification of labor akin to that posited by feminist theories of motherhood:[12] affluent mothers, more than in the past, intervene continuously and "shrewdly" in their children's institutional lives, constructing long days of highly scheduled, adult-controlled activities which instill and optimize cultural capital.[13] Working-class mothers, in contrast, intervene much less and allow children greater autonomy and relaxed time; they engage in a parenting strategy of "natural development" as opposed to the middle-class "concerted cultivation." Lareau's conceptual frame partly inspired my notion of maternal vigilantism, particularly in emphasizing the singular, unrelenting attention required as mothers engaged in both transmitting intangible class advantage and managing a high-need child.

Among those I interviewed, Rick and Judith Lowenthal exemplified parents engaged in the transmission of cultural capital accrued over several generations. The couple had met, Judith emphasized, while attending the same prestigious university at which her parents had long been affiliated researchers. After graduation, Rick pursued graduate training in information technology, the couple married, and for a time relocated to further his career. Judith at first planned to do freelance work in science writing, but at home with their first baby she quickly became too immersed in motherhood, explaining, "We always wanted [a bunch of] kids and we wanted them young." Some years into the marriage, with Rick well established, the growing family returned east, choosing to relocate very near the town in which Judith was raised and her parents still resided: "For me, first of all, my parents are here. Rick's parents live in [a nearby state]. We're still incredibly close with our group of friends . . . and they're all back here. And so it just felt like it was so *much* easier." This last statement referred to the practical, emotional, and non-commodified assistance with multiple, mundane aspects of family life[14]—but importantly, it also referred to having increased "social capital," a greater network of highly resourced kin, neighbors, and friends, to tap for access to densely bureaucratized specialists. In the following discussion, comparison with the accounts of other affluent mothers suggests the difference such high social and cultural capital can make in raising a needy child, but also in supporting marriages facing such challenges while immersed in the transmission of class advantage.

Husbands and Cultural Capital

Judith was voluble in praise for her husband, perhaps her key asset and a form of cultural capital, along with heterosexual privilege, which neither Bourdieu nor Lareau fully considered.[15] Rick Lowenthal also brought ample economic resources, enjoying high earnings but also flexible control over his time: as a successful IT consultant, he could pick and choose assignments and often work from the third-floor office of the family's large home. This, along with their close kin and grandparents to babysit, made the affluent Lowenthals downright time-wealthy at a time when many American families face harsh time shortages.[16] Judith recounted that she and Rick carved out lots of separate time as a couple, enjoying afternoon bike rides and evenings at local restaurants. In her view, they required this relaxed time alone to talk through parenting issues, particularly with such a high-need son as Allan. As already "chatterers," she laughed about the money they had earlier spent trying therapy to together address Allan's needs:

> We are best friends and we have communication. . . . The few times we've tried therapy, it's almost like, why are we paying this person? . . . Better yet, we can take the money we're spending to pay you to sit there and listen to us talk and spend it on a really nice dinner. And eat well *and* talk. So you know, personally, I am very blessed. . . . I know why many couples don't survive this sort of thing with their kid because you've got to be so strong, both of you. And then you've got to have communication.

Rick and Judith's marital success also stands out in light of the larger body of research, quantitative and qualitative, on the prevalence of negative outcomes among families with disabled children; such studies find that having a needy child, particularly if behaviorally oppositional, is associated with higher rates of marital strain, divorce, as well as serious depression for mothers. Yet when explaining how she had coped over years with her troubled son Allan's "anger and bad behavior [when it] would become just overwhelming," Judith strikingly explained, "Rick and I spent a lot of time together, just enjoying ourselves." With three typically developing kids and their activities, she added this as well: "I was also probably having a reasonably good time."

Judith's emphasis on a husband's friendship while she supervised the large child-centered household might reflect the twentieth-century ideal of companionate marriage, with its gender-divided breadwinning and homemaking but rejection of the nineteenth century's "separate spheres." Their wealth of time and money, however, allowed the Lowenthals to also enjoy aspects of the exclusive adult and self-development focus of what sociologist Anthony Giddens characterized as the postmodern "pure relationship," the competing ideal for the twenty-first century.[17] The Lowenthals' commitment to both ideals, child- and partner-centered, was evident when, a bit later in our conversation, I had the opportunity to meet Rick myself when he ambled down from his office to fix a mug of tea. Judith chimed in gaily to introduce us: "This is Linda who is writing a book on kids and special-ed parents." Rick slyly smiled: "Oh what fun!" Appearing unhurried and eventually offering a few heartfelt observations on navigating the medical system, Rick remained for close to twenty minutes, an unusually long time in contrast to the several other husbands I met in the course of visiting the homes of my research participants. While in a sense this episode was a display of privilege—in Rick's command of his time in the working day and the cultural symbolism of his involvement in a son's disabilities—this interaction also seemed to demonstrate their commitments to each other and both a child- and adult-centered marriage.

Comparing having a disordered child like Allan to "always just a very low-grade stress on the family" or a "very low-grade fever," Judith's expressions of marital satisfaction also rested on an ongoing sense that she was successfully transmitting cultural capital to her children. For as Lareau makes clear, such familial class transmission of intangible cultural assets is never an automatic process, or in our era, one with clear guarantees.[18] Critical episodes of Allan's volatility were interwoven with references to the sort of "high-brow" activities carrying the sense of class distinction and "distance from the common amusements" which Judith strove to inculcate in her four children.[19] For instance, as opposed to family trips to Disney World or a nearby shore, Judith detailed skiing and hiking expeditions, sailing, and overseas vacations:

> At the end of [Allan's] third grade [a particularly difficult year] we went to London with the kids. And then we went at the end of fourth grade, too. It's funny to look back on that trip because, yeah, things were harder . . . but at the same time, we did pretty well . . . it was like it didn't stop us . . . He [Allan] made life ten times more challenging; but at the same time, I don't feel like it held us back.

Judith then hesitated, explaining, "It [Allan's outbursts and anger] did in subtle ways, but you know, not on this *really big* level." These terms suggest she was assessing the costs to the family, weighing whether she and Rick had done enough to make a summer vacation fun but also distinctive. By hesitating and adding that the family was in fact held back "in subtle ways," she did concede a bit. However, the earlier reminder that the family actually had made *two* successful summer trips to London, and that Allan was "ten times more challenging" than his siblings during each, seemed to mark her maternal accomplishments and overall success. Because in Bourdieu's framework cultural capital is asserted by distancing oneself and family from "the vulgar crowd," the geographic distance of the Lowenthals' two summer trips abroad is telling, suggesting they had sought to strengthen their children's internalized sense of boundaries and superior taste.[20] Many upper-middle-class parents now do the same, with global travel nearly obligatory in "good" schools and selective universities, even if such trips, a bit like fathers' involvement, may furnish more in symbolic display than in practical payoff.

It may be easy to look harshly at privileged mothers like Judith, particularly in the terms of much popular and academic talk condemning over-involved, over-invested, "helicopter" parents unable to let their children suffer so much as a skinned knee on their own. I believe, however, this is too simple and again only blames mothers for much larger social and institutional problems. In my view, Judith's anxieties are real and rational, her efforts at class transmission to protect a precarious child more imperative, for he *will* enter a world of more precarious and globally competitive opportunities.

Judith's maternal boundary-making also involved cultivating her kids' "body capital"—for Bourdieu, elite forms of embodiment and assured bodily deportment signaling class advantage—as the Lowenthals invested considerable time in athletic, outdoor activities including skiing and sailing. According to Bourdieu, such "bourgeois sports" carry prohibitive price tags, but also "hidden entry requirements" in early training and access to exclusive locations which work well to reinforce social distance.[21] Such sports—including "back to nature" activities like the Lowenthals' hiking trips—also inculcate an elite embodied sense of individuated mastery and self-control. The low-brow popular sports, in contrast, accentuate rough physical contact, group bonding, and team competition, shaping a body holding itself differently from that of the individual who "makes his body a sign of its own ease" and self-assurance in the social world.[22] Bourdieu might have also added, as scholars of neoliberal risk culture suggest, that a corollary requirement for investment in such elite body capital is extensive engagement as a skilled consumer of the medical sciences.[23]

One of Judith's most exemplary and detailed stories of family life and class transmission with a disordered child revolved around a particularly challenging trip to a Canadian ski resort—a story that was at once about inculcating elite body and cultural capital, with social and geographical distance from the "common amusements," but also about elite engagement with the medical sciences. Put differently, the story provides a useful lens to illuminate the impact of Allan's issues on Rick and Judith's marriage, on their efforts to continue elite activities, but also on Judith's skills as an affluent neoliberal health consumer. Judith began with the offhand yet telling quip that all four of her kids were so expert at skiing and snowboarding that she had needed to locate a family orthopedist for their various knee issues. In particular for Allan, Judith boasted of his body capital, "It's an activity he loves so much, I mean he loves snowboarding a lot." Yet the trip brought disruption of Allan's daily routines just when they had been considering changing child psychiatrists and medication regimes. Allan's angry behavior was so exaggerated during the trip that, according to Judith, "everyone was freaked out, Rick was freaked out, the other kids were freaked out," and "I just felt like I couldn't go on." Beginning with the food he hurled across the kitchen as the family packed their SUV, "[Allan] had just lots of aggression, lots of fits and rages."

Judith, in fact, recounted that she spent much of the trip on her cell phone with their new pediatric psychopharmacologist, Dr. P. She described frantic calls, some while stuck in a huge holiday traffic jam: "I had been paging him and he had been calling back. But then . . . there was no cell phone coverage. He finally got me and I was so relieved that we were stuck in traffic [laughing] because it meant that I was going to stay in cell phone coverage." She also called Dr. P. from their rented condo and while in restaurants: "I *had* to talk to him . . . we were in pretty rotten shape as a family from this. . . . We all needed a little hand-holding." While unsure if Dr. P. would take calls about medications he had not prescribed, Judith and Rick had lost all trust in the child psychiatrist whom they had dubbed "the Witch Doctor." In contrast, the two spoke of Dr. P. as "a genius," and Judith was given hope when he confirmed that Allan's excessive irritability was likely due to side effects that SSRI Prozac-type antidepressants sometimes manifest in children.[24]

Despite this hope, Judith admitted that during the trip—as in similar moments of crisis with their young son—she and Rick experienced some marital strife:

> That was a very challenging trip, and we had a good time. But you know Rick and I *were* fighting. . . . It was mostly just frustration[but in such instances] we'll fuel each other. . . . Neither one of you know what to do, you both respond differently. My response is often to call the doctors and to lean on them . . . And Rick's response is to [say] . . . "You know, this is hopeless."

The incongruous phrase "and we had a good time" embedded in this frank acknowledgment of conflict underscores, yet again, Judith's ultimate sense of marital and familial accomplishment. She was dogged in efforts to salvage the trip and accepted the gendered responsibility for seeking expert guidance and restoring family order. Similarly, Rick's response—like that of many of the fathers I learned of in my research—was to distance himself emotionally. To his credit perhaps, others might have called off such a demanding excursion—or had their own anger badly provoked. But as in earlier comments on the London trips, Judith's tenor in recounting this story suggested that she was less irked with Rick than proud of her different response. She had alluded several times to her belief that most mothers inherently or naturally have more insight into their children's needs—for example, in the earlier comment that she was a "highly attuned mother," or at another point observing, "I'm a very instinctive mother. You know, it comes to me very intuitively." She had also offered that even the best fathers, like husband Rick, would sometimes "throw up their hands" when dealing with a troubled child. Good mothers, she suggested, were different: "You go through periods where you blame yourself . . . It's not so much blame as it's a *constant* reevaluation of what to *do* to get [Allan] better. . . . You know, it wasn't as much blam[ing myself] as it was looking for solutions and *not* being willing to accept the fact that there were none."

Perhaps sociologist Arlie Hochschild would suggest Rick and Judith had a sufficient "economy of gratitude" to sustain their relationship. That is, they seemed to offer or exchange ample appreciation for the other's contributions despite a highly gendered division of practical and emotional labor. Such appreciation of separate contributions was ironic for Hochschild because it led to reinforcement of persisting gender inequality in the homes of those she studied.[25] Yet the presence of a high-need, disordered child puts such stress on a marriage, and demands such expertise and additional labor, that the gendered "ways of knowing" Judith described are more likely to be seen as innate traits wholly unavailable to men. Under such circumstances a husband's generous acknowledgment of a mother's efforts may have to be enough.

Judith's readiness to "lean on" elite medical professionals in order to restore family order is another marker of her class-linked mothering; that is, the desire to model class-based entitlements to her children interacts with the gendered imperative to perform women's emotion and health-consumption work for the family. For Lareau, modeling such interactions with elite professionals for one's children is itself a core part of "concerted cultivation": she argues that affluent children thus learn "how to be assertive and demanding" and "how to make bureaucratic institutions [and professionals within them] work to their advantage," to "accommodate their individual needs."[26] The following additional comments Judith offered about Dr. P., the pediatric psychopharmacologist, exemplify the entitlement she aimed to transmit at the same time that she secured much-needed emotional comfort to restore family order: "He was very good with me in that crisis situation ... it wasn't [just] that he was telling me about the medication and the actual chemistry behind it [the antidepressant Allan had been taking]. It was more just him being there to support us and being patient enough to support us." Moreover, Judith had only originally secured a spot with Dr. P. by dropping her parents' names, respected members of the same university community. In activating this network of social capital, Judith occasionally referred to Dr. P. by his first name, another sign of the ease and entitlement associated with class privilege. Yet she playfully explored the limits of her entitlement in such nonreciprocal, client-provider relations of support by joking about Dr. P.'s availability: "He has this really annoying habit that he goes away completely, like totally unreachably, for the months of July and August. It's a horrible habit [laughs]. I'm going to have to fix that about him. I'm going to work on it [laughs again]." Similarly, she quipped about the costs of such experts, perhaps expressing both discomfort and pride in securing such high-end commodified support: "I mean, we spend a *fortune* on this kid. *This is like the multimillion-dollar child.*"

Certainly nearly every mother I met in the course of this research would have wished to call on similar resources to protect a precarious child. This was expressed most vividly by low-income single-mom Vivian Kotler as she had burst out with her best advice to other mothers: "You need to be rich for these kids. So my advice would be to become rich!" But in some respects Judith's additional cultivation of Allan's body capital, her added maternal efforts to ensure the fit, attractive appearance of a precarious child along with her typically developing children, differed less from mothers with fewer resources. All, for example, shared gendered responsibilities for feeding their families,[27] perhaps ramped up by neoliberal health campaigns individualizing responsibility for the obesity "epidemic."[28] Judith Lowenthal expressed some of this preoccupation with weight issues and pride in the fitness of all four of her children: "None of my kids are *really* thin, like you know those scrawny, scrawny kids. Like my kids are always very dense; when you went to pick them up, you were, like, you really had to lift. But they are *not* fat. They are very trim looking. I mean in other words, they look really, really healthy [chuckles]. They just have a good look. You know, they are just the perfect weight for their height."

Judith, like most mothers, may not have consciously considered the ways that cultural capital can be embodied to help maintain or improve class standing. Yet most women understand the significance of physical attractiveness in terms of gendered, if not of classed identities; and most of those I spoke with expressed a commitment to instilling or cultivating their children's fit, gendered bodies and body images. This is more challenging in several respects with struggling children, as the very invisibility of their issues and the opportunity to pass must continually be weighed against the need for recognition and support, though the latter risks bringing a good deal of stigma. This conundrum was clear in the 2012 incident in which a mother and her three-year-old autistic son, described as "crying inconsolably," were ordered to exit a plane which had been taxiing on the runway; according to the *New York Times* upscale Travel section, others traveling with autistic children have "survival strategies" such as to "dress their children in brightly colored T-shirts that declare 'autism awareness,' trying to make the *invisible* disability *visible*."[29]

Because no parent, and especially no mother, wants a child to be stigmatized or treated as tainted goods, Judith took extra pride in Allan's "trim looking" body and his lack of marking as different or disabled. Paradoxically, the atypical antipsychotic he had been on during one school year to quell his irritability and make his behavior less marked or visible has been found to cause significant risks of diabetes and substantial weight gain.[30] In her vigilante research combing the Internet, Judith had learned of the unfortunate side effects shared by this class of drugs before they were publicly acknowledged by pharmaceutical firms, "I think, 'Wow, I did the right thing [to take him off the antipsychotics].' He's not taking these potent drugs . . . and he's healthy and he's *thin*, because a lot of the antipsychotics make you put on weight. And you know, he looks great . . . if he had stayed on it I bet he would have filled out."[31]

Judith also emphasized obtaining fresh, low-fat foods, combining her efforts at class transmission with those to mitigate Allan's issues.[32] Judith owned shares in a local community farm to obtain vegetables in season and she shopped at expensive organic grocery chains for other items. In her earliest attempts to "chip [away at] the puzzle" of Allan's issues, she had tried modifying his diet to eliminate likely allergens: "[I] tried diet for awhile. I decided, you know, it was soy and citrus [which] bothered him, and we needed to keep that from him." These diet restrictions had not seemed to lessen his mood swings, but Judith still suspected that various nutritional deficiencies might be somehow involved in all such brain differences:

> The way to help these kids is not by *just* giving them drugs, but to really look at correcting some imbalance . . . [whether the] result of our diets, our genes, who knows? . . . [or the] interplay between the two. . . . [This] revolution in psychiatry [means that] the more we learn about the brain, the more we learn about cells, the more we learn about neurotransmission and metabolism . . . and the [entire] neurological system.

At our second meeting, while Judith finished a lunch of roasted vegetables and grains, she was more lighthearted and self-deprecating about feeding her family. Sidling to the sink to scrape ample leftovers down the garbage disposal, she smiled broadly: "My kids hate my cooking." She also gently mocked her own love of candy, not exactly acknowledging it as low-brow, but remarking on a slight recent weight gain for which she had been teased by family members.[33] Actually, Judith had been heavily invested in other boundary-making, class-enhancing notions of embodiment: those prescribed by proponents of "attachment parenting" and extended breastfeeding. With each baby, Judith had practiced the home births, years of on-demand nursing, "child-led" weaning, and shared family bed which these groups advocate.[34] Such practices, if posing some challenge to medical authority, may actually be complicit with neoliberalism and help shape such mothers into better privatized health consumers. Epitomizing a mother who takes individual responsibility for assessing information and calculating risks for her family, expecting no public or collective responsibility, Judith offered this explanation of her "attached" parenting:

> I always make a point of telling them [healthcare providers] that I had a home birth. . . . If their reaction is, "Oh my God, you were crazy, and that's unsafe and ridiculous," then chances are this isn't a doctor that I want to work with . . . I knew what I was doing, I knew the risk involved . . . I also make a point of bringing up that I nursed my children extensively: well beyond what many Westerners consider normal . . . I don't want it to come out in terms of how I fed my kids or how I parented my kids and have them look and blame me. . . . So I'm always up front about the attachment parenting and the sleeping and everything. And I always say, "We did this . . . after careful research" . . . I don't want to hear that sort of parenting being blamed for my son's problems because I knew it wasn't. I had three other kids [so] I knew that that parenting was not to blame.

A Second Affluent Mother, Abby Martin

Other mothers I came to know might have envied Judith's successful marriage. While just under half of the mothers I met in the course of this research were in (heterosexual) marriages, more often than not they described relationships strained by their challenging children. Most recounted accepting a stingy economy of gratitude, with little acknowledgment of their onerous care burden or vigilante efforts, as long as a husband simply recognized rather than denied a child's issues. Abby

Martin's case, because it followed the opposite trajectory—from a more equitable division of care to divorce because of a husband's denial—brings the pattern into stark relief. For fifteen years Abby enjoyed a marriage with greater shared childcare and breadwinning than most, if in a relationship she described as "short on intimacy." What finally drove her to divorce was her husband's persistent denial of their daughter's serious struggles, unusual given his involvement in shepherding her through daily life (more typically, husbands who were in denial were relatively absent from such care work).

Abby and ex-husband Ted were the white Euro-American parents of two children, a typically developing younger son and an older daughter with, to Abby's eyes, serious troubles. They were both employed as research scientists, with advanced degrees from prestigious universities; and, in contrast to the Lowenthals, they had waited until Abby had secured a professional position to begin their family. A small blonde woman with pretty but tired eyes, dressed in well-worn shirtdresses and loafers, Abby came from a family less sophisticated than the Lowenthals, though solidly middle class and college educated. Abby's home was also less impressive, though nestled into a hillside yard in an equally advantaged neighborhood. Stepping inside the 1960s split level, it was hard to ignore the dishes, newspapers, toys, and school projects strewn everywhere. I couldn't help but think back to the Lowenthals' finished basement, with its walls of built-in shelves and organizers, and a special desk just to keep Allan's projects undisturbed.

When I first met Abby she was still married, but she complained bitterly about the relationship and the burden of dealing single-handedly with Jessica, then fifteen, diagnosed first with obsessive compulsive disorder and later with an autism spectrum disorder. Abby confided that she was angry being left to consult specialists "entirely on my own." While she sought help to cope with Jessica's rigid intractability, Ted, in her account, remained oblivious, "in a romance with his daughter" rather than his wife: "He never admits it, that Jessica needs help. But then his mother was alcoholic and he never admitted that either. It's overwhelming, just overwhelming for me."

Abby went on at length describing Jessica's irritation when other kids touched her schoolbooks and when her food was not kept separate from the family's meals. Although Jessica was academically gifted, she had recently failed several subjects at the town's public high school. With Ted maddeningly calm, Abby worried that to school personnel she appeared hysterical: "They'll think I have Munchausen syndrome by proxy," she quipped with dark humor, referring to the infamous diagnosis for mothers so monstrous that they invent and induce their children's symptoms, endangering them out of their own perverse need for attention.[35] Ted Martin might have been described as a good father and partner in many other respects: he regularly transported the kids to and from school and was more likely than Abby to disrupt his workday for their activities or illnesses; though he wouldn't cook, he was home in the evenings so that Abby could fit in the swimming she needed for recurring back problems. Abby acknowledged grudgingly at that first meeting that Ted had always supported her career and that the two had enjoyed (high-brow) cultural activities with season tickets to the symphony and museum memberships. Yet she lamented, "I just needed reassurance that I had not invented these problems of Jessica's." Abby sadly concluded that after several long years without that acknowledgment "there's not a lot of the marriage left."

Over the ensuing years I kept in contact with Abby through occasional e-mail and coffee dates. I was not surprised when, a year and a half after our initial conversations, she demanded Ted move out and initiated divorce proceedings. Despite the new constraints on her schedule, Abby emphasized being better able, as a single mother, to care for her typically developing son—to make regular suppers, arrange for his rock-climbing classes, and calmly supervise his homework. Most of all, she felt she was better able to buffer him from his sister's verbal abuse. But Abby could not prevent Jessica from dropping out of school, nor when she turned eighteen, from moving away with funds provided by her father. Relieved that by nineteen, Jessica had received a high school equivalency diploma through a community college program, Abby had to sharply lower her aspirations for class transmission. Though she and Ted had ravaged their retirement funds in the divorce to protect the kids' college money, Abby was reduced to slim hopes that Jessica might continue to take even community college courses.

Highly educated mothers expressed sadness over children unlikely to attend the prestigious universities from which they themselves had gained so much, as in this observation from Abby: "It's too painful to talk to people with normal kids anyway . . . What do I say when they ask, 'Is Jessica in advanced math? What colleges is she looking at?'" The class difference from the blue-collar Hardestys and Gregorsons, in particular, were reflected in different and arguably more suitable aspirations for precarious kids. Both Rosemary Hardesty and Blayne Gregorson spoke with great satisfaction of their troubled sons' practical accomplishments, such as finding a part-time job or learning to drive. Rosemary Hardesty, for example, reported at length, "He just got his license. I gave him a [used older] car. Which was scary, it was very scary. I said, 'My God, he's on the road [sigh]. Is he going to be under control?' He's doing fine . . . I think he's overly cautious . . . [and] he just got a job at the mall!"

In the postindustrial knowledge economy with its (misleading) ideal of college for all, many middle- and upper-middle-class families may hope their kids will retain an advantage by graduating from more selective, competitive universities and colleges. With precarious children, however, this can lead to excessive pressure for mothers and kids, as well as a greater sense of failure in maintaining class transmission and family order. This was much like the final, bitter blow to Abby Martin's marriage, as she was convinced Ted had aided and abetted Jessica's decision to drop out of high school. Other mothers, particularly those with teens, also spoke of fears that their disordered children might face downward mobility and more precarious opportunities—and this was perhaps most difficult to swallow for affluent mothers whose kids' differences were accompanied by forms of academic giftedness. Socially advantaged, married mothers Angie Thompson and Colleen Janeway each offered wry observations expressing similar anxieties about class transmission: Angie, contemplating a battle with her local school for more special-ed services, sighed deeply, "I'm thinking, 'Oh my God . . . but *if* that can be the difference between her working at CVS and going off to college, I have to do it!" Colleen simply exclaimed, "My son will either end up at MIT or working at Blockbuster!" Such dark-humored quips are remarkable for their awareness that New Economy job growth, while spawning the innovative high-tech sectors, has nonetheless been concentrated primarily at the bottom, in minimum-wage retail and service jobs. And even these prospects are more precarious, as since the time of these interviews Blockbuster has gone bankrupt.[36]

A Third Affluent Mother, Theresa Kelleher

White Euro-American Theresa Kelleher provided another vantage point on raising a troubled son in the context of class privilege. Unlike Abby Martin, who remained in full-time employment, Theresa sacrificed a valued career and reverted to highly gendered nuclear-family arrangements to better manage her vulnerable son.[37] And unlike Abby, Theresa held on to her good-enough marriage. As Theresa described it, the inequitable and somewhat impoverished relationship seemed to offer sufficient shared acknowledgment of a young son's vulnerabilities and gratitude for her care work. Yet unlike Judith Lowenthal, who embraced full-time homemaking, Theresa reported having "loved" the career she clung to for the first seven years of her son's life. The mother of a younger typically developing daughter as well, Theresa and husband Peter had worked long hours in banking and finance, relying on the au pairs, babysitters, and house cleaners which Theresa would arrange. Their son Colin's difficulties emerged in preschool, prompting a series of caregiver and school crises, but Theresa had turned to flex-time scheduling and then to reduced hours to cope. She had finally resigned from her financial management position only when, in Colin's second-grade year, his issues "were actually getting worse: . . . it was all because of his needs. I don't think I would have quit otherwise. I mean because I *loved* working . . . I would *not* have been a stay-at-home mom."

When I met her, Theresa had been a "stay-at-home mom" for three years, and described the experience quite differently than Judith Lowenthal's "reasonably good time." For Theresa, "it was very lonely actually" and "that first year was very sad." Colin's needs had also taken a toll on her marriage, in another contrast with Judith's household:

> The hardest part was getting him [husband Peter]—he's always looking at money, you know, money was always an issue. Does [Colin] really need all those services? Does he really need to be tested? . . . I'd be reading all the books. I don't think [Peter] read *any* of them. . . . Clearly, he's concerned and worried about [Colin]. And he went with me to look at all the schools and to meet with the psychologists and therapists at the schools. But he doesn't want to be a part of the parent support group. He feels he doesn't get anything out of it.

These comments, with two main areas of complaint, reveal another somewhat stingy marital bargain. First, despite husband Peter's high-flying salary and the decade or more of high earnings which Theresa had contributed, Theresa was discouraged from making Colin the "multimillion-dollar child." She suggested her voice might carry less weight in decisions about Colin's needs than her husband's, a situation quite different than that suggested by Judith Lowenthal. In this sense, Peter offered "concern and worry" about Colin, but failed to fully appreciate the extent of Theresa's painstakingly gained expertise as the parent who was "reading all the books." Second, Theresa evidently felt unsupported in navigating clinical uncertainty. She had explained to me that Colin's diagnosis had shifted from ADHD to "anxiety disorder not otherwise specified," and then to a possible high-functioning autism spectrum disorder. However, here she added that Peter—in marked contrast to Rick Lowenthal—questioned pursuing further evaluation. On balance, Theresa credited Peter for helping her inspect special-needs private schools, yet this was only after their wealthy school district had agreed to cover much of the tuition. And in her somewhat flattened comments about his refusal to attend parent support groups, Theresa signaled resignation to a husband's emotional distance and authority because, she explained, she would not attend without him. She also recounted sadly that the entire family including the dog had just had new haircuts—she was the only one still "shaggy," lacking a reason to spend money on herself.[38] But then she joked, "We're the West Haven Hillbillies," and explained, "We just don't have that discretionary income." While this may seem, from a larger sociological perspective, the relatively trivial complaint of a still quite privileged mother, I will later return to more troubling implications in Theresa's use of her son's medication; this was likely, she had admitted, an attempt to self-medicate for clinical depression.

A range of voices now seek to blame harried employed mothers in affluent households, mothers ostensibly expecting perfect, high-achieving kids, for inducing or exacerbating issues in vulnerable children, or for seeking out diagnoses for typically developing kids simply to treat their underperformance. But comparing the in-depth narratives of three privileged mothers, each with distinct work-family arrangements, suggests that such arguments may often be oversimplified, based on little sense of the families affected or the complexity of their children's issues. I found that despite mothers' divergent employment decisions, each child's issues or vulnerabilities seemed similarly distressing, persistent, and difficult for their families. In Judith's account, neither early "attached" parenting nor making Allan the "multimillion-dollar child" had significantly mitigated his emotional struggles, though being full-time at home certainly allowed Judith more time to carry on her vigilante efforts. Theresa's account painted a contrasting picture because at the same time as she pulled back from an absorbing, demanding career, by her description son Colin's troubles worsened. It was difficult for me—with my own commitment to absorbing, demanding work—to hear Theresa's sadness without wondering how she and her family might have fared with different policy options—for instance, had she been able to take long-term family leave instead of abandoning her career.[39] And yet Abby, who remained employed full-time, never spoke of cutting back at work, only mentioning the difficulty of taking phone calls from specialists while supervising lab work; indeed, she described work as a type of respite from Jessica's challenging behaviors and school problems.[40]

Although my interviews are limited in number and represent only those willing to volunteer their accounts, such in-depth perspectives offer a richer sense of the lived experience behind burgeoning rates of childhood medicalization than either aggregate statistics or media punditry. The narratives of the ten highly resourced mothers instruct that even those fortunate enough to cut back or quit paid work faced a dilemma, with no decision on their employment outside the home a panacea able to absolve them of guilt for falling short. Moreover, the intangible aspects of class and cultural advantage so important to transmit in the New Economy remained as core challenges for all ten.

Stigma, Communities, and Class Transmission

If much of class transmission occurs within families, communities and neighborhoods also play a vital role in the accrual of intangible assets. For the affluent mothers, the stigma of a burdensome, unruly child disrupted such class-enhancing community ties as it also disrupted family order. In the anxious context of economic transformation, both rational and irrational fears for a middle- or upper-middle-class community's standing, particularly for its schools, may be heightened. A child whose disabilities are not immediately perceptible and whose disruptions are episodic may be more disturbing than those traditionally and visibly disabled, although both tax community and school resources. Less stable, unmarked impairments may evoke more mother-blame and spark greater irrational fears of contagion, of stealthily invading a neighborhood and classroom so that other innocent kids "catch it."

An affluent community, in contrast to such fears, might be expected to provide many advantages for those raising vulnerable kids—not just better schools and less dense, stressful physical environments but the educated population typically predictive of greater tolerance for difference and inclusivity. Researcher Colin Ong-Dean has pointed out that the original class-action suits establishing disability rights in the educational system in the 1970s attempted to make such inclusivity a broad social goal, though with little success. Policies instead have "enabled parents to raise individualized, technical disputes over their children's disability diagnoses and needs" without affecting regular-ed classrooms.[41] Now several decades later, with transmission of class privilege threatened by New Economy change, families with typically developing kids may have even greater fears of inclusion. The findings of Indiana University experts on stigma, Bernice Pescosolido, Jack Martin, Jane McLeod, and their students, in large-scale surveys of attitudes toward children's disorders, suggest such a trend. The team found levels of social rejection two to three times higher for a child exhibiting symptoms of ADHD or depression than for a hypothetical child with asthma or "normal troubles"; 20 percent admitted preferring that families with children exhibiting symptoms of ADHD or depression not live next door or share their children's classrooms; and between 25 and 30 percent reported preferring their children not befriend such kids.[42] Over two-thirds of those polled expressed negative attitudes toward medicating children, with many agreeing that child troubles may actually reflect poor "parenting."[43] Those with greater education, as well as women, were slightly less likely to express such discriminatory attitudes; however, those who were *married* were *significantly more* likely to desire social distance than those unmarried, perhaps because, as I am suggesting, those married have substantially more cultural and economic capital to protect and transmit.[44]

Among the highly resourced group I came to know living in affluent communities, research scientist Abby Martin was among the most
isolated. Abby acknowledged readily that some of her isolation had
been self-inflicted as she withdrew before others in her community
might stigmatize the family. She recalled with regret that she had sacrificed even "a minimal social life" because of a vulnerable daughter's
unpredictable turbulence. While inviting colleagues over for dinner
had been a routine pleasure in her early married years, such evenings
were now out of the question. Abby explained that—as mentioned
earlier regarding dashed class aspirations—"it's too painful to talk to
people with normal kids anyway." Abby had thus removed herself from
the "communities of judgment" which, according to philosopher Jennifer Nedelsky, assist and reassure in the "daily decision making of
motherhood"[45]—as well as from exchanges which, according to sociologist Lareau, provide important strategic information for developing children's cultural capital.[46] Yet evidently more important, Abby
protected herself from the likelihood of communities of negative
judgment such as those found in the Indiana University research, as
judgment can always cut both ways. British sociologist Ann Oakley
referred to something similar in noting the power of gossip in communities of mothers.[47]

Judith Lowenthal was much less isolated than Abby Martin, but living
in a similar town she had faced just such stigmatizing judgments because of Allan's troubles. For example, she recounted a recent exchange
of angry e-mails over Allan's exclusion from a neighborhood-wide children's party:

> I was actually writing an e-mail about Allan's mental illness [because] this
> party issue, it's *not* going to be OK . . . and [instead] I started to list the
> people that *were* supportive of me through all of this with Allan. And *who*
> *were* supportive of Allan, who believe in him, who aren't just saying, "Al-
> lan's a bad kid." Or you know, that he's mentally ill and [then they] don't
> want to talk about it.

But Judith, after thinking of those who were supportive—mainly kin
and old college friends—also reported the stinging rebuff by another
mother with boys on her block. Judith's vigorous "push-back" to such

incidents undoubtedly carried important personal and psychological dimensions, but it also revealed important social or sociological dimensions of class transmission in well-to-do communities:

> I had a really hard time with my best, closest, closest friend here. . . . She has two boys, same ages as two [of] my boys. We vacationed with them. We've skied with them. We've hiked with them. . . . [But] she got very upset with me for not going—she did this volunteering, it's part-paid, part-volunteer thing at the school . . . And I didn't attend her presentation. And she got really upset with me and was very hurt. And I couldn't believe that she was hurt. I was like, "You have no idea what I'm going through in my life." And this also fueled a bunch of insensitive comments about Allan, like, [they] don't really want to be around him . . . We hashed it out, [but] I don't think she will ever understand the total impact that it [Allan's disorder] has on our family.

The prevalence of intolerant views among those with generous economic and cultural resources was also evident in Theresa Kelleher's narrative. Previously I touched on Theresa's sense of isolation after leaving a high-flying career. Though she withdrew to better manage troubled young son Colin's schooling and therapeutic treatments, she also withdrew to counter his social rejection, thinking it stemmed from her career. She explained sadly that she had been wrong:

> One of my reasons for quitting . . . he wasn't having play dates or friends . . . and the au pairs, our nannies, would say, "You know, nobody ever calls and asks him to come over." I was thinking, "Well, a lot of this neighborhood is stay-at-home moms . . . and maybe I need to be here and become friends with them."

But once home and volunteering at Colin's school, she discovered the stigma extended further:

> There's one mom and son I have a hard time with . . . And the son was a bully really[and] this boy at the cafeteria would have the kids raise their hands if they were friends with Colin. I didn't find this out until much later, [but] at the beginning like a bunch of kids raised their hands. And

then by the end, none of them were! . . . And [if they did] he [the bully] would say, "You *are*? . . . [But] he's a kid with *problems*!"

Theresa eventually found out about these repeated, ritualized incidents of harassment from other mothers, realizing that Colin's troubles—and thus her own—had become a topic of neighborhood gossip. She described confronting the "bully's" mother: "So I called the mom. . . . She was saying to me, 'Oh thank you for telling me this! Our kids are *so* sheltered here, they're just not—.' I mean she all but said, 'They're not used to dealing with kids with problems.'"

These peer troubles seemed to occur across levels of social advantage and in wealthy schools. New research suggests that students with invisible disabilities are far more likely to be bullied than typically developing kids;[48] and Theresa's account of the bully's mother indicates why particularly among affluent "sheltered" kids, "different" children might be singled out. Theresa protected her son Colin by gaining the private school placement mentioned earlier, but she herself was less shielded. Some two years later, she disliked being back around the local school with Colin's younger sister because it "just brings back a lot of *bad* memories." And she faced intrusive questioning about Colin, "because it's normal to go to private school in this town." Other mothers asked, revealing their communities of negative judgment, "'Oh which one?' 'I haven't heard of *that* one'; and I just say, 'Oh, it's really small.'"

Colleen Janeway, who quipped that her son might end up at "MIT or working at Blockbuster," was one of just three full-time homemakers among the ten highly resourced mothers. Colleen's choice to leave the workforce had been more positive than Theresa's, made when her third child, son James, was an infant, long before she had any inkling of his special needs. Like Judith, Colleen had four children, three of whom were typically developing, successful, and popular in the local schools. Nonetheless, Colleen described very painful, stigmatizing situations in those same schools. One incident two days prior to James's last day in elementary school was emblematic. The entire class, most of whom had progressed though the K–5 grades together, was caught up in celebrating their imminent passage to middle school: "One of the room mothers calls me [after the fact] and says, 'Colleen, this is horrible. I can't believe it happened, but the class picture was taken and James is not in it.'"

James, she was told, had had one of his episodic "meltdowns" when jostled by other kids and had been removed. But to Colleen, it was "completely unacceptable" and "absolutely outrageous" that they had not immediately phoned her and postponed the photo shoot. "I said to the principal, 'Somebody could have called me. I mean you've called me when he needs a napkin at lunchtime!'" Significantly, Colleen immediately drew out the comparison to a traditional, visibly disabled child: "If that child were in a wheelchair, everyone would be all over themselves to make sure he was in that picture! You would be placing him there ... There were about one hundred things that could have been done. And *none* of them were done.... This child is a huge part of this class! Even if nobody else wants to sit next to him, he feels part of this class!"

The work of feminist ethnographers Alison Griffith and Dorothy Smith, while not concerned with those whose children have special needs, can help illuminate such episodes of resistance to genuine school inclusion experienced by Colleen, Theresa, and others who shared their stories with me. Griffith and Smith, scrutinizing intersections of class and gender, demonstrated that both working-class and middle-class communities required mothers to sustain and supplement local schools; but the crucial school-supplementing work of middle-class mothers also reproduced class privilege by "enabl[ing] the school *as a whole* to function at a higher level."[49] To Griffith and Smith, then, middle-class mothers act on the community level to further the class transmission occurring in their homes, both together increasing the odds that their children retain "special access to middle-class occupations" and creating an unavoidable reliance on other families.[50] Particularly with New Economy competitive pressures, mothers with kids in regular-education may understandably perceive the disruptions of "kid[s] with problems" and kids having episodic "meltdowns" as taxing school resources and personnel—and as threatening the enhancement of the school as a whole.

Several highly resourced mothers, seeking greater social acceptance and more appropriate academic instruction for their vulnerable children, simply opted for private schools. Yet private schools present their own obstacles and generate their own communities, some even more intent on protecting class transmission. Indeed, highly educated, Afri-

can American, and married, Virginia Caldwell-Starret reported bringing work home and losing sleep to maintain young son Henry in an
elite private school. When his teachers questioned his disruptiveness, his
ability to keep up academically and to fit in with other students, Virginia
obtained a formal diagnosis for the ADHD previously suggested by a
specialist and began administering Ritalin. In this process, she sought
out therapists and child psychiatrists, private tutors and special summer
camps, all the while increasing her presence at school activities.[51]

In addition to containing their own communities of judgment, private schools do not stand completely apart from the local organization
of education and the families involved. Students will move between the
two settings, as amply illustrated in Judith Lowenthal's account of moving Allan and his siblings across settings more than once; and many
families also have typically developing kids, siblings of their invisibly
disabled children, in regular ed. Special-needs independent schools, in
addition, rely on public districts for referrals and for at least part of their
tuition funds.[52] Moreover, their high costs—higher than many independent schools for typically developing kids—impel coordination with
public schools in the hope that children deemed successful might transfer back. Even Theresa Kelleher expressed hope that at the high-school
level, with the gossip and bullying further in the past and the addition
of students from other K–8 schools, her son Colin might transfer back.
But neighborhood talk and gossip might persist longer than Theresa
wished, as other mothers indicated. A few found such gossip paradoxically useful.

Judith Lowenthal exemplified such paradoxical use of neighborhood
talk: while causing her pain in some instances, she had also found such
informal information useful when transferring son Allan to a special-
needs day school. Judith was, notably, the only mother to report simply
paying the full tuition "out of pocket" for such a placement. Ferreting
out local information on who had such placements, what their diagnoses were, and what, if anything, they received from the district had
been crucial in making this decision. (Virginia Caldwell-Starret also
paid full tuition, but her son was enrolled in a prestigious independent
school known for its academic standards.) Although tuition for special-
needs day schools can be comparable to a private college, the Lowenthals elected to bypass any battle for limited town funds, making it all

the more true that they spent "a fortune" on Allan. Judith spoke plainly
of what she had learned; but she closed by pointing to what may be a
conflict for many families with kids in regular ed as well, illustrating the
permeability and interdependence of public and private settings:

> It was going to be a very hard case to fight. And . . . it's not worth it. Since
> [Allan's start], one of those families [also paying out-of-pocket] finally
> did take it to court . . . and I don't know how much they won, because
> obviously all of that has to be kept hush-hush by the family. I know they
> *didn't* win the whole tuition . . . [Allan's school] is a *ton* of money, but
> when we put him [there], we put our others back in the public school.

To battle was thus "not worth it" in several respects: the costs of a
court case,[53] the stress of fighting an uphill battle over Allan's level of
need, and the fact that the drain on district resources only taxed the
regular-ed schools attended by his three siblings. Avoiding a battle may
also have shielded the Lowenthals from further local stigma and gossip, with kids receiving such funded placements decried as "budget-
buster[s]" that drain regular ed.[54] Indeed, three affluent mothers who
had gained public funds for out-of-district placements for vulnerable
sons—Theresa Kelleher, Colleen Janeway, and Angie Thompson—each
worried about the rancor of friends and neighbors (and none revealed to
me whether they received "the whole tuition").[55] Angie Thompson, for
example, worried that the alternate school transportation called attention in the neighborhood to her son's special-needs placement: "There's
a lot of people that see that van pull up. And they're like, 'Why is he getting special treatment?' . . . The special-ed parents . . . we're the big, bad
guys . . . But I have nothing to be ashamed of. I pay my taxes, you know,
just like everybody else."

Privileged parents with invisibly disabled kids, according to Ong-
Dean, are likely to garner a disproportionate share of higher-cost public
special-ed services compared to similarly impaired children whose parents have less cultural and economic capital.[56] Without policies emphasizing the social benefits of inclusion, parents are left to compete over
each child's technical level of need—and, as I also found, privileged "parents" are likely to compete better. Yet they also cannot escape a culture
pervaded by mother-blame.[57]

Judith Lowenthal confronted this at perhaps its most extreme when initially seeking to exercise her high cultural capital to "customize" Allan's education in his second-grade year in public school.[58] When he was still not reading but in a class of twenty-six with "the stress of spelling tests," she worried that frustration at learning differences might be fueling the volatility at home. Yet Judith was stunned by the response of school specialists, who overlooked such possibilities in favor of mother-blame: "In second grade I had him cored [evaluated]. And the core exam came back and they told us that he was *very* bright, which we all knew, and that he had *major* psychological issues revolving around his separation from me. . . . They told me he had major separation issues *and* it was *my* fault and that's that. Oh yeah, it was *total* blame on me: mom blame."

Judith was one of just four mothers to report such seemingly dated, Freudian-style mother-blame, and the only one among the ten most advantaged mothers. Ignoring the child's possible innate vulnerabilities or the context of larger class sizes, standardized testing, and ramped-up academic standards, such terms echo mid-twentieth-century understandings that children's troubles were primarily caused by the mother's psyche: "The oversolicitous or overprotective mother [is] a common cause of abnormal, antisocial behavior on the part of the child."[59] Nearly all the mothers I spoke with reported feeling blamed by others and nearly all spoke frankly of the times in which they blamed themselves for their children's struggles. Yet nearly all understood their blame as more proximate or secondary than the Freudian model, placing themselves in interaction with neurobiological, genetic, and environmental factors. As I have argued, this leads to a more expansive notion of maternal responsibilities, in Judith's terms, to "constantly" reevaluate and relentlessly seek solutions to "the puzzle" of a child's issues. Judith also exemplified a mother's need to manage schools and school settings according to her knowledge of her child's brain, as in observations such as "Allan, because he's got so much muscle power in his brain, he could do the work they were handing him [in school]. He *could* do it, but it was not like what he *really* could do . . . It was like he was running ten miles and he was coming home totally drained." Only one mother, married working-class Lucy Nguyen, held on to something resembling a Freudian approach, placing the primary blame for a son's struggles on her own "nurture"; but intriguingly, this was not, in her account, because she had received such direct twentieth-century blame from others.

I will return to the other few mothers accused by specialists of directly causing their children's issues because, without Judith's class and marital privilege, such accusations could be more harmful. Judith herself was well insulated by the resources allowing her to transfer Allan's school settings and the evidence that her other children were thriving (as in her earlier defense of attachment parenting). Nonetheless, she did blame herself for some initial "ignorance": "There wasn't a single kid left back where [Allan] was in terms of the reading . . . [but] I didn't know about the field of learning disabilities. I just did *not* know." Yet Judith turned to a neighbor, a child psychologist—in Bourdieusian terms, activating her elite social capital, the network available through her well-off, highly educated community—for a second look at Allan's core test results. In short order this led to a referral for a neuropsychological evaluation and to a diagnosis of, in Judith's words, "*glaring* dyslexia."[60] For the next two years, in her account, Judith continued framing Allan's invisible needs through this label, focusing her vigilantism stubbornly on researching alternative school environments.[61] It was only after moving him to the costly independent special-needs day school that Judith, in some desperation, turned to the medical system to address his continuing emotional turbulence. But before turning to such negotiations of privileged mothers with the medical system, I return to the efforts of highly resourced mothers who remained, or remained longer, within public schools.

Negotiating Public Schools

For the large majority of mothers managing invisibly disabled kids who remain in the public school system, their energies focus on the Individual Education Plan (IEP), the individual contractual agreement for accommodations and services required by disability legislation. I discovered that the IEP process, ostensibly meant to include parents, was more often adversarial and mired in the paperwork of quarterly progress reports, annual reviews, and three-year reevaluations.[62] In contrast to Ong-Dean's portrait of the relative successes of college-educated parents in this process, I found such mothers more likely to be frustrated by the expectation that they "raise the bar on being a parent professional."[63] Put differently, Ong-Dean may underestimate the challenge posed by the individualized, technical approach, even to mothers with ample cultural capital and economic resources.

Among the highly resourced married mothers, most voiced surprising feelings of inadequacy. While Judith Lowenthal bemoaned her "ignorance" about learning disabilities, Theresa Kelleher described being intimidated entering IEP meetings with school personnel, "I'm not a psychologist. I wasn't a, you know, physician; and I wasn't a teacher of special ed . . . I thought, 'All these people are taking care of my child, that's their job.' . . . [But] I was so naive and idealistic . . . I never thought people would put cost over children's needs."

Elaine Irving came closest among the affluent married mothers to having such relevant professional credentials, with recent certification as a special-ed teacher. Yet Elaine depicted very similar frustrations advocating for her gifted but troubled son Micah. Married to a young math professor, Elaine had been employed teaching only part-time, with another "half-time job . . . mediating for Micah with the public school." Like others I interviewed, Elaine praised particular teachers whom she "really trusted." However, team meetings were, she complained, "very alienating":

> You know, I'm a very intelligent person, but I don't know much about the WISC [Wechsler Intelligence Scale for Children] . . . and scaled scores and the Peabody Picture Identification Test, and the test of receptive vocabulary. I mean what the hell! . . . And I just felt like this was the most surreal experience . . . [Micah] was just being pathologized by people who have had such minimal contact with him . . . plus there's this use of very advanced jargon . . . "Well, I ran the Beery Test of Visual Motor Integration . . . " Don't hide behind your jargon!

Elaine's observations, though she was being sarcastic, illustrate her fluency in the ability to mimic and mock the use of the technical names for each assessment measure. However, when she next complained, "I felt that they weren't listening to me," she echoed the sentiments of many others I came to know across educational backgrounds. Moreover, if Elaine possessed the higher cultural capital brought by a white, highly educated husband, she explained this was a resource requiring activation and only fully effective if he could be more frequently present:

And always the default seems to be, "Well, if a dad comes, too, then we will sit up straighter." So he [husband Phil] comes to the annual review, but . . . he wouldn't come to those kinds of meetings [about day-to-day problems] . . . it would have generated a long discussion about, "Are you sure I need to be at this one? Can it wait?"

Elaine concluded that with a husband worried about earning tenure and leaving her to be "the one with the three-ring binder about Micah," she was left to confront the labor-intensive daily management alone: the never-implemented homework accommodations "assigned in the ed plan," Micah's unfair removal from the "gifted and talented reading group," or his teacher's favored punishment of lost recess time. Elaine caustically summed up her work with the school: "So, who's finally getting punished? Me!" To clarify that this anger was primarily directed at the school, she laughed, "I have to add to the tape [I recorded interviews], 'I love my husband very much. He's a good guy.'"[64]

Others opted to locate commodified support specifically to bolster their ability to negotiate the IEP and to be less alone in this process. Sandra Barbieri, for instance, complained about the IEP process and worried that her vulnerable son Chris was more than a year behind academically due to insufficient special-ed supports. Among the married, highly resourced mothers in my research group, Sandra was lower in cultural capital, with only two years of college, though enhanced by many years employed in local government and marriage to a high-earning civil engineer. Sandra, much like Elaine Irving, knew that her effectiveness was hampered by a husband who could seldom be present because of his work demands:

I was doing 90 percent of it [advocating at school meetings] myself. And it was really tough because my husband, you know, he—I finally got to the point, "You need to come to meetings with me!" . . . But basically I was the driving force to get all of this to happen. And if I had [not] . . . my son, who knows where he would have been?

Sandra activated her privilege and economic resources to hire a stand-in, a professional educational advocate. Though it seems unlikely that such women specialists fully replace the symbolic weight of a husband's presence, Sandra explained the heightening conflict over her son's IEP and placement: "They weren't saying 'Oh sure, let's look out for the best interests of your child.' No, it was, 'Let's look out for the best interest of how we are going to save money!'" She spent over a thousand dollars for the advocate's intervention, "which my husband did *not* want me to do at the time. And I just said, 'Guess what? . . . That was *the best* spent money that I ever spent!'" Sandra also alluded to having purchased much-needed emotional support: "I was getting to the point that I felt like I was being, you know, banged down into the ground. Do you know what I mean?"

The words of mothers like Elaine Irving and Sandra Barbieri suggest two important revisions to the work of researchers like Ong-Dean: first, it may make little sense to speak of parent involvement in special-education in gender-neutral terms. Instead, it may be more fruitful to disentangle the impact of fathers' masculine authority, to test Elaine's contention that "if a dad comes, too, then [school personnel] will sit up straighter." In a second corrective, special education today cannot be understood outside of its increasingly medicalized context and the challenges this presents for parents. Sandra indeed underscored that navigating the educational system was only *half* of a mother's gendered and isolated vigilante responsibilities: "I didn't know anybody that was going through any of what I was going through because it was a medical problem *and* then the school problem . . . I needed to help my son and . . . I was doing the medical thing as well as the school thing. So it was a combination that I was doing from two sides. And I didn't really have anybody to talk to."

Into the Med System: Paradoxes of Labels and Pills

Mothers of varied class and race location share the paradoxical experience of both relief and dread in obtaining a medicalized diagnosis for a troubled child. Such labels frequently (but not always) offer access to school services and to health insurance coverage. Just as important, they offer recognition and a name, allowing mothers to begin making sense of distressing, largely hidden family experiences. Colleen Janeway, among others, emphasized this: "I think diagnoses are helpful . . . [each] is a *starting* point for an explanation." Most labels, however, also bring the stigma, pain, and fear involved in acknowledging a child's abnormality; and in an era of high-tech medicine and neuroscientific breakthrough, most bring charged questions of whether to administer psychoactive drugs. The model twenty-first-century mother may be expected to gain fluency in this brave new world, and some display of this expertise may be commendable. However, as the exchange between "Stephanie" of Boston and the etiquette columnist highlighted, she should not be too engaged—and perhaps must judge this according to hierarchies of more and less fearful disorders only beginning to emerge. Moreover, she will have to manage her own ambivalence, caught between dependence on and wariness of medicalization itself.

Elaine Irving exemplified the discernment involved in managing labels. She drew out a detailed hierarchy, describing son Micah's depression as much harder to speak of or publically acknowledge than his Asperger syndrome; but she suggested that these were both more shameful than ADD or dyslexia. Moreover, Elaine contrasted these invisible disorders to a much "more obvious" "physical handicap," with only such traditional disabilities bringing sympathy:

> Something like a physical handicap, I think people would be more sympathetic about. It would be more obvious . . . and I would probably be less reluctant to talk about [it] . . . People are really not talking about their kids who have depression. You know, they'll talk about ADD or a learning disability or dyslexia . . . But you know, kids with mental health issues, I would say people tend to be much less open about it. *Much*. And you know, I do the same thing myself . . . I'll talk about his Asperger syndrome and his behavioral stuff, but I won't say, "Oh you know, he's on lithium because he probably has manic depressive disorder."

In this thought-provoking commentary, Elaine seemed to be ranking by the degree of medicalization with which she must contend. For example, "learning disability or dyslexia" seldom involves medications (or at least not yet). And while she might have intended the label ADD to be synonymous with ADHD or to refer to the milder category of distractibility without hyperactivity, either way the ubiquity of such diagnoses and the Ritalin-type drugs might make those conditions seem enviable next to her son Micah's troubles. Elaine nonetheless placed Micah's Asperger syndrome and "behavioral stuff" as still less stigmatized than his "mental health issues," with the use of this latter term just a step away from the heavily freighted "mental illness." "Mental illness" was a label very few mothers used—and experts themselves debate its suitability for the em-brained disorders. Finally, however, Elaine signaled by the phrase "but I won't say 'Oh you know, he's on lithium . . .'" that the most shameful maternal acts involve administering psychoactive medications, particularly those less commonly associated with brain imbalance and more with mental illness.[65]

Many mothers turned to alternative approaches to prevent or minimize the use of pharmaceuticals and perhaps to engage in valorous practices they might embrace without ambivalence. While this was not an issue in which mothers differed significantly across class divides, it was clearly easier for those with ample economic resources.[66] Judith Lowenthal had expressed pride in being "very, very resistant to any type of medication" and, like many practicing attachment parenting, being "a very cynical user" of Western "allopathic medicine." Judith had also rarely been without a psychodynamic, "talk therapy" provider (though avoiding those based in Freudian perspectives). After an "earthy" "feel-good" family therapist, followed by an educational psychologist, she had turned to a behavioral-cognitive therapist to teach Allan self-control and anger management. Nonetheless, she was particularly shaken by the then ten-year-old's frantic response to this approach and decided to try medications: "He was very tearful and *very* upset . . . And he said to me, 'It just doesn't work, Mommy . . . Dr. R. tells me to just stop and think. But I just get this anger—and I just *can't think* when it happens!' . . . So that was the point where I decided I *had* to call a psychiatrist."

Sandra Barbieri displayed an extensive engagement with both biomedicine and alternative practices. With her young son Chris having serious "behavior problems" at school on top of his "dysthymia" and "processing problems," "We were seeing psychologists [and] we were seeing neurologists"—and "like three or four different psychopharmacologists." Yet much as she had with the educational advocate, Sandra purchased extra support from a "homeopathic doctor," speaking of their work together for "almost three years now," their use of "cranial sacral massage" and of diets restricting food dyes, sugars, and red meat. Sandra was decidedly ambivalent about medications, rejecting stimulants because her son's attentional issues were just "borderline"; his persisting emotional and behavioral troubles, however, drove her to lengthy drug trials researching and managing two antiseizure drugs. Sandra detailed questioning dosages, monitoring Chris's responses, challenging providers, and finally seeking out different specialists to "wean" him from the higher doses of the drug (Depakote), which seemed to exacerbate behavior problems. On lower doses of the other, Lamictal, with the homeopathic and alternative practices, she reported that the ten-year-old had "finally" become "kind of stable," his challenging behavior "almost in half of what it was." Sandra had thus come to depend heavily on an entire team of medical specialists, continuing to send the neurologist, psychiatrist, pediatrician, and homeopathic practitioner "all the stuff I get from the school" even with Chris's improvement. If she fell short of her original goal "to keep him [Chris] from having to be on *any* medications," she seemed proud to have contained his treatment to just one drug.

Judith Lowenthal's vigilantism took on a related but somewhat different set of psychiatric medications from those Sandra managed; yet like Sandra, Judith in the end selectively redefined her dependence to better vindicate her original beliefs. Judith's engagement had begun in the hope that "a little bit of an SSRI, a little bit of an antidepressant" for a few months might allow Allan to benefit from the cognitive therapy. These Prozac-related antidepressants were familiar and seemingly benign to many of the women I met; and Judith admitted to briefly trying them herself for premenstrual syndrome.[67] In contrast, such trials with Allan were far from benign; and rather than the widely assumed image of parents facing just one major decision point, about one drug, Judith detailed a tough process of ongoing decisions about multiple drugs, a process that so escalated that Rick and Judith referred to their prescribing child psychiatrist (Dr. S) as "the Witch Doctor."

Judith became, in her depiction, "obsessed" with consulting Internet and print sources on psychiatric medications, including articles in medical journals, while rigorously tracking Allan's reactions in "detailed log books." Eventually, in the space of seven to eight months, Judith managed trials of two SSRIs (Celexa and Zoloft), two antiseizure medications (Trileptal and Neurontin), and one atypical antipsychotic (Risperdal), in varied combinations. She displayed impressive fluency with biological psychiatry and respect for the paradigm, but coupled with outrage with its ties to the pharmaceutical industry. For example, Judith mimicked savagely how psychiatrists succumbed: if "his [Allan's] behavior actually got worse . . . then . . . I'd call her up [Dr. S.] . . . And she would say, 'Oh, OK' . . . And the next thing I know I had a prescription for yet another drug!" She also instructed me on unscrupulous industry practices which heavily promote psychoactive medications unapproved for specific use by kids, despite strict prohibitions against promotion of any drug for un-approved use:[68] "Here's this antiepilepsy drug, Neurontin . . . last year's drug of the century, their new fantasy drug . . . I don't know if you've read in the paper, [but] the company is being sued."[69] Risperdal, another drug Judith administered, later received federal approval for youths, but, as discussed earlier, like all the atypical antipsychotics, it brings risks for elevated blood sugars, diabetes, and weight gain.[70]

During their home-based drug trials, Judith, like many others, ac-cepted some risks while rejecting others, and not always on the most rational basis. For example, while Judith had carefully researched spe-cific drugs, she had also administered drug combinations; this increas-ingly common practice also lacks specific government approval.[71] Rick Lowenthal, joining us, framed the larger dilemma well, caught between the wish for a solution and skepticism toward psychoactive medica-tions. He contrasted the draining "*emotional* reality of everyday [life]" with Allan and the wish to ease his and the family's troubles, with the troubling "*intellectual* experience" of questioning the very authority on which they had become so dependent. He went on at length, expressing a sense of betrayal to which Judith readily agreed:

> You think that there is some *science* behind this. Or that there are years of valuable clinical experience [in prescribing off-label]. . . . [But] it's all just hit and miss! . . . We began with expectations of a certain level of competence, professionalism, *knowledge* . . . But . . . "No, we don't know what the side effects are. We don't know what the long-term health effects are . . . We don't know *what* it does or *how* it works!"

And Judith was even blunter: "This [has gone] against everything that I've ever believed in as a parent. Pumping my kid with random drugs, putting my faith in this medical establishment!"

Surprisingly, Judith did not walk away from child psychiatry or psychopharmacology, but redefined theirs as an alternative involvement when turning to Dr. P., the specialist offering "hand-holding" by phone during their distressing ski trip. Dr. P. was, according to Judith, not only a "genius," but "on the outfield" of the profession, offering an experimental treatment of megadose nutritional supplements for adolescents like Allan. As opposed to "pumping my kid with random drugs," Judith referred to the megadoses as "a multi-food product" consisting of "vitamins and minerals." Perhaps this better reconciled the rigorous management of Allan's daily dosages, like the drug trials of the preceding months, with more valorous, class-enhancing maternal practices like feeding her family healthful, organic foods, cultivating their embodied fitness, and practicing attachment parenting. Indeed, Judith casually slipped in that lithium had been added to Allan's megadose mix; and only when I asked if she could tell me more about that decision, did she get a bit defensive: "Look, lithium is a mineral. And you know when we've talked to Dr. P. about the massive list of ingredients that are on the side of the [supplement] bottle, he said quite clearly to us that he thinks it's probably the minerals more than the vitamins that are in it that are doing something. So anyway, lithium probably should be in that initial formula."

But lithium is both a naturally occurring alkali metal and a powerful psychoactive; lithium salts were used in patent medicines as early as the 1870s, and a century later they were approved by the U.S. Food and Drug Administration for prescription treatment of the manic depressive adults who would now be classified with bipolar disorder. Belying Judith's depiction, moreover, lithium carries high risks of toxicity, requiring strict monitoring through blood tests because of what is termed its "relatively narrow treatment index," with effective doses only slightly below those that could become poisonous.[72] Only three other mothers had administered lithium, and their attitudes were less sanguine. All three spoke of the needles and blood work as continual reminders of daunting risk, framing lithium with other psychoactives.[73] Judith, intriguingly, was the only mother I met to redefine a psychopharmaceutical as a natural supplement in attempts to calm her perhaps well-grounded fears of Big Pharma.

Privileged mothers faced with "pumping kid[s] with random drugs" under the care of well-trained specialists simply found that psychopharmaceuticals, contrary to much popular imagery, do not work all that well. Abby Martin, the science researcher whose husband denied their daughter Jessica's issues, might best exemplify this. Abby had concluded, after managing a series of unsuccessful home-based drug trials, that medications were no "panacea." She alleged that rather than appreciating her frustration with the medical system, her resigned attitude was misread by school personnel as "giving up" on her daughter:

> The SSRI, Celexa, exacerbated things . . . then Zyprexa, the antipsychotic, knocked her out. We tried Ritalin for a while, two or three months—but she lost *so* much weight. Then we needed Risperdal to calm her down, to sleep. We tried Buspar [anti-anxiety], but something was causing a tremor, a neurological problem . . . so she's been off all medications for a year. I get accused at the school of giving up. What *do* I have to do? They see medication as a panacea.

I met only one mother who voiced genuine enthusiasm for our twenty-first-century wonder drugs, affluent at-home mom Colleen Janeway. With her son James so stigmatized at school, Colleen's vigilante struggles had led to perhaps more apt labels (rather than the initial ADHD, Colleen had accepted later diagnoses of nonverbal learning and anxiety disorders). She relied on a drug combination—an atypical antipsychotic and an SSRI antidepressant—similar to those tried but rejected by both Judith and Abby. Colleen announced to me, unprompted, "I'm a *huge* believer in pharmaceuticals. I really am"—statements surprisingly free of ambivalence. Yet Colleen still described an earlier "traumatic" two-year period of struggling to manage stimulant medications: each had induced too many "crashes," and she had despaired, "We're *not doing* this anymore."

Mothers' Well-Being and Work Environments

Another kind of ambivalence about medications and high-tech medicalization was evident in the stories of mothers about their own well-being and use of psychoactive medications. Fewer married mothers than single mothers reported relying on such medications. This may have been because their good-enough marriages offered important emotional protection. But two affluent married mothers, Angie Thompson and Molly Greer, along with middle-income Blayne Gregorson, suggested a less positive interpretation. Angie and Molly each indicated, if obliquely, that married mothers ought to resist turning to medications themselves because they must continue to literally embody family order. Angie tried to employ humor: "I've got [laughs] three out of four of us on medication. I wouldn't be able to remember to take it." Molly was more serious, reporting that although she spent many years in psychotherapy and suspected depression, she rejected being formally diagnosed: "I was too busy to, to reach that edge, 'cause you know I had Andi, Nicholas [her kids] . . . So who had time to think about [whether] there was something wrong with you?" But Blayne was most direct, perhaps because she had less class standing to protect: "My God, what kind of family *is* this *if Mom* is on meds?"

Affluent Theresa Kelleher's story of turning to her son's medications might underscore several of the paradoxes confronted by privileged mothers raising disordered children. Recall that Theresa, of "the West Maple Hillbillies," had finally quit the career she had "*loved*" to better care for her vulnerable young son Colin. Padding around her dining room in comfortable jeans during our three hours together, Theresa depicted her final working years as deeply disquieting. When Colin had been in kindergarten and his younger sister was a toddler:

> I was feeling so stressed with Colin [when I worked] . . . I remember trying to get him to school. And he was having *so* many problems. I remember being in the car, and having my daughter in the car seat, and giving her a pill by mistake that should have been for Colin. Like being in this rush and—I mean, I made her spit it out right away, and she did. But then I remember saying to my doctor, "My gosh—I'm so distracted that I'm giving my wrong child the medication!"

This moment shook Theresa enough that she implored her family physician to prescribe Ritalin for her right away: "It just bothered me *so* much that I'm giving a five-year-old a brain-altering medication that I had him give it to me too . . . [because] I came to the realization that if my son has it [ADHD], I probably do too." Theresa seemed a bit embarrassed, revealing this only near the close of my long visit. But such adult use is increasingly common, driven by parents of children diagnosed with ADHD, but also by those coping with New Economy workplace demands.[74] Theresa perhaps reassured herself as she justified her actions, emphasizing that she took just "the minimal dose": "I started talking to some adults who were taking it. Like my roommate from college, her children had ADD . . . she started taking it. But you know, I took the minimal dose. And I said to her, 'Well, how much do you take?' And she said, 'Boatloads!'"

Theresa explained that workplace demands had become nearly unbearable without Ritalin, despite the fact that in the effort to retain her, her firm had allowed a condensed work schedule: "I got up at like 5:30 in the morning, and was at the office at 7:30 and left at 2:00 . . . But . . . everything was like dominoes, and if one thing went wrong, it was like everything went wrong: traffic or a client was late, then the meeting went late, it could be anything." And with the need to wield complex financial data while charming clients, she described Ritalin in the terms of a cognitive performance enhancer: "When I would take it [Ritalin], if I went to a big board meeting or an investment committee meeting, it would really help me focus."

Paradoxically, Theresa, at home full-time, still took Ritalin. She admitted this hesitantly, emphasizing that her use was occasional. Yet she observed, "Maybe I am depressed"; "I probably should have this evaluated . . . because [a speaker at my son's special-needs school], he said . . . when adults have a hard time focusing it could be depression [rather than ADHD] . . . I just wanted a blood test that said, 'Yes, you have it, no you don't.'"

From a sociological perspective, depression may be a very understandable response to a truly "no-win situation" for high-earning mothers like Theresa, mothers who "would *not* have been a stay-at-home mom." Without policy options or federal protections, privileged women with jobs on the high-flying side of economic transformation may ironically face more difficult, zero-sum choices if also managing a high-need child than mothers earning far less. High-end work with its 24/7 demands and largely male-dominated environment can be particularly family-unfriendly, a point well illustrated by the mother and financial manager character Kate Reddy of the British novel *I Don't Know How She Does It*—played by Sarah Jessica Parker in the 2011 Hollywood film version.[75] A less successful husband than Theresa's, a husband like Richard Reddy, might become a "de facto househusband left to bring up their two young [typically developing] children." The novel and film instruct, however, that such an arrangement is no prescription for marital health.[76] Moreover, research finds that women become hyper-visible in such "coolly rational" masculine business environments, requiring them to skillfully display finely tuned body capital and just enough sexual allure.[77] Theresa sighed sadly remembering such investment in her own body capital, yet she was keenly aware that such a "lifestyle" was nearly, if not completely, impossible to combine with care for a high-need child.

Other work environments may be more manageable for those with vulnerable children. Abby Martin, for instance, found that a science lab, though still a masculine environment, represented a quiet respite from family disorder with fewer postindustrial demands for 24/7 availability or embodied display. Lower-stakes, lower-paid jobs, those traditionally held by women in the "pink-collar ghetto," counted as good choices to many mothers, though not always alleviating the felt-need for psychoactive support. Jobs within the hierarchies of nursing, social work, teaching, or other paid care work fields at least required only familiar interaction styles and less investment in body capital. Elaine Irving, for example, reported excitement to be moving from part- to full-time middle-school teaching; and when we exchanged e-mails a year later, she remained happy with her decision, with her son Micah stable and no worse off. Even some seemingly bad jobs appealed to a few of the overwhelmed mothers I met, providing respite for those with few worries about protecting class resources or transmitting cultural capital. Middle-income Blayne Gregorson, who dismissed the suggestion of ever being "a mom on meds," had a two-year college degree and long experience at a technical firm. But after years of living with "turmoil" at home, Blayne traded down to sales work in retail housewares at a nearby strip mall. She sighed deeply, "I just want to fold towels."

Conclusion: Almost Like Botox?

Despite the self-mockery in Theresa Kelleher's nickname for her family, "the West Maple Hillbillies," the affluence of the high-income families *almost* makes mothers like Elaine Irving, Theresa Kelleher, Abby Martin, and Judith Lowenthal look like stereotypes of smug upper-middle-class entitlement—with only glaring differences in life experience from middle-income mothers like Blayne Gregorson or Rosemary Hardesty, or particularly from low-income Vivian Kotler. Such stereotypes of affluence, like the epigraphs which began chapter 1, suggest mothers who too easily follow parenting fads, and in medicating a disruptive, underperforming child, aim to minimize their care work while maximizing family status or cultural capital. Administering powerful psychoactives would seem, in such a flattened caricature, little different from other investments in cultural display, from keeping an attractive home, a toned, fit body, or a Botoxed face. But such popularly circulating images or "folk" theories are too glib to account for the relentless, sometimes painful efforts required to care for a troubled child. Although their class transmission reproduces glaring social inequalities, on an individual level, such mothers aim only to protect and strengthen vulnerable children—and in this, they differ little from mothers in diverse race and class locations. Most never expected to resort to psychopharmaceutical treatments—and despite the continuous popular suspicion, most find that medications rarely minimize care work and don't offer any quick fix. Moreover, all ten affluent mothers worked concertedly, often in considerable isolation and with stigmatized identities, to patch together services and treatments from ever-more specialized, fragmented sources within densely bureaucratized educational and medical systems.

While three of these advantaged mothers were committed to full-time mothering, the other seven continued to be employed outside the home. Some conservatives argue that such employed mothers induce or exacerbate disorder in vulnerable children while others imply that blame lies more squarely with high divorce and partnership "metabolism" rates. If both arguments may be partially correct, they still cannot account for children like Micah Irving, Henry Caldwell-Starret, or James Janeway, raised in modern nuclear rather than postmodern or "recombinant" households.[78] In addition, it would be shortsighted to blame even very affluent individual mothers, or fathers, for the larger neoliberal politics and postindustrial capitalism shaping caregiving and family life in the twenty-first century.

I would argue instead that the ten advantaged mothers with high cultural capital and ample resources confronted a string of paradoxes.

Rearing troubled children was certainly easier with the money to pay for specialized services or schools—and when a mother had internalized an elite sense of entitlement, she might better deal with highly credentialed specialists. However, compared to those with less social privilege, life with a "multimillion-dollar child" created additional class-based expectations and obstacles. For mothers committed to cultivating a sense of distinction and optimizing the transmission of intangible assets, unruly children threatened a well-internalized vision of family order. This order centers perhaps most of all on (heterosexual) married, companionate partners and a father/husband with generous earnings; yet, as Angie Thompson put it, a troubled child "definitely puts a strain on a marriage." If Abby Martin was the only one of the class-advantaged mothers to divorce in the course of this project, others faced a striking paradox: because marriage brings significant status, economic resources, and, most of all, a respite from isolation and stigma, mothers endured inequitable, even strained marriages for recognition of their vigilante efforts.

Judith Lowenthal may have been a happy exception to this marital paradox, but she did not escape the remaining ironies of class advantage. She had confronted head-on the paradox of community stigma. While residing in an affluent community would seem to offer many advantages to those raising high-need children, with better-resourced schools and better-educated neighbors, such communities may in turn be less inclusive and increase the stigma faced by mothers and their households. The affluent mothers all spoke of spoiled public identities and loss of social ties; and survey research suggests such patterns as well, with the highly educated little more tolerant or inclusive, and those married more likely to desire social distance for their own families, anxious to protect their own class transmission.

A third paradox confronts highly educated mothers like Theresa Kelleher, whose high-status earnings originally allowed the family to purchase a home in West Maple and to feel at ease within the town's privileged boundaries. Yet such demanding, round-the-clock work is difficult to sustain for all mothers, even those whose kids are temperamentally easy, as volumes of academic and popular writing attest.[79] Theresa's class advantage in this sense only led to a set of bad choices: to watch the struggles of a very young son worsen while succeeding near the top of the New Economy; or to endure isolation, loss of status and income in the hope that full-time vigilante efforts, along with her increased presence, might mitigate his issues.

This leads to the fourth paradox I observed: though a few mothers like Judith Lowenthal enjoyed a relative wealth of social support, with a network of friends, family, and kin in the area, such support was scarce for most when stigma led to shrinking social ties. With few established public or institutional spaces to turn to, particularly in a neoliberal era of declining social provision, mothers fall back on private resources. But purchasing commodified support, while itself a decided class privilege, remains a hollow, instrumental transaction compared to genuine relations of care and support. Moreover, even these instrumentalized sources—the compassionate psy-sector specialists, educational advocates, and alternative practitioners—were often difficult to locate, and class advantage often did little to alleviate the sense of personal responsibility weighing on each mother to find more and better sources to manage a disordered child on her own. In fact, mothers with very low resources but access to public services and family interventions may have been better off on this score. Sandra Barbieri had been all too aware of this irony, recounting how she had been rejected by state social services for families, which would not even act as a referral service because she and her husband, a civil engineer, earned far too much: "I guess that's a good thing. It was a bad thing at [that] one point because, like I said, we couldn't get the services . . . It's like, 'Well, can you help us? Can you find programs for us?' . . . and they said, 'No, no, no,' and the doors got closed. So I said, 'OK, I guess I am on my own.'"

Finally, in the last paradox, highly resourced mothers like Sandra may have been better able to cope with their ambivalence about childhood medicalization than those with less class advantage. Sandra, like Judith Lowenthal and Gabriella Ramos-Garza, was better able to challenge medical authority and locate alternative practitioners. However, privileged mothers were no less likely—and perhaps were even more likely—to become deeply dependent on biomedical authority to help their vulnerable children. Though such mothers frequently described difficulties in obtaining providers who might listen to them—and some like Theresa Kelleher described months-long waiting lists for child psychiatrists—most navigated successfully, like Judith Lowenthal with the "brilliant" Dr. P., to specialists on whom they relied very heavily, administering psychoactive medications though they were never more than partial help.

When I last checked in with Judith in 2007, life in the Lowenthals' sunny home continued to have many ups and downs; and Allan, with a new passion for jazz, was an adolescent bringing, in Judith's words, "my most challenging parenting years." The family's resources, both economic and cultural, had only partially eased Judith's vigilante quest to resolve or ameliorate Allan's struggles; and the stakes for class transmission were ratcheting up as he moved through high school with thoughts of college on the horizon. As Abby Martin had expressed, everyday exchanges between mothers at this critical juncture became newly isolating for Judith:

> [A good neighbor] she'd talk about being so worried about her older son and I just want to scream. It's like, "Come on, he's thriving. He's doing well. Maybe he's not getting straight As, but so what? You know I'm worried about like my kid even making it!"

Nonetheless, compared to those raising equally troubled kids with fewer resources, the Lowenthals' ability to pay for schools and specialists, call on their network of neighbors and kin for referrals, and be on a first-name basis with such providers, created stark differences in daily life. Moreover, the presence of a husband, even if largely symbolic, counts as perhaps a most crucial cultural resource—as I learned from the many single mothers willing to share their experiences with me.

4

"I Think I Have to Advocate *Five Thousand Times Harder!*"

Single Mothers in the Age of Neuroscience

Michelle was a single mother, and school staff focused on possible problems in her home environment to explain Bethany's behavioral issues. According to Michelle, everyone assumed that, being a single mother, she could not be smart or a good mother. Once she was married, however, everything changed.
—Colin Ong-Dean, Distinguishing Disability: Parents, Privilege, and Special Education, 2009

"Two Classes, Divided by 'I Do': Marriage for Richer; Single Motherhood for Poorer."
—Front-page headline, Jason DeParle, *New York Times*, July 15, 2012

Vivian Kotler, a tiny white Euro-American woman with short curly hair and a no-nonsense style, was some dozen years older than Judith Lowenthal and considerably more care-worn. Although we had spoken by phone a few times, we first met in person on an early spring morning, just after she had seen her twelve-year-old biracial daughter, Isabel, to the school bus. I gathered that this was an often fraught process, with Isabel stubborn and oppositional and Vivian offering rewards as one might to a much younger child. We spoke all morning and into the early afternoon in Vivian's meticulously organized spare apartment in a low-slung housing project. Seated at a small dining table with neat stacks of books and mail to our side, I noticed a desk with an older computer and an additional neat stack of books and papers. Out a back window was a pleasant green space of grass and shrubs. Vivian revealed that it was difficult, however, to keep things tidy and organized with Isabel very impulsive, "run[ning]" on the furniture and "destroying everything." Diagnosed with ADHD, other learning disorders, and, most recently, the suggestion of possible bipolar disorder, Isabel was in her fifth school setting. She had finally received public funds for an out-of-district placement at an independent special-needs day school.[1] Vivian had a great deal to convey about the rigors of raising a special-needs child alone, and she frequently invoked her identity as a "single parent"—without any prompting from me—to explain her experiences and her point of view.

I had not been thinking of lone mothers as a group with categorically distinct issues and challenges beyond those more fundamentally rooted in economic and ethnoracial differences. Vivian's narrative, and those of the twenty-two other single mothers I met in the course of this research, prompted rethinking. In this chapter I compare the experiences of the single mothers with those of married mothers in comparable circumstances, and suggest that the presence of an unruly child together with the absence of a spouse puts such lone mothers in a distinct cultural location, in the context of attitudes, stereotypes, and suspicions raised by the rising rates of single motherhood in the postindustrial United States. I find indications that mothers heading fatherless homes with children labeled disordered may stand in for and suffer from our larger discomfort with postindustrial family change and New Economy threats to manhood.

Because the mothers I met described a range of changing life circumstances, it was sometimes a puzzle to decide if they belonged in this chapter. In addition to the four long-married mothers who revealed that they would be seeking divorces, several were in second (or third) marriages, having spent some years parenting alone.[2] For the most part I do not include such mothers here because their separations were so new or their time outside of a marriage minimal. Only one mother, never-married Dory Buchanan, was open about being a lesbian, with one biological child and another who had been adopted; while I might have asked directly if she had a partner or coparent, she had described herself specifically as a *single* lesbian mother. Never-married Brooke Donnelly also revealed the use of assisted reproduction to have a child by choice; though I asked every mother who resided in their household, Brooke volunteered nothing about her sexual orientation or partners, reporting that she resided alone with her young son, with frequent visits from a sister who had been like a live-in nanny during his infancy. May Royce described purchasing a duplex with a close friend after her divorce, the two women sharing one unit for several years while renting out the second for needed income. Though May clarified that theirs was a non-sexual friendship, it was easier to define May as "single" when I learned that this "Auntie" to her son had moved into the second unit with a lesbian partner. Yet "Auntie" clearly remained close to May and her son, in another set of linked nontraditional households.

In addition to such household diversity, the group of single-mother respondents contained significant, complexly intertwined class and ethnoracial diversity. None was "becom[ing] rich," as Vivian Kotler had advised, but eleven of twenty-three single mothers (three women of color and eight white women) earned a decent income, at or over the median for U.S. women at the time of these interviews;[3] and a few in this subgroup earned substantially more. But twelve (four women of color and eight white women) had below-median incomes, with several falling under poverty levels. Still, like other researchers studying low-income single mothers and visiting their homes, I found that only a small number came close to stereotypical depictions of "poor moral health," unable to maintain sufficiently settled, organized homes for their children, falling into what sociologists term "hard living."[4] Paradoxically, I found that some single mothers with among the lowest incomes, like Vivian Kotler, were among the most effectively organized, becoming skilled direct caregivers of their high-need children, and vigilantes engaging assertively with educational, medical, and state authorities.

My sample group is small, the evidence is more often suggestive than overt, and in every case single motherhood is entangled with varied levels of education, income, cultural capital, and ethnoracial privilege—but across such differences, the lone mothers reported greater suspicion of their maternal fitness than married mothers with comparably troubled children. Claudia Malacrida also found that single mothers of children with ADHD in Canada and the United Kingdom were considered in "poor moral health" compared to married mothers of similar kids.[5]

I also examine the effects of ethnoracial assignment as it intersects with the already suspect status of a single mother. I find indications that Euro-American single mothers could reclaim some of the maternal respectability lost in raising disordered children outside heterosexual marriage, and that they were protected from the worst aspects of state intrusion. Feminist and critical race scholars have argued that women continue to be disciplined along racial lines, though such lines can be difficult to disentangle from economic class—as anthropologist Karen Brodkin has argued, our construction of race "almost *is* the American construction of class."[6] Yet neoliberal mandates urging mothers to personally mitigate all risks to their children's health, well-being, and future success seem to fall hardest on the shoulders of lone mothers lacking full white privilege.

Many of the challenges faced by the single mothers—including suspicion of their moral fitness—were also faced by the married mothers: blame for the child's problems (from both themselves and others); lack of the time, knowledge, and money required to obtain needed services; the challenge of dealing with multiple authoritative bureaucracies; the wrenching questions of medication; lack of family and social support; racial and other stereotypes. For the single mothers, however, the obstacles tended to be higher and more concentrated, to the extent that their experiences emerged as qualitatively distinct from those of their married counterparts. As Vivian put it, invoking the Titan of Greek mythology who carried the weight of the world on his (not *her*) shoulders, "As a single parent, things are never fine at home because you're always having to be the Atlas."

In this second decade of the twenty-first century, single-mother households in the United States are more common than ever and include just over a quarter of households with children under eighteen. These households are headed about equally by never-married mothers like Vivian Kotler and by divorced mothers.[7] I explore the differences in the experiences and accounts of single mothers from those of the married mothers raising invisibly disabled children, and try to disentangle complicating and interlocking layers of gender, race, and class advantage and disadvantage.

Collisions of Work and Care: "Derailing, Constantly Derailing"

Both married and single mothers experienced conflict between the demands of raising a disordered child and the demands of full-time employment. For single mothers, without a partner's income, the conflict could be heightened enormously. Vivian Kotler and Susan Atkinson were among the few single mothers to withdraw completely—and very reluctantly—from paid work to devote themselves to full-time care of a troubled child.[8] Though five additional single mothers also lived outside the paid labor force, they had withdrawn for other, complex reasons, including their own visible and invisible disabilities. Eight others managed to remain in full-time work, while an equal number scaled back to part-time hours because of their high-need children.

Neither Vivian nor Susan wanted to leave paid work. Vivian was emphatic in her frustration: "Basically as a single mother of a special-needs kid, you end up sacrificing everything. You end up sacrificing your time. You end up sacrificing *even trying* to find a job . . . Every time I try to have a job, I get a call from the school!" Susan's financial need was less dire because of family support, but she expressed similar frustration: "Bottom line, I ended up quitting my job because I had to be home with my child . . . [and then] that *was* my full-time job." While Theresa Kelleher had also felt compelled to quit a much-wanted career, the devotion of single mothers Vivian and Susan entailed much greater financial sacrifice.

Vivian, for example, had been headed toward a middle-class life, and after college graduation she described herself in very similar terms to Theresa: each recounted enjoying an independent life before becoming relatively older mothers. But while Theresa emulated her father's business background, earned a related graduate degree, and began her ascent up the career ladder before marriage and motherhood in her thirties, free-spirited Vivian, with less affluent divorced parents, traveled, living and working in several states and abroad. Unlike Theresa, when she became a mother in her early forties she had neither a husband nor a solid career. Sorely disappointed by her African American boyfriend—according to Vivian, he originally sued for custody because he had not wanted a white woman raising his child—Vivian reorganized her life to raise biracial daughter Isabel on her own. She moved into the safe, if shabby housing project, turned reluctantly to state assistance, and ran a licensed home day care to make ends meet during Isabel's early years, assuming she would seek outside employment and leave the projects once Isabel was school-aged. Yet despite her college degree, Vivian described life with a high-need child as "derailing, constantly derailing" (in contrast, the Kellehers remained ensconced in their spacious "West Maple" home).

Large-scale studies indicate that experiences like Vivian's may be fairly common. The 2005–6 National Survey of Children with Special Health Care Needs, for example, found that nearly 30 percent of those whose children had ADHD reported cutting back or stopping work; and for autism spectrum disorders, this rate doubled.[9] Clearly, among growing numbers of lone mothers in the United States, the consequences of a child's special needs can be particularly dramatic, exacerbating the divide between married and single and increasing the odds that single mothers will fall into poverty.[10]

Because of her straitened economic circumstances, Vivian was forced to be even more inventive, persistent, and resourceful than married vigilante moms like Theresa in "doing everything I can to make her [Isabel's] life better." She took pride, for example, in the bartering arrangement she had set up when Isabel reached school age, trading her labor so that Isabel might attend a liberal, nondenominational Christian academy outside the projects: "I sent her [Isabel] to a private religious school up in [an adjacent suburb] because I wanted to get her out of the projects . . . but . . . I couldn't afford it. So what did I do? Not only did I get a scholarship, I said, 'Look, I'll work for you.' So I worked without any monetary [reward]."

The arrangement, which lasted for three school years, went beyond the private school administration, also requiring creative dealings with the state welfare system. Teaching gym and serving as a classroom aide and substitute covered the balance of Isabel's tuition, but it required closing the home day care that had supplied her only cash income. This could also have run afoul of the workfare requirements imposed by newly implemented Temporary Assistance to Needy Families (TANF) reforms, which increased the work requirements (and imposed time limits) for receiving public assistance.[11] Vivian, however, explained that she crafted her work at the school to "double count" for both tuition and workfare: "I was on welfare so basically, what I did was I created my own job [at the academy]. . . . I knew in kindergarten [that] she had ADHD, the diagnosis was coming up. So I *had* to do these things in order to support my child . . . I was able to do that for kindergarten, first, and second [grades]."

While this tenuous arrangement left the family with minimal funds, it provided not only an education for Isabel and a kind of employment for

Vivian, but also a familiar and supportive community. Yet, over time, Isabel's turbulence threatened the carefully constructed arrangement and both the school's head administrator and the pastor began recommending Ritalin. There was no explicit ultimatum, but Vivian felt the "more subtle" pressure was clear. Despite grave doubts, and after seeking medical guidance, she finally complied. "I struggled to stay there because she'd [Isabel] been christened there too. And you know, one thing about these kids is you don't want to uproot them." After several months during which Isabel experienced loss of appetite, dizziness and heart palpitations despite changing stimulants, Vivian stopped the medication, turned to homeschooling and broke with the close-knit congregation.

The feelings she expressed about these events went beyond concerns for Isabel or dismay at the collapse of her work-welfare arrangement to a real sense of betrayal. The community, she emphasized, ought to have supported her more: "Why can't the church come around like a fellowship? . . . Really I find that very sad. Because you know, I think the religious organizations should be even more responsive in that way. And they weren't and . . . I find that really contradictory . . . Help me more, I'm a single parent, you know? I'm a single parent with a special-needs kid."

Many aspects of Vivian's story—the breakdown of fragile arrangements under the stress of a child's behavior, the conflicts over medication—could and did happen with married mothers, too. But for Vivian the consequences were more severe, because as a single mother she had come to rely on the arrangement with the church for everything: not only Isabel's schooling, but also her own job and daily social life. The loss of adult (though unpaid) work and community took a toll on Vivian's health (as did the stress of dealing with various state agencies for meager resources, as I detail below). "Physically my blood pressure has gone up, I've lost a lot of weight," she explained. As she described a grueling routine while homeschooling, rising at 5:00 a.m. to exercise, prepare lesson plans, and do the work of "ten different people," I asked where she had found social support. Vivian blurted out, "I didn't go anywhere! . . . Nobody wants to be my daughter's friend. But nobody wanted to be my friend either . . . even at church."

Other mothers, both married and single and from across the socioeconomic spectrum, spoke of similarly fraught experiences with disruptive children within religious organizations. About a quarter of those I interviewed still reported finding important support in faith-based communities. And like Vivian, who later joined a larger church with a Sunday school "disability unit," single mothers seemed less likely than married mothers to walk away because of an unruly child.[12] This might indicate single mothers' greater needs for formal communities of care and support. Research on the shrinking of extra-familial ties and friendships outside of marriage in the United States today does suggest that unpartnered adults may be left in the cold.[13] Divorced mother Lenore Savage, who had no religious affiliation, stated bluntly that her family's "isolation" was her "biggest problem," bigger even than her son's troubles. Lenore observed, "I sort of wish I were religious or something so that I would have a church group." Indeed, divorced mother of three Shauna Lapine spoke of the support she received from her faith community: "That was my one little sanctuary . . . They absolutely knew me and it felt very good to be there . . . That community really kept me together." It was so important that when Shauna's oldest son's disruptive behavior threatened his participation, Shauna drew on her master's degree in social work and insisted on conducting trainings on ADHD for religious education staff.

Concerted Mothering as a "Team of One"

Vivian had grown up with white ethnoracial privilege and graduated from a local state college; but she had been raised by divorced, lower-middle-class parents and lacked the cultural or economic capital of those from the professional elite like Judith Lowenthal. Her plainspoken demeanor, however, concealed an insightful perspective on what she admitted was a life of "sacrifice." Lacking a kin network or strong ties to other mothers, and having sacrificed paid work to care for Isabel, Vivian had invested instead to become adept at scouting for resources on daughter Isabel's behalf while also providing nearly constant, attentive care. She exemplifies the vigilante mother, taking the law into her own hands to raise and advocate for a vulnerable child, and seemed to excel in her often lonely crusade for her daughter's well-being. Vivian was well aware of the irony of her unrecognized skills: "My [BA] degree is actually in history. But I say that anybody that deals with a special-needs kid, they've earned their degree already in something [else]. [Chuckling] I've put it on my résumé!"

Apparently some of the school professionals were as impressed as I was at the effectiveness with which Vivian, while raising her daughter in a housing project, navigated educational and medical systems and the dense bureaucracies administering public assistance. Vivian re-counted with relish that after a particularly frustrating special-ed team meeting, a supportive counselor had praised her, "Vivian, you're a team of one!"[14]

She was, however, keenly aware that she often provoked more nega-tive responses. In one poignant observation, Vivian clarified that she had *not quite* been blamed directly for her daughter's troubles: "I saw the blaming thing. OK, it wasn't, it's *close* to the word 'blame,' but it takes a different flavor . . . it was a way that they treated me . . . I was left out on my own . . . I didn't feel like the school was *behind me* in any kind of way." Moreover, she clearly perceived a special stigma associated with being a single mother: "[As a single mom] oh yes, I am looked at dif-ferently, very differently. [Chuckles] I can't describe *how* because I'm *not* really looked at . . . I get . . . ignored . . . So I'm a single parent, and OK, . . . I have to struggle for everything, I have to advocate. I think I have to advocate *five thousand times harder!*" This is, of course, Vivian's perception; I cannot verify that she actually received less support than the married mothers. But I am inclined to give considerable weight to the perception of such an astute informant, particularly given culturally pervasive stereotyping of single mothers and the reminder of sociolo-gists Carol Heimer and Lisa Staffen that such bias against lone mothers is worsened when professional staff under heavy workloads must rely on quick judgments.[15]

Divorced white mother Lenore Savage, who navigated educational, medical, and juvenile court systems on behalf of a troubled son, echoed Vivian's analysis. After ten years as a married mom and another eight single, Lenore was in a position to make a direct comparison: "It's in-teresting along the gender lines. If the guy leaves and you're the main person there, I think you get much less respect with all these systems!" Shauna Lapine was also acutely aware of being stigmatized since her divorce, though she maintained that her home was safer, calmer, alto-gether better for her children:

It's so much stigma to your parenting skills the minute you admit your kid's having trouble. They *assume* you have a troubled home. So I knew after my divorce, they would assume *all* Leo's issues were from that. "Oh well, he is from a broken home": some school person actually said that! I blew up: "*Excuse me? Our* home is fixed now!"

Vivian might have been summarizing many such experiences I heard from divorced mothers when she noted wryly that perhaps she was better off never having married: "Divorces happen a lot when you have a special-needs kid. You know, the husbands bail and the woman is left. That's my take on a *lot* of it." Her darkly humorous observation resonates with the narratives of those who endured considerable marital strain. Vivian may have been relieved to have never had to contend with this "patriarchal" burden, able to organize her household from the start around daughter Isabel's needs—but at the same time, she was all too aware of the downsides.

All the mothers I interviewed, regardless of marital or socioeconomic status, wrestled with the stigma of raising an emotionally or behaviorally challenging child, the sense of blame, whether explicit or implied, from schools, other parents, and even family, and few if any escaped some sense of self-blame for their child's difficulties. Yet I found in stories like Vivian's and Shauna's striking suggestions that the lack of a husband added another layer to an identity already spoiled by a burdensome child.

Divorced Lenore Savage volunteered that, because her ex-husband appeared to be the quintessential "good provider," she was held singly responsible for a depressed, turbulent adolescent son. Lenore reported, "With a lot of people at the high school, I felt very judged," seen as the "vindictive" "crazy," ex-wife—though before her divorce, she explained, she had been the model "at-home mom," "very active in the schools."

Susan Atkinson was the only mother who actually sued her school district, borrowing from family to cover the sizeable attorney fees, and ultimately coming to a settlement in which the school fully covered her daughter's outplacement tuition as well as the legal costs in exchange for Susan's public silence.[16] Even though she prevailed, Susan indicated wholehearted agreement with Vivian, Lenore, and Shauna that it was because she was a single mother that the negotiation had become so fraught and extended in the first place: "I strongly recommend for [a] divorced person [to] hire an advocate!" Susan became tearful thinking back, wishing she had acted more stridently sooner: "How much is my daughter scarred by this experience?"

Surprisingly, single mothers who emphasized genetic factors expressed the most explicit sense of guilt for their children's issues, a sense I rarely heard from married mothers. After all, there are many possible contributing factors to their children's disorders. Experts explain that "the causes of ADHD are not completely clear . . . [it appears to] involve various combinations of neurological, genetic, cognitive and other factors" including "events that compromise the nervous system before, during, and after birth."[17] One would think that genetics would have little to do with marital status.[18] Still, never-married Kay Raso told me "I think that my poor son got the worst-of-all genes and that he has a more severe case of anything that anybody in my family or his father's family had." And she added sadly, making herself a proximate cause for her unintended part in this genetic lottery, "I don't feel guilt except [for] the genes that we each gave him."

Two divorced mothers, also white Euro-Americans, reasoned similarly. Lenore Savage exclaimed, "I think it's a real genetic thing . . . I felt very guilty, like, 'Wow, I've doomed my children . . . because both their father and I are—'" alluding to histories of depression. And Susan Atkinson questioned sadly, "Is it because [of] my ex-husband and the combination of our genes? Oh God, I blamed myself."

Lenore, Susan, and Kay were all highly educated, but less-educated single mothers similarly invoked genetic causes for their children's embrained troubles and their own proximal guilt as unwitting accomplices in their transmission. Long-divorced, high-school-educated African American Patricia Gwarten, while blaming herself for failing to pursue greater early intervention, also cited genetics: "I know that my [ex-] husband's family has a lot of learning disabilities." High-school graduate Jenny Tedeschi was married when I first interviewed her, and confessed her marital breakdown only in a follow-up phone conversation. Although she had only begun to identify as a single mother, I include her here for the similar sense of guilt she expressed. Citing what she perceived as overwhelming odds for the heritability of invisible brain disorders, Jenny extended her maternal responsibility to containing the family's future genetic transmission. She explained she would dissuade her son from having biological children and squelch her own "selfish" desire for a second child:

> He [son Will] kept trying to tell me, "My brain is shutting down" . . . It's something . . . you know, in the brain . . . And it would be selfish of me to have another kid I think. Because I *felt* like having one: but guess what? You might have this—and how selfish! No way, no! And I'm going to tell him [thirteen-year-old Will], I haven't told him yet, but "You're adopting. You're not"—He has a 75 percent chance of his children having his issues, 75 percent! That's a given. And he meets a girl, I'll tell them, "Don't, don't. Either go for genetic counseling or you adopt."

Regrettably, the popular literature that mothers turn to for advice and support often reinforces the dominant negative imagery surrounding single mothers. Few works on our Amazon top parenting books list were as extreme as *Brain Rules for Baby*, which threatened that mothers who do not "stay married"—flouting one of the author's top five "rules"—risk causing neurological harm: marital discord and divorce may "lower your baby's IQ," "inhibit your baby's future motor skills, attentional states, and ability to concentrate," even "shrink the size of your baby's brain."[19] But others also circulate such controlling images, as the authors of *Welcome to Your Child's Brain* in a (rather promotional) *New York Times* piece glancingly put "single parenthood" on par with "criminal behavior" and "drug dependence" in the list of negative outcomes befalling children whose parents do not properly develop their offspring's prefrontal cortex.[20] Another instance was captured in the newsletter of the nonprofit Federation for Children with Special Needs: a brief review criticized *The Common Sense Guide to Your Child's Special Needs* for presenting medications with depiction of just two families, a married couple who "researched and hesitated" and a "single mother [who] sought a quick fix." This "disappointing" discussion, the reviewer noted, "added to the stereotype of children from single parent homes experiencing additional struggles."[21] While first astutely pointing to the negative images surrounding single *mothers*, the reviewer next substituted the term "single *parent*," like so many others ignoring the very gendered core of the issue.

The sheer absence of single mothers in much popular childrearing advice might also speak volumes and be just as troubling and guilt-inducing for lone mothers as the circulation of such pejorative images. Most books we analyzed from the 2011 top parenting books on Amazon made little mention of single-mother or even "single-parent" homes, despite their increasingly common demographic presence. Popular works like *NurtureShock*, *Mind in the Making*, and *The Whole-Brain Child* did not mention single-parent households at all. While the 2008 fourth edition of *What to Expect When You're Expecting* included a brief section titled "Pregnancy and the Single Mother," the best-selling follow-up, *What to Expect in the First Year*, ignored the possibility that any parent in the United States raises a child outside a heterosexual union.[22]

Negative images and assumptions about single mothers also pervaded a provocative 2012 Sunday *New York Times* article.[23] On the front page of the country's leading newspaper, the article featured two families and explained the growing economic gap between married and single mothers more from private relationship choices than from the larger structural transformation of the job market.[24]

Intriguingly, the *Times* noted that the ten-year-old son of single mother Jessica Shairer has Asperger syndrome. Indicating that the boy was prone to "sharp mood swings," he was depicted unfavorably as yelling at his mother when she could not afford to give him money for snacks, but perhaps more sympathetically as an "isolated" kid who "cried and cried and cried" when no classmates came to his birthday party.[25] Although journalist DeParle never explicitly blamed the boy's troubles on his mother, the contrast with married mother Chris Faulkner could not have been more pointed. Ms. Faulkner's sons were also depicted as emotionally needy, but no medicalized diagnosis was mentioned; and both were said to be "blossom[ing]" thanks to their "awesome" father.[26] An unsettling racial subtext also deepened the contrast between the good married mother and Ms. Shairer's suspect lone motherhood. While both mothers are white, Ms. Shairer's son is biracial. Her personal irresponsibility, we are told, began when she became pregnant and her boyfriend, an African American fellow college student, wanted to start a family; both quit school and she stayed with him long enough to have two more children, though he "earned little" and treated her poorly.[27]

With single mothers so often portrayed negatively—when they are not erased altogether—there is good reason to credit the sense expressed by the single mothers that it is especially difficult for them to navigate professional waters on behalf of unruly children. This sense was well captured in Vivian Kotler's pained observation that as a single mother she was "*not* really looked at," was "ignored" by school personnel, and was thus impelled to "advocate *five thousand times harder*." The single mothers I spoke with recounted many instances in which professionals, who could be potential allies and sources of support, echoed the negative cultural images exemplified by the *Times* article and advice literature.

From Vigilante to Concerted Cultivator

Even as they struggled against these stereotypes, some of the single mothers provided striking examples of an effect I have discussed in a previous article:[28] Through the process of vigilante mothering—researching, advocating, petitioning, demanding on the child's behalf—even mothers without extensive cultural or financial resources shifted toward a style of interaction and childrearing characteristic of more affluent, educated parents. Thus a child's invisible disability may partly override the stark class distinction in parenting style described by sociologist Annette Lareau, in which working-class parents rely on less intrusive strategies, deferring to institutional authorities and showing little assertiveness in confronting professionals in the educational and medical systems. According to Lareau, working-class parents allow children more autonomous "natural growth" in contrast to the "concerted cultivation" of cognitive, cultural, and body capital pursued by intrusive affluent parents.[29]

I found instead that many single mothers, even those with limited education, responded to the needs of their vulnerable children by redoubling their efforts, describing how they became more demanding and began to feel more entitled.[30] As their children's special needs propelled mothers into more interactions with professionals, those with lower cultural capital received something of a crash course in the more assertive, informed demeanor of the middle class. At the same time, their tireless search for a combination of educational, medical, and alternative resources that would enable their children to thrive often moved them across the fuzzy and porous boundary that divides therapy from cultural enhancement. While the opportunities single mothers arranged for their vulnerable children may have been solidly middle-class compared to the elite activities pursued by the affluent families, whether ballet classes, summer enrichment programs, or health-food regimens, they extended well beyond the special-education services offered in schools and the pharmacological treatments endorsed by most physicians.

Divorced mother Shauna Lapine "case managed" her son Leo's treatments, including at age five managing his medication, but also finding a psychologist to conduct "play therapy," and negotiating a reduced-fee arrangement to enroll Leo in the "fancy" Montessori school in a nearby "rich community" for his first three years of schooling: "They gave me a little scholarship, and we set up a payment plan, and we were off and running." In retrospect she laughed at the cultural contradictions, describing herself as a "hippie" Montessori mom "with a [new] baby in a Snugli," yet recounting how at their "lefty" food co-op other mothers would stare as she gave Leo his Ritalin, "crushing it up in his organic yogurt."

When I met her several years later, all three of her kids attended public schools, but each was involved in additional family and educational therapies, children's choruses, religious education, and summer day camps. Even so, Shauna expressed awareness and regret over the enrichment activities she couldn't provide: "So I was working three days a week and . . . trying to ferry kids back and forth to shrinks and OT [occupational therapy] and speech therapists . . . and Hebrew school and Sunday school. God forbid they should take piano lessons or be involved in sports! I mean I can't even go there . . . Isn't that terrible? I'm not even encouraging them. . . . I couldn't conceive of how I could juggle that. And I feel really guilty."

Vivian Kotler also scrounged and bartered to provide daughter Isabel with middle-class sessions of (at various times) ballet, gymnastics, fitness training, summer arts enrichment, and ice-skating. Isabel particularly needed such enrichment, Vivian reported, for the "social skills" and "to help her motor skills." "I do feel that she definitely needs [more of] the physical component," in addition to the "educational component." No doubt such activities do serve a therapeutic function, but they also build the embodied self-assurance important for middle-class standing, even if not at the elite level of the Lowenthals' skiing, sailing, and hiking trips. Vivian also stressed the importance of being "very nutritionally oriented," like Shauna with her organic yogurt but also like affluent Judith Lowenthal with her shares in a community farm: "If she [Isabel] doesn't eat properly, you can tell." And Vivian felt it important that she was "modeling" such habits, "like eating lots of fruits and vegetables, [chuckling] at my age you have to do that. [And] eating protein . . . [but only] chicken or any kind of meat that does not have the hormones."

Patricia Gwarten, in contrast to Vivian and Shauna's higher education, had only a high-school degree. Yet she was tracking many aspects of her six-year-old son's development, including working to "increase his exercise" and "change his diet," hoping to prevent or forestall the need for medications: "I'm giving him more fruits and vegetables, and more fish because of the omega-3. Also I would love for him to take olive oil . . . It's hard [laughs] to get him to take vitamins. But I'm trying, because I don't want the medication." To social theorist Pierre Bourdieu the attention surrounding expensive fresh foods believed to be particularly healthful also reveals their high cultural status as distinct from foods oriented for mass consumption.[31] For single mothers raising vulnerable children, such purchases take a bigger bite of the household budget compared to affluent married mothers—yet they seem to represent the same intertwined desires to ameliorate a vulnerable child's troubles while inculcating culturally superior "good taste," perhaps optimizing their chances of a middle-class future.

It is possible, of course, that the less-advantaged mothers who agreed to share their experiences with me were exceptional, but some related research suggests similar tendencies. One qualitative study of low-income, immigrant Asian mothers of children with special healthcare needs, for example, noted that those whose children had "chronic conditions . . . were more forthcoming in seeking out and utilizing services" including special education, with some "actively campaign[ing] for access."[32] In a larger study, Heimer and Staffen found that nearly all the mothers of premature infants in an urban neonatal intensive-care unit developed skills to provide "confident," "competent care" after their baby's release, despite the staffs' "discomfort" with single mothers.[33] Admittedly it is a long way from monitoring a child's blood oxygen flow to ballet lessons. But the shift from acquiescence to experts to assertive advocacy is similar; and in the middle range of the most frequent invisible disabilities, the distinction between needed therapy and "concerted cultivation" can be very muddy, particularly in an era when every good mother is exhorted to engage with neuroscience, foster brain development, and push cognitive achievement.

The complex class positions of the single mothers I interviewed also resonate with the arguments of feminist sociologists like Judith Stacey and Karen Hansen that New Economy restructuring and household diversity together make many women's class positions difficult to capture with categories originally based on male breadwinners. Women's class positions in "postmodern families," Stacey maintained, are increasingly "ambiguous and contradictory"; and Hansen similarly emphasized that varied gendered family-household arrangements and accompanying variation in household assets like home ownership complicate the meaning and experience of class position.[34] The accounts of the mothers I interviewed suggest that the presence of a troubled child adds further complexity, as mothers across a range of backgrounds draw selectively and assertively from the treatments and services deemed necessary by professional authorities, and often go further, turning to the higher-status alternatives and extracurricular enrichment more often associated with Lareau's affluent "concerted cultivators."

Paradoxes of Engaging the Neoliberal State

Sociologist Jennifer Reich has argued in a somewhat different context (that of parents under scrutiny by child protective services) that the inability to rely on one's own private service providers can be a serious problem for parents who must engage with the state.[35] Having such providers, or the personal networks to such providers, can help cut through the bureaucratic hurdles that go with raising invisibly disabled children, as we saw in Judith Lowenthal's narrative. Many of the un- and under-resourced single mothers, in contrast, were engaged with tightly constrained state bureaucracies and without such resources. They confronted the associated delays and bottlenecks, rigid rules and petty intrusions, in pursuit of the professional treatment, services, and family support to care for a needy child solely or primarily through public channels.

Expert opinion is sharply divided on whether this engagement with arms of the state is advantageous. While some suggest advantages for troubled children covered by state benefits, others argue that state coverage brings further stigma and limited, second-class treatment. The experiences of those I met suggest that both may be true to some extent—an interpretation which extends the work of many feminist scholars of the U.S. welfare state.[36] In particular, sociologist Sharon Hays has demonstrated that public assistance since the 1996 Personal Responsibility and Work Opportunity Reconciliation Act continues to express our larger cultural ambivalence, torn between desires to punish and yet to genuinely help struggling single mothers.[37]

Vivian's experience exemplifies both sides of the coin. She was keenly aware of the punitive side through the harsh workfare rules she had negotiated for minimal, time-limited cash assistance and the paperwork so painstakingly organized next to her computer for other public benefits: "If I could harness this energy that I've got into a job [instead] that would be wonderful!" Yet with so few family-friendly jobs, lone mothers with high-need kids also find genuine help even in tightfisted state assistance. In addition to TANF, they turn most importantly to Medicaid for health insurance for their kids; but they also may navigate dense public bureaucracies for Section 8 public housing and rent subsidies, for food stamps, and perhaps the most convoluted and constrained, for Supplemental Security Income for eligible low-income families caring for disabled children.

Vivian had tapped several of these sources including Section 8. She exulted over their impending move to a "wonderful" state-subsidized, off-site apartment away from the projects: "Nobody [will] know that we're in the 'quote' projects anymore . . . it [the new apartment] gives the illusion that we're normal people. And that's what my daughter fights for is normalcy." Vivian's vigilante research had uncovered a detail in Section 8 policy allowing upgrades on medical grounds. She had filed a request using Isabel's latest (added) diagnosis of possible bipolar, though ironically this was a diagnosis Vivian largely rejected. The petition required supporting documentation, "a letter from an MD," to authorize that the move was "medically necessary." And while remarking proudly, "So I went out and I got it!" calling one after another of those they had seen through the public Medicaid system seemed a world away from those with private healthcare: "It's a fact that I'm going to *ten thousand different people* to get something that I [could] have done on my own! . . . Of course, I don't have [a] medical degree . . . [But] my gosh, the different people . . . you have to go through *so* many different people."

Paradoxically, a 2011 review specifically of children's mental health services found distinct *advantages* for those eligible for public coverage. The review's authors, a team of Boston-based journalists, noted that for those with private health insurance, nationwide shortages of child psychiatrists lead to lengthy wait times, sometimes of months, to receive an initial visit[38]—and this was certainly the experience reported by more than a few, like May Royce who had shown me the notebook logging her unreturned calls.[39] Publicly dependent mothers like Vivian, the report argued, gained more immediate care for troubled children. In addition, they may gain *better* care with access to social work teams, in-home family therapists, and crisis intervention counselors, all less readily available to those with more income. The director of the state's Society for the Prevention of Cruelty to Children pronounced, "If I had a child with a serious emotional disorder in the Commonwealth of Massachusetts I would do *everything* I could to have them on Medicaid [rather] than on private commercial insurance!" She attested she would "quit her current job if that . . . would qualify her child for public health insurance."[40] Indeed, several in my sample, like married mother Sandra Barbieri, lamented earning too much to access state social work services. Others, like single mother Shauna Lapine, had high praise for the counselors at their public community clinic. Vivian, however, had experienced the downside of state austerity measures in the high turnover of counseling interns at the clinic she and Isabel relied on, turnover which upset Isabel and may have cost her at least one summer program when she acted out aggressively against another student.

In addition to dealing with Medicaid and public housing, Vivian was one of the very few to succeed in gaining benefits from Supplemental Security Income. Administered by the Social Security Administration, SSI for indigent children began in 1972 as an afterthought to longer-standing work- and earnings-based disability assistance. SSI was intended to partially offset the costs and foregone parental earnings involved in raising an impaired child in a low-income home, though eligibility was restricted to traditional disabilities based on earlier state programs helping indigent blind children to avoid institutionalization. A 1990 Supreme Court decision expanded eligibility to social-emotional-behavioral disorders, but this was rolled back by the 1996 Personal Responsibility Act (which inaugurated TANF) to only those kids with "marked" or "severe [social-emotional] impairment."[41] The proportion of recipients nonetheless shifted dramatically, from kids with invisible disorders representing just 8.3 percent in 1990 to well over half in 2011.[42] These changed proportions, with the absolute increase in recipients, received widespread attention from investigative journalists for the *Boston Globe* in a 2010–11 series of front-page articles and online segments titled "The Other Welfare" and "The New Welfare."

Unfortunately, the *Globe* series played heavily into charged antiwelfare stereotypes, emphasizing an image of SSI benefits as undeserved handouts to an underclass of truly dysfunctional mothers—and provoking contentious congressional hearings.[43] The opening story was accompanied by photos (and online video) of a Black mother and son—and seven of eight mothers depicted in the full series were women of color—evoking images of the recipients as suspect racial others and "welfare queens."[44] Readers had to slog much further into an interior page to discover that "federal data show that roughly half [of children on SSI] identified as white."[45] And the series dealt only lightly with the fact that SSI is a badly underfunded program denying assistance to 67 percent of applicants and benefiting well under 10 percent of kids living in poverty.[46] The findings of sociologist Sharon Hays provide a more clear-eyed perspective. She finds that merely to apply for SSI disability coverage "requires a lengthy application process and is so complex that many law firms specialize in nothing other than helping people make disability claims."[47]

In a bold secondary headline, the *Globe* went further, suggesting that SSI creates "dangerous incentives for families to medicate the young" even as it acknowledged that many recipients "undoubtedly" deserve help with "exhausting," "deeply troubled children."[48] Large-scale studies comparing children on Medicaid with children on private insurance do suggest worrisome evidence of disproportionate psychoactive medication use.[49] The difference is small, however, and does not justify blaming low-income single mothers or assuming they are responding to economic incentives rather than seeking what is best for their children. It is just as plausible that pervasive images of suspect lone mothers, like those circulated in the *Globe* series, unwittingly inform the recommendations of educators and healthcare providers. Among the mothers I interviewed, the low-income and single mothers wrestled with the issues of whether and how to medicate no less than married mothers with greater financial and cultural resources. Moreover, other important evidence demonstrates that, in contrast to pejorative controlling images, children of color are *less* likely to receive psychiatric medications even in low-income families.[50]

Among the mothers in my research, the limited reach of SSI benefits was evident. Divorced Bev Peterson, for example, had her application on behalf of a daughter—diagnosed as bipolar and on and off medications—rejected because "it's *not* a disability in their eyes." Two "hard-living" single mothers, in contrast, reported children with similar diagnoses who were on SSI, perhaps indicative of the system's decentralized case-evaluation process. Vivian Kotler was unusual in pursuing an appeal when her initial SSI application for daughter Isabel was denied: "I had to go through the Social Security court system and get a lawyer [through legal aid]."[51] In the end Isabel was granted benefits and a lump-sum back-payment of several thousand dollars, though to tap these funds each item required medical authorization. To repair a "hand-me-down" computer, purchase educational software, even to cover Isabel's new glasses, "you have to ask permission . . . and to explain, explain, explain . . . how it relates to her disability!" Noting how this entrapped her in dependence on the state, Vivian added immediately, "And I'm not making any money here for my work . . . *Not* that I *want* to make money [for such maternal care], but you see the problem." And Vivian repeatedly emphasized that she would have preferred independence:

> I'm trying to look for a job . . . there's an outreach worker [at Isabel's school] that said to me the other day when *I* had to correct *her* [on how to access community-based therapists], she said, "You're unusual because you know everything to do and all the resources." I said . . . "Well . . . I do need help in other areas." Then I quickly said, "I need help in finding a job!"

Privatizing Dependence

Like Vivian, many of the single mothers I spoke with found it difficult to find or keep paying work while also caring for a disordered child—as Bev Peterson put it, "I couldn't hold a job and take care of Natalie. She *was* a full-time job." Without the income of a spouse or partner, each faced a dilemma: seek state support, despite its inadequacy and the bureaucratic hurdles and petty surveillance it entails, or try to rely instead on private support from family, friends, or boyfriends. In our neoliberal era with its drive to cut welfare rolls and demonize mothers seeking public help, our society conveys a clear preference for the private approach, but it, too, has its costs.

Kay Raso represents arguably the best-case scenario. She was able to keep her "good position" directing a large nonprofit agency serving at-risk children. Because her only child, David, was kicked out of successive schools and after-care programs for disruptive, aggressive behavior, Kay was often frantically scrambling to find care for him. Even as her home life, as she put it, made "a mockery" of her professional role as a "champion for children's rights," her employers accommodated her needs, allowing her to work late each night at home so she could leave work to meet David's school bus. Nevertheless, Kay averred that she was always "exhausted" and doing a "half-assed" job, adding that "being a single mother is, you know . . . *difficult!*"

A few others were able to maintain good-paying full-time work by enlisting kin to provide caregiving. Cara Withers, in medical supply sales, relied on her mother to live in the household and share care for a high-need son and typically developing daughter. Similarly, social worker Brooke Donnelley had a devoted sister serve as her vulnerable son's nanny in his first year. Other educated single mothers like May Royce and Dory Buchanan with decent earnings in similar "feminine" professions, reported struggling at times to piece together care for challenging kids even with close, supportive friends nearby—in May's case, just upstairs.

Susan Atkinson, like Vivian and Bev, did not have a paying job, but unlike them, relied entirely on private sources of support. Susan had become completely dependent on her aging middle-class parents and an ex-husband with "a very difficult relationship" with his daughters.

College-educated Susan had initially worked part-time after her divorce, moving with two toddlers into her parents' garage apartment only to "regroup." But ten years later—the latter five spent in full-time vigilante mothering for her troubled younger daughter—Susan remained in the same apartment with sharply dwindling resources. At some moments Susan sounded quite privileged and entitled, recounting, "I had hired an educational consultant; I strongly recommend for [a] divorced person [to] hire an advocate . . . I also hired a tutor . . . and I had [both] privately . . . [and] I paid for that." Yet, at other moments, the emotional toll of her privatized bargain emerged. Unable to leave her parents' home, it was nearly impossible to hide her twelve-year-old's tantrums and poor interaction skills from family members who chastised her openly, saying things like "If you just disciplined this kid more . . . " She bared her anger finally: "Many a time I'm thinking if I had the money, I would buy a house *out* of this town!"

Less educated mothers Jerri Dougherty and Patricia Gwarten, in contrast, had each cobbled together a sort of meager public-private bargain, enabling them to remain at home, getting by on a combination of public services—particularly Medicaid for their kids—and some pay from the state for in-home caregiving. Jerri fostered a developmentally disabled senior in her rented rural home, while Patricia provided short-term foster care for girls (one at a time) in her urban apartment. Both had received some short-term training for their paid caregiving, and yet it remained, as care work for multiply stigmatized others so often is, undervalued and underpaid, exemplifying our national devaluation of both familial and extra-familial care.[52] Although their arrangements gave them the flexibility to care for a needy child (and without Kay Raso's sleep deprivation), they continued to live in poverty.

No one, however, personified the conflicts and contradictions of the public versus private dilemma as clearly as Bev Peterson, whose daughter Natalie had been denied SSI coverage. Bev struggled for many years to take "personal responsibility" for her troubled daughter. Leaving an abusive first marriage armed with only a high-school equivalency degree and a few community college courses, Bev found full-time employment in office jobs. But legal fees from the acrimonious divorce, with mounting expenses for a young daughter "acting out" at school, drove Bev to food banks and local charities, and finally, to a boyfriend who promised to help with the bills. But that relationship ended over his large debts on her credit cards, and Bev, pregnant with her second child, was forced to file for bankruptcy.

When the new baby arrived, Bev somehow managed to run a small home day care to bring in minimal cash and still care for her kids. But for her efforts, she was denied any assistance by the county welfare office: "I made too much money!" Her comments on seeking welfare convey the important boundary work she engaged in as a single mother. In attempting to distance herself from the demeaning stereotypes, she largely echoed harsh images of those receiving public help as disreputable and undeserving. She labeled them "slum" or "sleaze," and, perhaps worst of all, "overweight":

> When I went to the [country welfare office] . . . it was the hardest thing I'd ever done in my life . . . and I said, "I can't even feed my kids this week." And she [the staff worker] said, "I'm sorry. I can't help you." . . . And I wasn't [looking like] a *slum* or anything. And I wasn't an *overweight* woman. I wasn't your typical *sleaze-bag* out to get some money from the state . . . It was awful! They made me feel like I was trying to get something for nothing.

While it was hard for me to listen silently as Bev invoked these negative stereotypes, as the interview extended over several hours Bev also raised significant challenges to prevailing neoliberal discourse. She illustrated again the contradictory pull sociologist Hays contends is shared by most Americans, between desires to punish dependency yet assist those trapped by circumstances beyond their control: "This government is so screwed up. There are so many wrongs and they are helping the wrong people!" And: "They [the government] are not thinking clearly when they are making these cuts on childhood issues and crisis issues in families." Yet she also continued to underscore her own boundary-making: "I think they are looking at these things [crises with troubled kids] as *all* welfare cases—and it's not the case. These are struggling families out there. You know, *normal* [families], too." When we met, in fact, Bev had fairly recently remarried in what she emphasized was a far healthier relationship. I dearly hope she was right and that she had not felt compelled to step back toward "normal" privatized dependency.

Hurtful as they are, the images of dysfunctional mothers, of "sleaze-bags" and "welfare cases" haunting Bev Peterson, and of "disturbing cycles of government dependency" written about in the *Boston Globe* contain a grain of truth. As Hays demonstrated, however, it is a very small grain and applies to only a small proportion of low-income single mothers.[53] Among those I interviewed raising invisibly disabled children, seventeen of forty-eight had low incomes, but just four recounted "hard-living" stories of family dysfunction. Each of these four lived well below the poverty line, with little education, limited ties to the paid labor force, unstable residences and homelessness, and long-run or even intergenerational issues of addiction, mental illness, family violence, and trauma. Each had had one or more children removed by the state, perhaps deservedly, although each had been reunited and was living with her focal, invisibly disabled child when I met them.[54] Such removal, the last major form of engagement with the state to be considered, is feared by many single mothers lacking class and ethnoracial advantage.[55]

Mother-Blame Taken to the Limit: State Threats of Child Removal

Nowhere were the mixed blessing and curse of involvement with the state and the stigmatization of single mothers more evident than in the stories I heard of families' involvement with child protective services or departments of social services (DSS).[56] DSS social workers are called to investigate whenever charges are made of suspected child endangerment including parental abuse or neglect—and they determine whether children should be removed and placed in foster care.[57]

Teachers, school counselors, healthcare and mental health providers, as well as welfare caseworkers, are legally required to report signs of abuse and neglect and most often will do so because they are deeply committed to children's well-being. But perceptions of abuse and neglect can also be shaped, imperceptibly, by the culturally controlling images or stereotypes that sort mothers into fit and unfit, respectable and disreputable. According to Reich, the task facing overextended social workers in child protective services is both weighty and complex: to sort parents, primarily mothers, into those worthy of being rehabilitated from those essentially so harmful or toxic that they are beyond rehabilitation.[58] When professional staff face greater workplace pressures, tighter budgets, and larger student-, patient-, or case-loads, these stereotypical pejorative images come into play more readily. So it is not surprising that, following national patterns, only four of the twenty-one married mothers reported ever being questioned by DSS (19 percent)—and of these, only "hard-living" Marilyn Chester lost custody of her children.[59] In contrast, ten of the twenty-seven single and separating/divorcing mothers (37 percent) recounted involvement with DSS.[60] Moreover, the white Euro-American lone mothers seemed to face experiences with DSS worse than those of their married peers yet substantially better than those of the single mothers of color.

Drawing the attention of DSS was invariably a traumatic experience. The mere suggestion of DSS charges was devastating to mothers of children with emotional and behavioral disorders, most of whom had already felt a great deal of proximal and sometimes explicit mother-blame. At the same time, however, DSS investigations sometimes led to the provision of important interventions and services aimed at family preservation (even if those resources were less generous than in previous eras). This double-edged nature of DSS involvement came out most clearly in the stories of the four "hard-living" mothers with sadly stereotypical issues like long-term dependence on public assistance. Arguably these mothers do bear more responsibility for their children's troubles, yet the questions of maternal fitness must also be understood in the context of highly constrained life circumstances.

Hard-Living Mothers

White working-class Marilyn Chester perhaps most closely resembled the cautionary toxic mother. Marilyn recounted a sad history of violent childhood abuse, leaving home and school at age sixteen and, over the ensuing decade, giving birth to three children. Marilyn was forty-one when I met her and she admitted to struggling with alcoholism, illiteracy, and poverty, living on a mix of welfare, SSI (for her post-traumatic issues), and intermittent low-paid work. Though Marilyn had eventually married the father of her younger children, the couple's "problems . . . mostly money-wise" had led to an ostensibly temporary decision to relinquish the three kids to foster care with relatives. In

Marilyn's cryptic, bitter account, DSS was involved only so that the kids' Medicaid could be transferred with them; yet she blamed the recalcitrance of the agency, its "[red] tape and paperwork," for the custody loss stretching to nearly a decade.

I ultimately included Marilyn only because she had regained custody of her middle child, an adolescent boy diagnosed with ADHD, over a year prior to our introduction. Despite evident attention to his sports schedule and school progress—she ticked off the courses he needed to complete and as I left she rushed to drive him to a team practice—Marilyn's narrative focused primarily on various kin conflicts and anger at the courts: "It still makes me mad. We should go right back into court and say, 'OK, this is bull . . . I want my kids back!'" And Marilyn described her oldest son, who had aged out of foster care, with a story sadly lending truth to pejorative stereotypes. She happily explained that he remained close though already married and a father: "He comes down quite a bit [to visit]." But when I asked whether he brought his young children, too, she added a bit sheepishly that her grandchildren were already in foster care: "I guess [it was] something to do with a fight with [his wife]; and he punched her or something, so the state took the kids."

Unlike Marilyn, the other three "hard-living" mothers were single; yet each, though mired in poverty, had lost custody of children to DSS for much shorter periods than Marilyn. Each might have been considered toxic, yet like Marilyn, each had been dealt a tough hand of constraining life circumstances. All came from troubled working-class families, and only Greta Roigerson had completed high school. Greta and Leesha Baker each reported surviving familial childhood sexual abuse, and Joann McGinnis bluntly described long years of drug and alcohol addiction shared with siblings.

Three years into recovery when I met her, Joann was mother to fifteen-year-old Thomas. She had lived alone with the boy in a series of tiny apartments until he was in middle school. Though she had been "drugging," she emphasized having been "clean" during her pregnancy and always providing for Thomas: "I've worked my heart out all my life, drugging and all. I've always been very responsible. I've always had a roof over my head for my child. I mean neglect, yeah, OK. Every crackhead does it. But my child has always been fed, a roof over his head, and much love . . . God forbid you try to take my child away . . . [be]cause I love him with all my heart. He's all I have." Thomas had been diagnosed with ADHD in elementary school, no surprise to Joann who told me with a snort, "I was also a Ritalin baby."

I gathered from a staccato account mainly filled with recovery-talk that Joann finally came under court surveillance when Thomas's irregular school attendance brought charges of neglect. She was ordered into drug treatment and relinquished custody of Thomas to her only clean sibling. When I met them, Joann and Thomas had been reunited for two years while she continued court-monitoring and drug-testing. She described Thomas's recent school expulsion with flashes of anger ("He really screwed that up!") tempered by sympathetic understanding ("He's really a great kid [but] . . . ").

In complicated ways, however, she also showed awareness that some issues were larger than her private struggles: Thomas, because he was biracial and strongly resembled his "jet black" Brazilian father, was viewed through a racialized lens in their largely white school district:

> Well, when I brought him up to school the first day for middle school, Thomas McGinnis, what kind of a name does that sound like to you? An Irish name, a white boy with red hair and blue eyes, you know. "Thomas McGinnis?" the lady says to me, "this is Thomas McGinnis?" I said, "The one and only." "Oh, we expected a white child." Why—how can you say that?!

She continued that the teachers had "never liked Thomas," who had been humiliated when held back a year: "Yeah he's the biggest kid in his class." Despite the recent expulsion, however, Joann boasted that a year earlier, "he took himself off" his medications. And I could not decipher whether this statement was primarily a show of bravado or she was genuinely unworried about his future.

In contrast to Joann McGinnis's pride that she had "never been homeless," Leesha Baker and Greta Roigerson each had experienced homelessness. Both mothers of three, they had each spent about two years in shelters, keeping some of their children with them while others were placed by DSS in foster care and residential facilities. Each had, for that stretch, lost custody of a son diagnosed as bipolar and expressed some sense that DSS had provided much needed treatment and respite (each mother and son had been reunited for several years when I met them; and despite the many parallels in their lives, I met them separately and they were not acquainted). Leesha and Greta each also expressed resentment about state involvement, with more reserved Leesha asking a very similar question to legal scholar Dorothy Roberts: "What I don't understand is why DSS had to have custody in order for my son to get these services?"[61]

In contrast to sensationalized images of single mothers of color unnecessarily medicating their kids in order to qualify for government checks, African American Leesha Baker reported weaning her bipolar son off the drug combination prescribed for him while in foster care. Leesha described the irritability now more widely acknowledged as a side effect, claiming that, without the medications, his behavior improved; and while that could have been due to the slow healing of the wounds of homelessness and family separation, Leesha announced, "I'm not a doctor but I do know my child!" Irish American Greta Roigerson, on the other hand, believed her diagnosed son needed medication. She spoke tearfully, however, of administering them being "the hardest thing" in a harsh life.

Greta's disheveled, dark apartment was quite unlike Leesha's tidy, bright second-floor flat, though all my visits, including two to Greta's home, were planned and at the women's invitation. Unfortunately, however, they shared with hard-living Joann and Marilyn the heavier body weight and cigarette smoking of the "slum" image that Bev Peterson had invoked so scornfully and defensively. At the same time, all four struggled with difficult health issues beyond their control: rheumatoid arthritis, bouts with cancer, a serious eye infection, and the toll of childhood trauma, familial sexual abuse, and violence. And while all four relied in part on government benefits, each also tried to work—in convenience stores, pizza shops, even assembling holiday trinkets, but they failed repeatedly to make ends meet.

Race and State Surveillance of Settled Single Mothers

In addition to the hard-living mothers just described, other single mothers whom I met led settled, organized lives yet still appeared more suspect to child protective services than those with marital privilege.

But the only settled mother to have a child actually removed (though custody was ultimately restored) was single mother Marika Booth, who described her racial identification to me as "Afro-American/American Indian." The fatherless homes of Euro-Americans Nora Jorgenson, Cassie Mueller, and Kay Raso made them vulnerable to public questioning of their maternal fitness. Yet, exemplifying national patterns in related issues of child (and fetal) endangerment, each was questioned less, and her privacy respected more, with children apparently no less troubled or burdensome than Marika Booth's daughter.[62]

Nora Jorgenson—a slim, blonde former attorney—faced the threat of charges of child endangerment from DSS amid an acrimonious divorce, which also undercut her economic privilege. Nora's younger son, Stephen, then in the third grade, had had a series of angry "meltdowns" in school on top of persistent learning and reading difficulties:

> The [County] Family Center said to me, "What are you [doing]? If you don't end this nonsense, we're going to charge you with neglect of your own children." You know, the nonsense of putting the boys in the middle of the divorce. . . . I mean they were basically saying what everybody was saying: "This child is in need and you've got something to do with it. Somehow you are responsible. Whether you put him in need or you didn't put him in need, you fit into the equation." So I really, I almost had a nervous breakdown!

Nora here vividly expressed the singularity of maternal responsibility: regardless of the causes which first "put" a son "in need," even if it was biological brain differences, she remained in "the equation" as the proximate cause. Nora's self-criticism was harsh in the face of this rebuke from quasi-public family counselors: "[When] I was stuck raising these kids by myself, *I* wasn't ready to do that. . . . So that's when . . . everything fell apart. So obviously Stephen's needs became exacerbated."

Her words also reveal the persisting gender divide, with no share of responsibility for a child's troubles apportioned to an ex-husband. Nora continued, instead speaking poignantly in her maternal confession: "When your children are so difficult, part of you *detaches* . . . It's so obvious that the child has problems, but some of the problems are worsened by the way [you] feel towards them . . . emotionally, *I was de-*

tached." Indeed, a mother who "detaches" appears unnatural and evokes the coldness of the "refrigerator moms" once thought to directly cause their children's autism.[63] In the age of neuroscience, according to best-selling advice, too much detachment still threatens a child's optimal brain development: "Research shows that the kind of care a child receives determines to a large extent how well those brain connections will be made."[64] But Nora went on to recount how, in her case, the threats from the state finally provoked such attachment: "I thought they were going to take him [Stephen] away from me . . . I mean, they could have filed charges against me! . . . [So] all of sudden something changed inside of me and I said, 'No, I owe it to [him]!' And I felt a much stronger bond."

In truth, if in-depth research on child protective services is correct, it may have been her display of proper deference to authority and the visibility of white privilege and class advantage which averted state surveillance rather than such deep internal change.[65] Nora herself mused that she demonstrated many of the right external traits, even if she lacked marital privilege, "You'd think someone who looks like me, who has an education and a nice family background, and you know, drives a [nice] car and holds on to everything, you'd think, 'Well, gee, she's got it made.'" Yet when her son Stephen "got kicked out of summer camp *two* summers in a row," Nora resigned from a downtown law firm for intermittent part-time jobs. In short order, while turning to Prozac to stabilize herself and food stamps to feed her boys, she lost her home to foreclosure and moved into a modest rental unit owned by her ex.[66] She also reported smoking more than ever, a marked detraction from her otherwise elite embodied demeanor.

Few of the married mothers, in contrast, expressed fears that state officials might take a child away. Even Judith Lowenthal, directly accused by a school psychologist of causing a son's separation troubles through attachment parenting,[67] was never questioned or even threatened with questioning by child protective services. Moreover, she was spared the distressing implication of sexualized harm that fell upon white, highly educated single mothers Cassie Mueller and Kay Raso.[68]

Cassie Mueller had abandoned funded university doctoral studies because her young son Ned was so "difficult to parent" and had been asked to leave several high-quality day care and preschool settings. She described her own life, when we first met, as "almost bizarre": "I'm strad-dling a lot of different worlds. I'm Ned's single parent and advocate, and in a work role that is not necessarily seen as all that important [part-time clerical]. And then in teaching [a night course] which I absolutely love . . . And that and being *poor*! . . . It's almost bizarre to feel like I have all these different images and roles."

With her contradictory resources, well-educated yet "poor" Cassie spent months researching Ned's issues and "going through the state's hoops" to obtain public coverage for expert assessments. And these proved inconclusive. Finally, the public school pressed for a diagnosis when Ned became aggressive with other kids, sending Cassie and Ned to a highly regarded child psychiatrist. As Cassie explained, she was "just so incensed" when he leveled direct blame at her for "this so-called Oe-dipal complex I was *giving* my son!": "He spent about fifteen minutes with us [in which] he asked me questions about my social life. And I thought, 'How irrelevant can that be?' And he actually said that my lack of a social life could be feeding into the Oedipal complex that was affect-ing my son . . . [since] I wasn't dating and I didn't have a man!"

Cassie's story also suggests an alternative explanation for the higher rates of medication among children of single mothers—besides the easy and stereotypical assumptions that it helps such mothers qualify for SSI or just makes a stressful daily life easier, single mothers may be more quickly pressed to medicate by providers unwittingly affected by nega-tive cultural imagery. After concluding from a fifteen-minute meeting that Cassie was encouraging a sexualized attachment with her seven-year-old son, the highly regarded (if likely overstretched) child psychia-trist also "pushed a prescription" at her for the antipsychotic Seroquel with the warning, "You *have to* get this filled . . . I'm serious. And you *need* to put him on this." The narratives of Vivian Kotler and May Royce reinforce the suggestion that some professionals may jump to hasty conclusions. Kay Raso, whose story I discuss next, was encouraged to medicate her eleven-year-old son with *five* psychoactive medications simultaneously (though she selectively drew from this advice, working vigilantly to eliminate or lower doses).

Cassie, anxious to keep her son off medications and to keep what she took to be a "severe" and unwarranted evaluation out of her son's records, was relieved when some of Ned's documents seemed to be lost in a move to a nearby town to save on rent. Eventually questions arose, but by then Cassie had turned to homeschooling, no doubt because she thought it best for Ned, but also to avoid the public scrutiny and state-medical intrusion that had already shaken her. Perhaps as a result, she avoided any DSS intervention.

Kay Raso, though known in her community as a professional children's advocate, did come under DSS investigation following the most explicit accusation of sexualized harm that I heard from my research group. The incident began when vulnerable son David at about age ten begged to be homeschooled and became, like Cassie's son, physically aggressive at school. According to Kay, at their "big special-ed" meeting to address the crisis, the district psychologist suddenly announced, in front of "the special-ed director, the guidance counselor, the principal," "I found out that David sleeps with you every night to satisfy your sexual needs!"[69] In Kay's account, he continued, "If you don't do something to control your son, I'm going to take him away from you and file a [DSS] petition!" Though the principal hesitated, declaring "Well, let's not go that far," some weeks later Kay recalled with distress, "The phone rings, and it's the DSS social worker who's investigating me!"

Kay was blunt and self-critical, observing that her parenting might have seemed "warped" just as she had earlier characterized her life as "half-assed": she had at times allowed David to remain home alone; she allowed profane language, especially if it defused David's turbulence; and she did lie down with him when he was too anxious to sleep at night. However, "everybody that the social worker interviewed gave rave reviews," and when experts concluded that "he [David] needs to be with his mother" charges were dismissed. Eventually the district was also compelled to pay for an outplacement, the accusing psychologist was sanctioned, and Kay remarked with evident satisfaction, "She's now one of my best friends, the social worker who investigated me!"

Stories like Kay Raso's, Nora Jorgenson's, and Cassie Mueller's offer only a suggestion that white, educated single mothers with invisibly disabled sons, though protected somewhat by their race and middle-class standing, may still be vulnerable to state scrutiny. They may be more visible than married mothers also raising burdensome children because of the cultural deficits associated with fatherless homes, once linked in the public mind to ethnoracial otherness. But such white Euro-American single mothers may ultimately be judged respectable enough *if* they can bear up under scrutiny and demonstrate other markers of class standing (difficult in Cassie's case, with little income). Yet, while their claims to respectability and maternal fitness may be fragile, their experiences may still stand in marked contrast to the experience of single mothers with volatile children who lack race privilege.

Black Mothers in Public

I first met never-married "Afro-American/American Indian" Marika Booth at a spring special-ed parent advisory council meeting in a diverse school district with a mix of working-class, immigrant, and gentrified neighborhoods. She smiled appealingly, but said little in the meeting, afterward chatting in an animated voice about her daughter's upcoming transition to high school. Marika, who had worked full-time in office jobs since completing high school, invited me to come by the nearby apartment she shared with her daughter that weekend. Over coffee in her carefully appointed kitchen, Marika shared a story that began like Kay's and several others, when overly sensitive daughter Geneva began resisting going to school at about age ten. Though Marika, with her mother and sister, had located a therapist for Geneva and enrolled her in a study of children with anxiety, school officials still brought truancy charges and reported Marika to DSS: "She [Geneva] was missing so much time in school. Then the court got involved with us. And then I just felt my life was taken away from me!"

What Marika had "taken away" was dramatic: her rights to privacy, to autonomous parenting of daughter Geneva, and to her daughter's very presence. For an initial six months she was threatened with losing her daughter, and this was followed by a fifteen-month period in which Geneva was placed in a residential group home for emotionally disordered girls. Throughout this two-year stretch, Marika herself was under court order to participate in rehabilitative services, undergo home checks, and report to the court every few months. When I met Marika, Geneva had been allowed home for weekend and holiday visits for about a year, but she had been living fully at home with her mother only for a month; and good school attendance and continued family therapy were stipulated before the family's case would be closed.

To me, a remarkable aspect of Marika's account of this serious and acutely painful public intrusion into her family was her acknowledgment that it also brought Geneva badly needed help. To illustrate her daughter's initial level of distress, Marika described dropping her at school on her way to work, but the young girl would "run off and I had to chase her." Even scarier, Geneva "attempted to cut herself:" "It was rough . . . as time went on, I was afraid of my child . . . [The] family therapist, the services, the [DSS] program, they built my strength back up . . . And if it wasn't for their support, I don't know what condition I'd be in today . . . And I think . . . [they got] her the proper help that she needed." At the same time, though, Marika remained angry at the intrusion and loss of control:

> I just *hated* going to court. The court was two years straight. We had to go three months, six months, nine months to report to the judge how things are going. "Mom's doing this, Mom's doing that." "The child's doing this, the child's doing that." OK, we did that for two years! *Fine!*

Much later in our day together, Marika's anger seemed to reignite as she remembered first learning that Geneva, not quite twelve years old, would be placed in the group home:

> I feel DSS should never have come down on me as hard as they did . . . we walked in the courtroom . . . and I was like a basket case . . . I said, "This can't be happening!" . . . The way the system did it, DSS . . . had this planned . . . they all decided that she was going to the group home. That's when I first found out about it . . . I said, "Is anybody listening to me?" . . . yeah, they all have the titles, they all have the power.

When I asked Marika if she had ever felt that being a single mother made things worse, she immediately responded, "I felt they were using it against me." She continued: "I had to go out and get an outside lawyer, which I could *not* afford. And that put me so behind in debt, but I *had* to do it. I just felt I could not walk in that courtroom by myself, even though my mother was there." Striking here is Marika's sense that the court ignored the presence of woman-centered kin ties in evaluating her maternal fitness—without a husband, she seems to say, she might as well have been "by myself." Marika also went on at length about the "annoying" ways in which being an *employed* single mother was ignored. Sociologist Reich discovered this was an all too common problem in child protective services, with difficult expectations for mothers' availability if they wished to retain or regain custody.[70] Marika, for example, recounted receiving calls at work, "'Marika, we're going to come make a home visit. Can you do it on your lunch hour?' 'Oh yes, I can'... *anything* so I could get my daughter back!" Marika also attended regular family-therapy sessions interrupting the workday, making the hour drive to the group home for such appointments as well as for team meetings, even through winter storms. With each session, "I was losing time at work," running through all allowable vacation and sick time.[71]

Right after describing her ethnoracial background, Marika admitted considering that race and skin color might have influenced DSS and the family court. Black Americans, she observed, are "look[ed] at" as "low-class," even "stupid." In somewhat disjointed remarks, however, Marika implied that she had pressed herself to dismiss this line of thought, perhaps to keep already inflamed emotions in check and sensing that she must display deference: "At first I did think that because my skin is black, they're going to really come down on me... I will admit that did run through my head. But then I said, 'Marika, you can't always think that. You've got to let that go.'" Nevertheless she sounded embittered when concluding, "I think that's what really shocked them, too, that I was able—I tell you I have *not* missed *one* DSS meeting, *one* school meeting, *one* group home meeting. I was at every court-order thing! We [Marika with her mother or her sister] were there! I never missed one thing. So I guess it took them two years to realize I was a dedicated parent and I *wanted* my daughter home."

Like Vivian, Cassie, and other mothers described, and despite her relative powerlessness in the face of aggressive and intrusive state intervention, Marika did not acquiesce in pressure to (in her view) overmedicate Geneva. In keeping with Canadian sociologist Claudia Malacrida's finding that marginalized mothers whose children were diagnosed with ADHD evidenced greater skepticism toward authoritative biomedical discourses,[72] Marika recounted struggling quite adamantly against overmedicating Geneva, even while she was in the group home. Marika insisted on being consulted on medication decisions and was acutely attentive to Geneva's reports over the phone and during visits. Amid repeated suggestions to increase Geneva's dosages, Marika finally demanded, "I don't want her meds changed!" Marika then explained what had occurred during the months of DSS supervision before Geneva's removal to the group home:

> At one time, they had her on a hundred milligrams. And I mean, you are telling me to give her this, but you want her to go to school? . . . My daughter kept saying, "Mommy, I'm so tired." . . . So I worked on it and I worked on it, and finally I got it down to twenty-five . . . But *every* time we would have a [team] meeting, I said, "That Seroquel's a problem." It was very, very frustrating, like, 'Can't you see this?" She's telling them she's tired, but they're thinking it's behavioral, because of her attitude [toward school]. *No!* It's the medicine.

Tragically, though Marika had not put Geneva through periods of homelessness, unemployment, poverty, or addiction, and mother and daughter seemed to enjoy stable loving kin support, their experiences with the state resemble those of the hard-living mothers like Joann McGinnis or Leesha Baker. Even more than Leesha, Marika might well ask why the public support services Geneva needed could be offered only when she had been removed from their home. Moreover, even if DSS involvement, including the group home, was ultimately of great value, it still seems fair to ask whether Marika might have been treated with greater respect. Certainly state actors accorded white Euro-American single mothers Nora Jorgenson and Kay Raso this respect, although their sons' behaviors were no less disordered than Geneva's. According to legal scholar Dorothy Roberts, Black mothers have been scapegoats since slavery and largely remain so: "A popular mythology that portrays Black women as unfit to be mothers has left a lasting impression on the American psyche," with single motherhood reviled primarily because it was considered "a Black cultural trait that is creeping into white homes."[73]

Conclusion: A Distinct Cultural Deficit

The accounts of these single mothers illustrate how the presence of a troubled child heightens the tensions experienced by all single mothers in an era and nation that—as it clings stubbornly to a married-couple norm—sorely lacks public supports for lone caregivers who are also their families' major breadwinners. Single mothers of burdensome children, I found, faced particular challenges, paradoxes, and contradictions. They were no different from married mothers in their sense of relentless, singular responsibility to improve their children's troubles and to go to great lengths, each largely on their own, to do so. Yet single mothers pursued this vigilantism facing a distinct cultural deficit because of their fatherless homes. While all the mothers I interviewed felt stigmatized by the very ambiguity, unpredictability, and invisibility of their children's disorders, lone mothers faced a "double whammy," coming from a social location of less respectability with which to navigate the dense bureaucracies of educational and medical systems and branches of state social services.

Yet, even in the face of suspicion of their moral fitness as mothers, and the lack of support that even a good-enough marriage could provide, several, including Vivian Kotler, suggested that without the burden of a husband's demands for family order they may be *better* able to cope with a needy child. Having other social advantages—economic resources, higher education and cultural capital—protected some single mothers raising troubled children from state intrusions and allowed them to enlist private specialists. Yet here, too, there is a paradox, as having those resources also excluded them from genuinely helpful aspects of state-run programs, such as the child mental health resources or family supports available through Medicaid and DSS. For the families eligible for state benefits, however, they came with burdens of additional bureaucracy, intrusive scrutiny, and even child removal, along with a stigma, exemplified by media suggestions that disreputable, racially other mothers might medicate their kids simply to get on the public dole.

Quite to the contrary, the single mothers I interviewed, no less than those in two-parent affluent families and across wide gulfs in income, household type, and ethnoracial difference, agonized over whether, how, how much, and for how long to medicate their children. Even the few "hard-living" mothers I met wrestled with these issues and worked vigilantly for what they believed was best for their children. As one such mother confided tearfully to me at the end of a morning together, "The hardest thing about that decision was, you know, I didn't want them to be medicating my kid to make it *easier for me*."

Some of the mothers' stories clearly suggest that, at times, mothers raising troubled children genuinely need and can benefit from constrained and often stingy public benefits. Even within the limitations of public resources, though, they could be more genuinely supportive if threats of punitive action were lessened, bureaucratic mazes made less opaque and surveillance less petty. Why couldn't there be more stories like the positive accounts I heard from the few *married* mothers who came under the scrutiny of child protective service workers: working-class Rosa Branca, who stayed on voluntarily in the mothers' group run by her social worker; and affluent Abby Martin, who after her initial shock at being reported to DSS, described the intrusion of social workers into her home as a huge affirmation, offering the support she had badly lacked? I found, like other analysts of child welfare and mothers' state involvement, a complex interplay tending to impose punitive actions rather than genuinely helpful resources precisely on those in greatest need. No doubt, as even some of the mothers agreed, state intervention or even child removal can sometimes be necessary and beneficial. At the same time, however, wrongheaded, negative, and often racialized cultural images of single mothers may be exaggerated or play a larger role when children are burdensome and exhibit episodes of disruptive, distressing behavior.

I will turn back to mothers like Marika Booth, raising children of color, to further scrutinize the difference race might make amid the tensions families face in our constrained postindustrial era. The stigma or threat presented by an invisibly troubled nonwhite child poses distinct contradictions and paradoxes within the long U.S. history of sorting between the "priceless" and the expendable or unwanted children of the less fit. Moreover, when such unwanted children are young nonwhite *boys*, the threat of dangerous masculinity looms large, charging mothers with far more difficult tasks in navigating the medicalization of childhood. I thus explore the ambivalence of those raising children of color to such medicalization, as well as how this intersects with class advantage and, as I turn to next, the gender of the vulnerable child.

En-gendering the Medicalized Child

We are medicating young boys with Ritalin in large numbers
and adolescent girls with antidepressant medications. In my
view, it's like we're medicating the resistance.
—Carol Gilligan, "What Do Feminist Experts Say?" *Ms.*,
July–August 1997

In my interviews with the mothers, we discussed fifty-five focal kids
with invisible disabilities—forty-four sons and eleven daughters—a
pronounced gender difference in diagnoses that is fairly consistent with
national (and international) data. Large-scale studies of psychoactive
medication use over the past two decades have shown some convergence,
with girls' rates increasing, but a gender gap remains; and when further
examined by age, diagnosis, and drug type, gender differences are all the
more striking. Boys are, for example, more than three times more likely
to be treated with a stimulant for ADHD.[1] The data on autism spectrum
disorders find more disparity, with only one girl diagnosed for every
four to five boys—and the higher functioning autism disorders, the
only ones I included in my sample, are even more skewed toward boys.[2]
Researchers critical of childhood medicalization, who see it largely as a
profit-driven trend toward *over*-medicalization, occasionally glance at
such gender differences,[3] but noted feminist researchers have had oddly
little to say about the gendered framing of those children medicalized,
treating them as a largely gender-neutral or gender-balanced group.[4] In
contrast, the gendered basis of childhood medicalization stood out strikingly to feminist theorist Carol Gilligan, who provocatively asserted in
1997 that we medicate kids who might challenge gender conformity. An
important exception among researchers has been Ilina Singh, who, if not
as romantic as Gilligan, has demonstrated that neither clinical research
nor drug advertising see disordered children as gender-neutral; rather,
if we might assert that there is something like a "medicalization indus-

try," it assumes that mothers are treating disordered *sons*, en-gendering thus not only most primary caregiving but also disorder as largely about boyhood.[5] I maintain, extending Singh's insight—and in a more modest sense, Gilligan's assertion—that gender norms and ideologies deeply shape experiences and understandings of the invisibly disabled child, with most emphasis on maternal accountability for sons whose potential for future manliness is precarious or disordered.[6]

A few scholars of masculinity and boyhood have argued that oppressive cultural forms of manhood are the actual or root cause of these disorders in boys. Psychologist William Pollack, following Nancy Chodorow's psychoanalytic theory of the reproduction of gendered identities, argued that boys are pushed too early into traumatic separation from mothers out of our cultural preoccupation with masculine differentiation and autonomy.[7] He maintained that this culturally driven process, exacerbated by fathers' relative lack of participation in early care, causes rising rates of invisible disabilities—though perhaps in interaction with individual, neurochemical vulnerabilities.[8]

More contentiously (and without Pollack's recommendations to increase fathers' caregiving), sociologist Nicky Hart, like conservative author Frances Fukuyama, blames employed mothers. For Hart, boyhood has been medicalized simply because it is more convenient for such women, whose careers force sons into the "early individuation [which] may impose unrealistic demands on the embryonic male personality."[9] Although my sociological research with mothers cannot directly address boys' developmental needs, it can provide suggestive evidence that mothers perceive that they are held accountable for sons' failed or shaky separation. At times they also hold themselves accountable for sons' lack of normative masculine strength and independence.

This is not to concede to Hart, or Fukuyama, who accuse employed mothers of preferring escape from the "female labor-intensive mode of early child socialization" which boys in particular so much need.[10] Indeed, the thirty-three employed mothers, the majority of whom worked full-time and provided needed household income, could hardly be said to have escaped labor-intensive family lives. Instead of speculating about the developmental needs of boys versus girls, I compare the narratives of mothers of sons to those with disordered daughters, demonstrating that all draw from shared cultural logics of gender and its binary divide.

The mothers of vulnerable daughters were indeed less preoccupied with the separation, boundaries, and muscularity that preoccupied the larger number of mothers of sons. In contrast, the mothers of daughters spoke of attending to the additional layers of invisibility which surround troubled girls and reflect larger cultural logics of femininity.

Although I delegate the issue of race and the medicalized child primarily to the next chapter, I do want to note that disordered sons and daughters neither live their daily lives nor appear in cultural imagery as race-neutral, just as they can never be considered gender-neutral. Put differently, socially assigned ethnoracial location interacts with gender to shape the meaning and experience of disability for both mother and child. In the next chapter, I analyze the more troubling, negative aspects of this intersectionality of race, gender, and the meaning of children's em-brained issues—making invisible disability most worrisome for those raising sons of color. But before I turn to this nuanced argument of differences and similarities in the racialized meanings of childhood medicalization, I first isolate for analytic purposes just one dimension of this intersectionality, the gendering of disorder and the disordered child.

Mothers Gone Soft?

Those perhaps most concerned with the imperiled masculinity signaled by childhood medicalization have been conservative critics and media pundits. Such voices embrace instead the need to instill manly independence and the individualism that Pollack and Chodorow find so problematic for boys. And though sometimes only implicit, those like Fukuyama as well as George Will, Thomas Sowell, Phyllis Schlafly, and Rush Limbaugh have pointed the finger at mothers who have gone soft on sons, who have, with lives busy outside the home, failed to produce the properly separated boys strong enough to uphold this modern gender divide.[11] The mothers' talk I analyze of sons' gendered development, in contrast to these louder public voices, is nearly all indirect and implicit. Nonetheless, I suggest it is also a form of shorthand tapping deeply embedded, shared cultural norms.

As I heard more and more from mothers, I began to see some partial truth in the conservative account of "mothers gone soft"—both tap shared cultural beliefs, with their imperative to reinforce the binary divide. Mothers worried they had made their sons' issues worse by encouraging overly close ties and dependence between them—and these were mothers with widely varied work-family arrangements. Some wondered about accusations that such ties might have even *caused* their sons' disorders. The less pronounced individuation, the less bounded relationship, was seen as provoking disorder and disability. Mothers of sons recounted performing a risky high-wire act with their young, vulnerable boys: as mothers, they should push, be "tough," and do all they can to encourage differentiation—but not too fast, not too coldly, or they may well inflict serious harm. Such mother-blame is, of course, doubly gendered, disciplining women's normative feminine caregiving while also holding mothers accountable for sons' budding masculine development. As Chodorow, Pollack, and others following feminist psychoanalytic models instruct, because of the intensity of the gender binary in our culture we accept or even encourage girls' slower and less complete break from mothers while expecting the repudiation of such ties from boys. Indeed, none of the mothers of troubled girls mentioned similar accusations of being inappropriately close.

Mothers used a variety of indirect terms and phrases to refer to maternal failings to promote sufficient separation in boys. Some reported being accused of "spoiling" or "coddling" boys, verbs that suggest weakening and producing effeminacy (or what used to be called a "mama's boy"). A few accusations were worse, with the starkest condemnations reported by Euro-American single-mothers Cassie Mueller and Kay Raso. Both were accused of direct rather than merely proximal blame for young sons' troubles by inflicting sexualized harm, being overly close out of their own frustrated needs for adult male partners. Both received these accusations from mental health professionals, with the implication that seeking more neuroscientific, em-brained explanations would be merely to cover their own guilt. Two other Euro-American mothers, affluent Judith Lowenthal and blue-collar Blayne Gregorson, also reported the sting of direct blame for keeping challenging sons too close, too feminized. Perhaps because each had the legitimating protection of heterosexual marriage, neither was accused of inappropriately sexualizing these ties. I might have expected Judith to have been the most easily targeted since she was open about her "attachment parenting" and extended breastfeeding; instead, she was only told that her six-year-old boy had "major separation issues *and* it was *my* fault." Blayne, who seemed palpably shaken recalling a similar incident, described the suggestion from a specialist that she was failing to assuage her adopted son's "severe separation anxiety, especially from me"—a suggestion that might have seemed only of proximal blame except that, as Blayne clarified, at the time he was ten and had been adopted at just six weeks.

These accounts of experts making mothers the root causes of their boys' troubles were the exceptions among the women's narratives. But most mothers described being surrounded by accusations of proximal blame from family, friends, and professionals. And many of these accusations of secondary blame were implicitly critical of sons' precarious masculinity. Blayne Gregorson sadly recounted marital strain arising because her husband thought she "spoiled" their son Brandon. This criticism, coming in tandem with that from the child psychiatrist, was painful to Blayne, who angrily declared that her husband had been often absent, working two jobs, and only years later acknowledged what she was dealing with. Single-mother Kay Raso reported, with equal sadness, that she'd lost close friends who believed she "coddled" her son David: "I went through hell hating myself because I couldn't be more strict with him." Angie Thompson, affluent and married, was exasperated with such criticism from all corners—expert and nonexpert—as was working-class homemaker Heather Dunn, whose two grade-school boys each had distinct special needs. Angie put it this way: the pediatrician said "to be firmer" and:

> Our families put their two cents in . . . and say, "If he was my child . . . he'd never talk back to me. If I had him for two weeks, I'd completely straighten him out." . . . [But] when my mom calls and asks about how the kids are doing . . . I used to pour my heart out to her and say, "What is wrong with him? Why does he hit people? Why doesn't he have any friends?" And my mother would say, "Oh, it's because *you* are *so hard* on him."

Angie tearfully wondered: Was she too "hard"? Or was she too soft to "straighten [Spencer] out"? Heather Dunn recounted similar contradictory reactions. Though she described a daily struggle with her sons, who were "like night and day" in their divergent vulnerabilities, the conflicting exhortations of special-ed teachers seemed only to highlight that she was far from getting it right in either case: "Most of the time the teacher would . . . say to me, 'He'll [Jared] be alright, don't push him so *hard*! . . . [But] Ms. M. said to me this year, 'Stop making excuses for [Terry]!' . . . [Then] they say I baby [Jared] *and* that I'm too easy on [Terry]!"

Historically, Freudian-influenced psychiatrists found both types of mothers, overindulgent and overly cold, equally at fault and directly responsible for sons' serious issues.[12] Freud himself had noted, if primarily concerned with fathers and sons, "The two main types of pathogenic methods of upbringing [are] over-strictness and spoiling."[13] In our neuroscientific era, however, strictures against "spoiling" and "coddling," according to mothers in my group, mainly fuel proximate blame for mothers' poor attempts to manage sons with neurochemical vulnerabilities. Like the four mothers just discussed (Angie and Heather, Kay and Blayne), many others I met shared similar worries and reported similar criticisms for mishandling sons' innate weaknesses. Strikingly, in addition to the array of medical, educational, and alternative treatments each cobbled together and laboriously managed for troubled sons, mothers embraced additional strategies to inculcate masculine body capital. As well, they described taking largely singular responsibility for promoting the toughening of sons' bodies and thus of (literally) more tightly bounded autonomy. This stands in fascinating contrast to Annette Lareau's ethnographic finding that, with typically developing children, fathers took the primary role in inculcating the "physical prowess" and "physical strength" so central to "masculinity."[14]

In a related vein, sociologist Michael Messner has demonstrated that athletics in contemporary American culture remains a major site for the production of gendered bodies and the maintenance of the gender binary. He writes, for example, that in boys sports, "Masculine styles and values of physicality, aggression, and competition are enforced and celebrated."[15] Thus mothers of troubled boys worked to inculcate masculine physicality in boys otherwise too "coddled," and in their very vulnerability, perhaps too effeminate. Mothers may have filled in for fathers who were unavailable or unwilling to play the part Lareau found in (largely married-couple) families with typically developing children.[16] In the long run such masculine demeanor and embodied assurance might also be helpful for high-need boys to succeed in New Economy volatility. As anthropologist Emily Martin has theorized, flexible postindustrial jobs may require such agile, resilient, assured, "flexible bodies."[17] I add—as did Bourdieu himself—that this body capital is gendered:[18] mothers of disordered daughters (like single-mother Vivian Kotler) also spoke of their attempts to engage vulnerable daughters in body-enhancing activities, but these were gymnastics, ice skating and ballet with (even in this postfeminist era) little mention of masculine-typed athletics or team sports.

Mothers of sons also expressed frustration around their efforts to inculcate such masculine physicality. Troubled sons could be stubbornly uninterested or too vulnerable or disruptive to participate without major incidents or meltdowns.[19] Mothers' frustrations were heightened when they were surrounded by expectations that their efforts should be unrelenting, but they themselves often made athletics a high priority. Renee Riverton expressed such frustration with one of her sons, Bobby, who had been diagnosed with ADD and other learning issues. At first she emphasized sharing the responsibility with her husband, explaining that both loved outdoor sports and had tried many: "Well, we tried T-ball, baseball, you know? And basketball. And that just didn't work!" Later, she added, "My husband and I coached cross-country and indoor and outdoor track, for three years I think. And Bobby ran track for a *little* while, *but* he didn't like it." Adding that only "the one-on-one sports were good," she proudly noted Bobby's turn finally to rigorous cross-country skiing, rock climbing, and mountain biking. It was clear that these became her singular responsibility to manage, for example, driving him to the various competitions: "I would take him to the different cross-country competitions at different inns. They had it [the ski races] from inn to inn, and so I did that with him." Renee laughed perhaps a bit ruefully, though, that some of these activities might be "a little *too* rough," especially when Bobby at twenty-one was threatening to try hang gliding after having just recovered from a serious climbing injury. Her somewhat embarrassed, half-sad delivery suggested that taking on increasingly risky athletic challenges was Bobby's way to *over*compensate for a more timid, even effeminate boyhood. Family efforts to promote his physical toughening, in this case, may have been almost *too* successful.[20]

Angie Thompson, who agonized over whether she was too hard or too soft with son Spencer, was another who expressed frustration trying to instill masculine physicality. Angie repeatedly brought up the topic without my prompting. She seemed distressed when telling me of her efforts to involve Spencer in team sports and of her family's disapproval when she finally quit trying. Angie shared with Renee Riverton a white Euro-American working- or lower-middle-class background; each had attended some college and worked part-time. But Angie's husband was better educated with significantly higher earnings than Renee's—and transmission of gendered class privilege through cultural and body capital may have felt more urgent and imperative to Angie, particularly with Spencer entering high school and almost fifteen years old:

> Alright, alright, we're *not* going to soccer practice today because I've got this kid in the backseat of my car, he's absolutely hysterical, he won't get out of the car. . . . I [had been] thinking, "OK, I have a boy. He's got ten fingers and he's got ten toes and he's going to be a jock . . ." *nope* . . . I got pressure from my family, 'You have to bring him to hockey practice. He's gonna like it if you say he's gonna!'"

Later, after she had spoken of several negative peer interactions and school issues that Spencer had endured, Angie reiterated, "You know, my father is very athletic and he *can't* understand why Spence doesn't like the Patriots [New England's pro football team]," and here she added near tears, referring to the core dilemma of how to recruit support when a child's issues are so invisible: "[be]cause he *looks* normal!"

Cara Withers, divorced Afro-Caribbean mother of two, seemed to have found a workable alternative to team sports and was less frustrated than Angie Thompson: Cara took her "extremely sensitive" and emotionally disordered son Michael for before-school gym and weight workouts—and this, she carefully explained, was without his younger sister, though both attended after-school karate classes. Tellingly, Cara explained that the extra early-morning sessions were to help Michael, twelve, to "build himself" and to deal with "boys [who] can be very rough," even "brutal." When she immediately added, "I need to teach him the right way," I thought she might have been about to fill in something like "to be a man." But before I could ask, Cara had quickly continued on, measuring how much Michael needed to "build himself" by comparison to his younger sister. In again emphasizing the term "rough," and even "extremely rough," she framed Michael's issues through the opposition or gender reversal with daughter Delia: "Michael is the sweetest child . . . but he tends to get upset about everything and cries . . . he just breaks down immediately . . . His sister . . . [Delia] is rough, extremely rough. Michael is more passive. She's the aggressor, he's the passive one . . . and he gets embarrassed very easily. He's extremely sensitive, extremely!"

It seemed that Cara knew she must take action against such gender-reversed traits in her children, her daughter being the "extremely rough" one while her son "embarrassed easily" and was "the passive one." Michael and Delia's father, Cara's ex-husband, was not absent, but like many divorced dads he was removed from his kids' daily life: "Every other weekend he has them. He's a good dad."[21] Because she took it upon herself to build her son's masculine physicality, Cara reported following a stringent daily routine, rising at 5:30 each morning. Mother and son were at the gym by 6:00 a.m. to work out, though as her household's breadwinner, she worked "forty to sixty hours a week." Perhaps as Michael became older, he might reject having his mother as workout coach, but for the time-being the joint investment in body capital seemed to be paying off—as Michael built muscularity, Cara reported having slimmed down. Moreover, Cara brought in relatively good earnings as a medical-supplies saleswoman; and in such interactive, New Economy employment, gendered body capital and embodied self-assurance matter, perhaps all the more so for a woman of color.[22]

Some mothers making efforts to also instill masculine body capital to help volatile, troubled sons reported additional, surprising obstacles. Sadly, some of the psychoactive drug treatments, the atypical antipsychotics used as "mood stabilizers," also often cause blood sugar problems and significant weight gain. This was a major worry for single mother Kay Raso, who like Cara Withers had started early morning exercise with her son. If less vigorous than Cara's regimen, Kay might have had to start gently given the depth of her thirteen-year-old son's anguish about his body:

> He [son David] wouldn't even discuss his weight. So it was so deep . . . [and] I think once he found out, when he got weighed just three weeks ago and found out how much he weighed, it really shocked

him. . . . It turns out that 0.25 milligrams of Risperdal is all it takes . . . [it] does something to your hypo[thalamus] or whatever it's called[23] . . . [So] I wake him up at six and we walk for forty-five minutes and that's really helped.

Kay reported that on top of the weight issue, at five foot one, David was self-conscious about being short for a young man in early adolescence; and the extra weight, she reported, made him literally "obese" at 180 pounds. With such a large weight gain, David may also have suffered the feminizing effect of added fat deposits in the breasts, a less common but noted side effect of these medications.[24] Kay added still more poignant details: "The thing that breaks my heart and makes me admire him is that, as fat as he is, when I tried to take him off of Risperdal three months ago, within four days, he pushed me against the counter . . . this [was] just out of the blue . . . after perfect behavior. And then he started to cry and he said, 'You know what? I'd rather be fat than act like this.'"

Affluent homemaker Colleen Janeway also reacted to the threat these medications posed to her twelve-year-old son's gendered body capital. After listing other worries about James's future, Colleen added her distress over a much less dramatic weight gain than that confronting Kay Raso:

My God, he's so sweet. He's so happy. He's so *dependent* on us. How independent is he going to be? . . . You know, will he [ever] be married? Will he have a job?. . . . I feel emotional . . . you know, he's really not in the norm. Our child is really not in the norm . . . When I'm really honest I have those feelings, too [fear for his future]. I get the lump in my throat because there's my little boy who's cute and funny and smart, and you know, twenty pounds overweight from the Geodon!

Colleen struggled to explain further, perhaps to justify why this minor visible marking of difference bothered her: "He looks normal. But you know that was also the feeling of— . . . It [his disorder] *is* invisible but it isn't. I mean . . . when you look, he looks different than other kids, and yeah, still a *little* different. It's *not* entirely invisible." Colleen expressed here a sense of anxiety about a vulnerable son's ability to pass or to live as a young man just "a *little*" outside "the norm," about his continued dependence and its not being "entirely invisible." Colleen herself, on the warm summer morning we spent talking in a coffee shop, appeared quite fit and well ordered, tanned and relaxed in crisp light shorts and blouse. I wondered, but could not guess, if this appearance reflected actual ease and assurance in the world, a form of compensation for a son's disorder, or both at once.

Bullying and Boys Post-Columbine

Several mothers added a sense of urgency to sons' needs for masculine toughening because their sons had been either bullied or threatened with physical violence. Cara Withers was the least direct, but she may have been alluding to bullying or threats of violence when she lamented that boys could be "brutal" to her "extremely sensitive" son Michael. She had also lamented that it was her daughter Delia, the "rough" one and "the aggressor," rather than Michael who was "streetwise," an important trait for boys, Cara made clear, in their diverse urban neighborhood.[25] Her further observation pressed the point, implying again that Michael had confronted aggression: "The hardest thing [for Michael] is we live in the city. You *can't afford* to cry . . . and he just breaks down immediately." Heather Dunn was more direct. White Euro-American and married, Heather and her family lived on a much lower household income than Cara but resided in a similarly diverse urban neighborhood. Heather referred to several specific instances as evidence that Jared, eleven, had been "pick[ed] on all the time"—and this without my prompting. Jared, by her account, usually managed to suppress any reaction when "this kid kicked him," or even when "body-checked right into the radiator" at school. Yet when Jared finally had endured too much, he had become uncharacteristically aggressive, striking back against one particularly abusive boy. Heather expressed vigorous approval for this unusual instance of aggression, suggesting relief that Jared had finally responded in a tougher, streetwise manner. I say this because she employed terms far coarser, more stereotypically working-class and male, than any used in the rest of our nearly three-hour interview: "You know what? I'm sorry to say it, but I'm glad that he [Jared] did it because now the little bastard will leave him alone! Because he knows Jared will kick his ass!"

African American Patricia Gwarten, another astute single mother, shared similar unprompted concerns with me, if less vividly, perhaps because her son had not yet experienced the same level of violence as had Heather's somewhat older son. Nonetheless, Patricia mentioned bullying as another reason for regularly exercising with six-year-old Jake, "to build up his muscles." Though Jake was just a first-grader and too young for the added muscularity of even early puberty, Patricia had begun to strategize:

> I do [work with Jake] because he has to exercise to build up his muscles. So we, we'll walk [all] around the area or I'll take him to a park . . . winters are the hardest because we're inside all the time. I have to find a winter sport so he can maintain the muscle tone and . . . to address the bullying.[26]

Just at this point my expression must have changed, and picking up my surprised look Patricia immediately added:

> I know! You wouldn't believe that a first-grader is bullied. I couldn't believe it myself. I'm like, "Whoa—you're talking about little kids here!" But it's a different generation, I tell you. So just to make Jake feel good about himself.

Researchers have confirmed trends indicating that the preoccupations of such mothers with boys' muscularity and bullying are well-placed. Psychologists find that normative masculine body ideals depicted in media and action-hero toys have grown larger and more muscular in past decades, influenced by the steroid-induced hypermuscularity of so many athletes and celebrities. And such pop culture images influence boys at young ages.[27] At the same time, the prevalence of serious bullying seems to be increasing—or at least it is gaining greater public attention with new forms of "cyberbullying."[28] Cyberbullying seems to occur across gender lines, as in the sad case of Phoebe Prince—the already troubled young woman who committed suicide in western Massachusetts in 2010 after being harassed by fellow high-school students, male and female alike, as the "Irish slut."[29] Such peer harassment, however, is generally expressed in forms which are still differentiated by gender, exemplified in the Prince case with the "slut" label only applied to young women. And when physically aggressive or violent forms of bullying are considered, it becomes decidedly masculine, highly concentrated among boys and young men.[30]

The Phoebe Prince case also reveals that young disordered bodies tend to be seen through both gendered and racialized lenses. This tragic, vulnerable young woman was targeted as a recent immigrant to the United States from Ireland and too easily cast with the disreputable sexual promiscuity long attached to nonwhite and "not quite white" women.[31] In contrast, the bodies of disordered boys have been understood as deficient in masculinity, feminized or gay, yet potentially violent.[32] (For young men of color, potential violence is emphasized, though in contrast to white youths they may be cast as too masculine.) The reality may be nearly inverted: at least one nationally representative survey of parents along with school principals and staff found very high rates of victimization (as opposed to perpetration) among those diagnosed with masculine invisible disorders.[33] And researchers at Indiana University concluded that there was very little evidence to link such disorders to violent behavior, despite the unfortunate public perception.[34] It seems the reality may be closer to Heather Dunn's account of her son Jared's continual bullying: vulnerable boys, if sufficiently taunted and physically harassed, may be provoked to defensive violence to prove their manliness. Lucy Nguyen's account of her adolescent son Ken's harassment was perhaps more revealing. It was explicitly racialized and involved an explicit attack on the young man's masculinity:

> My son says "I'm half Asian." Someone [in the neighborhood] called him a "chink." My daughter said, "What's a chink?"Actually my son, someone called him, I forget, either a "fag" or a "fairy." That was worse. He [Ken] beat him up. He broke his nose and cheekbone. I was afraid they'd call the police, that they'd be at my door; but they never did.

Both mothers, while proud that vulnerable sons had defended themselves, were emphatic that neither young man had previously been violent.

Sociologists Michael Kimmel and Matthew Mahler, in an influential analysis of two decades of school shootings, made a very similar argument. They discovered from a systematic review of the evidence that young men's violence in these tragedies came after being "mercilessly and routinely teased and bullied."[35] Moreover, the string of twenty-eight terrifying school massacres between 1982 and 2001 were carried out by adolescent boys without severe mental illness—and all but one were white Euro-American. Kimmel and Mahler maintained that rather than a recent form of extreme deviance, violent aggression and physical dominance have been the long-standing norm for American masculinity: a century ago, for example, regular fighting was prescribed by psychologists to promote boys' healthy development. Therefore they understand school shootings as a defensive reaction, a way to counter victimization and reassert manly honor. In our current era, we are more ambivalent about boys' aggressive physicality: we formally prohibit it in public spaces, yet it continues to be celebrated in media and popular culture.[36] Mothers rearing vulnerable, "extremely sensitive" boys again perform a high-wire act promoting masculine toughening as a result. While wishing to protect "shy, bookish," "nonathletic, 'geekish' or weird" sons from bullying,[37] mothers risk leaving young sons open to harsh public sanction if they go too far to encourage toughened responses, particularly as boys grow and become more physically imposing. The delayed outbursts or explosive reactions of such boys to victimization can also be far more visible than the controlled, even calculated aggression of those doing the bullying, as the next two stories suggest.

The narrative of divorced Euro-American mother Lenore Savage exemplified the dilemmas mothers face rearing less normatively masculine sons amid our cultural ambivalence about boys' aggression.[38] Her son Noah was diagnosed with emotional disorders, and in adolescence he eventually faced serious sanctions in both the schools and the juvenile courts. Following neoliberal dictates, Lenore blamed herself to a significant extent, as for example in this piece of her narrative pinpointing when serious issues began. Poignantly, in this confession of "let[ting] him pull away" following her own mother's death, Lenore failed to mention that she also managed to work full-time and care for Noah's younger sister: "I actually fell into depression like two years down the road after things [custody battles] had sort of settled down. But my mother died, the divorce was final . . . it was like then I crashed. And I think that's when Noah really started to have problems. I think he was at that stage where boys pull away, you know? And I let him pull away. And I should have tried even harder to be more involved then."

Lenore also wondered whether she should have been tougher and really "cracked down" on Noah in high school when his academic performance became uneven (initially he had been a strong student who won prizes and took Advanced Placement, college-level courses). Lenore also spoke of social isolation: "He was really withdrawn by that point." But again self-blame entered when she noted that all three (herself, Noah, and his younger sister) were "really isolated" and "pretty much loners." Tellingly, Lenore noted that there was "a lot of bullying" at the high school Noah attended, observing unprompted, "You know, I think a lot of kids really gave him [Noah] a hard time. And certainly, he had things stolen from him. You know, that's pretty common. Where it's not exactly a mugging, [but] it's *an intimidation*."

Noah's first provocative behaviors, perhaps partly in response to this "intimidation," resulted in only short suspensions from school. But, according to Lenore, these behaviors were worrisome and "so weird," including creating art pieces which included blood, that school officials became fearful. Noah was then expelled, "suspended sort of forever" in Lenore's words, for throwing a chair in a crowded classroom. She elaborated: "[This] was considered an assault, although he didn't throw it at a human being and it didn't hit a human being. And at the time he was in a music class that had not had a teacher for two days." Importantly, Lenore interpreted or contextualized Noah's acts quite differently from school officials, seeing in the unsupervised classroom the defensive reaction of a nonconforming young man, an introverted artist, to the "hard time" he was given by his peers. Her next comment emphasized this peer context: "And other kids were throwing things—and Noah one-upped them all by throwing a chair instead of whatever the [smaller] things were that they threw."

Kimmel and Mahler similarly concluded that the effects of "hectoring," "bullying," and even less serious "teasing" in provoking boys' violence "should not be underestimated."[39] The "retaliatory" school massacres they analyzed were of course horrific and exceptionally rare incidents compared to the more everyday acts I heard about. But the shootings have had a wide impact on public attitudes, school cultures and policies, as well as on our perceptions of boys' physicality and aggression.[40] Lenore Savage brought this up with me, despairing that Noah's high school years were caught in the aftermath of Columbine. Columbine High School in Littleton, Colorado, was the scene of one of the deadliest school shootings, where fifteen individuals, including the two young perpetrators, were killed; the tragedy occurred in 1999, just four years before I met Lenore.[41] Lenore linked the severity of school sanctions to the fear sparked by Columbine and was very critical that Noah was expelled without an attempt to understand what (or who) had provoked his actions:

> Actually I think that they were judging him in a very, very harsh light; and that they really didn't understand who he was and how hard it was for him: Not that he didn't do awful things. But . . . I just don't understand why they were so freaked out by him . . . This was also right around the time of Columbine—which I think colored *everything* greatly.

Because Noah desperately wished to return to his local public high school, Lenore turned to two sympathetic counselors for help. And each of these, one inside the school and one in a community center, confirmed her suspicion of the impact of Columbine:

> The woman down there [the counselor in a community youth guidance center] said, "You know, I hate to say, but this is happening *a lot* since Columbine." And a lot of things that happened to Noah in high school, his special-ed counselor said, "Ten years ago, this wouldn't even have ruffled a feather."

Boys, Invisible Disability, and Gender Policing

It may also matter that the bullying and harassment of boys with embrained disabilities often includes gay slurs. The stigmatization of less than immediately perceptible, not-normal brain differences may have some important similarities or parallels to nonnormative sexualities, raising similar questions of passing or remaining closeted—though rapid generational change in attitudes surrounding gay and lesbian rights may soon make this comparison obsolete. Nonetheless, significant research has found the rampant bullying and peer harassment of nonconforming boys to be pervaded by gay-baiting—even of boys not, in fact, gay. Sociologist C. J. Pascoe found such gay-baiting pervasive in her influential ethnography of a California high school, though she argued differently from Kimmel and Mahler that such taunting or hectoring no longer represents rampant homophobia. Instead, Pascoe emphasized that gay-taunts marked boys' policing of masculinity, of masculine embodiment and demeanor, combined with a matter-of-fact acceptance of most gay students whose embodied demeanor did not violate the binary divide.[42]

In either case, whether representing deeper fear of homosexuality or the policing of masculinity, gay-taunts may be particularly noxious for neurodiverse boys. The hectoring in Lucy Nguyen's narrative of her son Ken, for example, had led to the young man's violence, and according to Lucy, it was "worse" than his being confronted with racial slurs. I heard nothing like this in Lenore Savage's account of life with her son Noah; however, Noah's acute episodes of depression and anxiety after regaining admission on appeal to the public high school, his subsequent truancy, and thus his landing in the juvenile court system may have been related to a school climate pervaded by gender policing and bullying. Research has found greater anxiety, depression, social withdrawal, and truancy among straight and gay students in schools with higher levels of such harassment.[43]

There were enough glimpses in the narratives of others to suggest the ubiquity of gender policing and its threat to boys already vulnerable and stigmatized. I discuss the first of these incidents at some length as it also involved boys at school. It was supplied by Judith Lowenthal, one of the affluent homemakers, who described a gay-taunting incident from four or five months prior, at her son Allan's private middle school (a day school focused on language-based learning differences). The incident had led to his brief suspension and was very upsetting for Allan and Judith because, for the most part, the emotional fallout was expressed in private, at home and with his family. According to Judith, a known "troublemaker" was hectoring a small group as they waited to be picked up at the end of the school day:

> There's this one boy in Allan's grade who is a real handful, he's very high energy, often a troublemaker . . . and this boy was railing, I don't know why, last spring. I guess he thought it was a big deal to call kids "gay." And

he was picking on this one kid, and he was saying, you know, "Oh you're gay, you're a fag!" And he was really being obnoxious, and of course Allan [has been taught] . . . that you don't joke about being gay, it's a serious racial slur. Ah, anyway, Allan wanted to stop him. . . . [later] my parents told me that when they were there for Grandparents' Day, this kid was calling other kids "gay" and names. So . . . I was like, "Whoa, why hasn't anybody told this kid to—? It's not OK." It's the equivalent, you know, that's in my mind the equivalent of a racial slur.

Here Judith importantly defends Allan's intervention as virtuous: he had been raised in a conscientious liberal environment of tolerance and sought to stop "the equivalent of a racial slur." And, as she had earlier pointed out, Allan's issues tended to make him very literal, absolutist in interpreting such rules, even at age twelve. But perhaps Allan also identified with the "kid" being targeted or felt he might be next because, as Judith continued, he broke an explicit school rule in being physical:

I guess all the kids, they were all standing around. It's a crowded space. There was lack of teacher supervision, and K. [the troublemaker] wouldn't stop, and the kids kept telling him to stop. So Allan put his hand out and covered K.'s mouth. And nobody saw this except the kids themselves, but apparently that's what happened. The next thing that happened K. runs to his [parents'] car and he's got a bloody nose and is crying that Allan hurt him and punched him. So [the school] has a very strict policy . . . if a child physically touches or hurts another child, they get a day's suspension.

This "very strict policy" seems similarly to reflect national educational system changes like the adoption of zero-tolerance policies post-Columbine. Judith did not refer directly to Columbine as Lenore Savage had, but she similarly complained of the mishandling of an emotionally disordered boy's response to a form of bullying: "He [the school principal] had already talked to Allan about having this [suspension] happen, he didn't consult us! He didn't consult Allan's therapist, he didn't consult the school counselor. He failed to realize that he was dealing with a child with a serious emotional-behavioral disorder. The whole thing threatened Allan's stability."

In Judith's account, like Lenore's, such zero-tolerance policies ignore the context provoking aggression and may too readily single out more vulnerable, already victimized boys. Judith's account of Allan's experience with such one-sided school sanctioning was also heartbreaking:

> Allan came home and cried and cried. It took us two hours to get his meds into him because he said, "This isn't better. This world isn't better. You told me that taking these meds would be better. This isn't better. Look what happened to me." I mean he was a wreck. I spent two days solid on the phone with the therapist and the principal.

The second glimpse of the pervasive policing of gender conformity among boys came from a mother on the other side of wide gulfs of race and class privilege. African American single mother Leesha Baker (one of the four hard-living mothers) provided this glimpse, assessing the young men "hang[ing]" on the "streets" with her vulnerable son Dion rather than in an account of school bullying. Leesha's words emerged, like those of Afro-Caribbean Cara Withers, as she spoke of fears for a vulnerable Black son's future. While Cara had not referred explicitly to young men's sexuality, both Cara and Leesha responded to a social structure sorely lacking positive routes to Black manhood. Indeed, Leesha's words and tone hardly framed being gay as admirable; yet, she held it up as outside the street life leading to entrapment in the criminal justice system for so many working-class sons of color. Anxious that her troubled son at age eleven looked up to his male cousins, Leesha observed:

> Well, the older kids, they're either locked up or they're gay. And the ones that ain't gay, and the ones that ain't locked up, they're out there smoking weed trying to be a thug on the streets. And he [son Dion] hangs with his cousins. I tell him, "Keep on hanging out there with them, somebody's going to shoot a bullet and you gonna catch it. Or the police gonna find you . . . if you don't want to listen to me, you think your cousins know more than me and you wanna be cool, you gonna pay the consequences."

Leesha expressed no hope that her son might be gay or learn from gay Black men who had avoided becoming "thug[s] on the street." An already vulnerable son facing poverty and racism did not need another strike against him—and Leesha perhaps understandably practiced a form of gender policing much as Cara took her vulnerable son to the gym, to help him survive in an unfair world not of his (or her) making.

I almost hesitate to add a last form of verbal hectoring which emerged from mothers' accounts. Taunting or name-calling boys for being in special-ed classes may seem minor compared to gay-taunting and bullying, though sociologist Valerie Leiter also alludes to its seriousness.[44] Such name-calling may be less gendered as well, as I heard from both mothers of struggling daughters and sons that their "normal," "good-looking" children were taunted by peers as "sped kids" or "speds." Donna Simon, a Euro-American divorced mother, reported that her youngest daughter, diagnosed with ADD, had suffered badly from such harassment. Donna observed that taunting a "child" as a "sped" was a terrible insult: "You know, they use that 'sped' word like, ah, it's the plague. . . . It's a *very* negative comment!" Two mothers of sons shared very similar observations, and it is possible, because of the policing of masculinity, that for boys such taunting carried greater risks of escalating into physical violence. Affluent, married Angie Thompson was worried when neighborhood kids singled out her son Spencer for riding the "sped van" rather than the regular school bus. And Theresa Kelleher, also a white, affluent mother, recalled with distress that her son Colin was labeled by a neighborhood bully, if not as a "sped kid," as going to a school "for kids with problems."

Such accounts suggest that "sped" labels may share at least one aspect of gender policing, as each creates boundaries and distance from a stigmatized form of difference. Intriguingly, one mother, never-married Brooke Donnelly, briefly alluded to this parallel between invisible disability and homosexuality. Explaining why she had responded to my notice in an online newsletter, she confessed she had told only "a handful of friends" that her young son's diagnoses had moved to a more serious level from ADHD to possible bipolar disorder: "This was kind of a nice first step for me to have you over and talk to you. . . . I feel like I'm this close to going to a support group for parents . . . But I have some kind of fears and reservations around doing that, kind of *outing myself,* if you will." While this language of "outing myself" and coming out of the closet has been the dominant discourse of lesbian and gay rights movements, Brooke invoked it to describe revealing the hidden stigmatized difference of a young son's invisible disorder.[45] Brooke's use of this discourse was all the more remarkable because, she revealed, her own family had always been open about a brother's physical and intellectual impairment.

Daughters and Disability: "She Was So Inward, She Was Like *Invisible!*"

The ten mothers with struggling daughters—like Donna Simon, whose daughter had been harassed as a "sped kid"—confronted challenges both similar to and different from those raising disordered boys. If facing the stigma and the resented cost to the community were points of similarity, the largest difference was simply that girls' troubles seemed to be shrouded in greater layers of invisibility. Though mothers of sons also struggled to obtain accurate diagnoses, mothers of daughters reported greater obstacles and longer years of distress before the relief of at least some name for their daughters' invisible issues. Navigating the educational system with the kind of post-Columbine *over*-visibility and fear inspired by sons who act out at school may be equally distressing, as Lenore Savage's and Judith Lowenthal's stories instruct. But mothers of daughters going years without recognition or validation of their experiences were less likely to garner the professional support on which mothers of boys like Judith relied—and without diagnoses, they were largely unable to access special-education services. Three of the ten mothers, raising eleven disordered daughters, across wide gulfs of economic and cultural privilege, offered firsthand testimony of this gender disparity.[46] Each directly compared school negotiations on behalf of typically developing sons to those for needy daughters—and in each case, they concluded, *less needy* boys better captured the concern of school personnel.

Affluent, Euro-American Abby Martin was the mother of a son and daughter—but it was daughter Jessica who had demonstrated repetitive, isolating, and at home, quite volatile behavior since early childhood. In middle school, Jessica had become increasingly unable to function despite being academically gifted. But an (ex-)husband's denial coupled with Jessica's withdrawal left Abby alone, her concerns perhaps seen by school staff as her own disorder: "They must think I have Munchausen syndrome by proxy!"[47] Several years later, I learned that Jessica had dropped out of high school.[48] But Jessica's younger, typically developing brother Matt, according to his mother, did well in school, in friendships, and at home. Matt was the child, however, to unwittingly capture the concern of school personnel—the very same professionals who had resisted acknowledging Jessica's struggles:

> [At eight years old], Matt's hair was long, and they thought he was crying too easily. His teacher sent him to the guidance counselor, and she spoke with the principal and the nurse. They thought it was poor hygiene and child neglect . . . So the guidance counselor called me, "We have a complaint and we have to report you." So with my daughter, *nothing*. I have been trying to get them to see something was wrong from the fourth grade [five years before this conversation]. But with my son, they turn us in to the DSS![49]

Notably in this account, after years of "trying to get them to see" Jessica's troubles, it was Matt's visible violations of masculine gender norms, his "crying too easily," his long hair, which led school personnel to request the intervention of child protective services. Abby lamented that, in contrast, the multiple requests she had made to have the school psychologist meet with Jessica had been rejected. She admitted that Jessica's struggles were almost wholly invisible at school, yet such actions dismissed her years of experience of Jessica's excessive irritability and stubborn resistance to sharing in normal routines at home: "[Jessica] was never a behavior problem *in the* classroom; she just doesn't get the homework in . . . so the teachers *don't get it*."

Paradoxically, Abby found her maternal honor vindicated *only* when state child protective services investigated. This made her one of very few whose dealings with DSS, if at first disconcerting, actually became quite positive—perhaps not surprising, because those few with positive experiences were notably white and well educated. Although Abby admitted initial shock at such intrusion, her high cultural capital, racial (and initial marital) privilege, and quiet home in an advantaged community immediately conveyed respectability. And social workers, in making home visits on behalf of her son Matt, instead supplied long-denied recognition and naming of Jessica's more serious troubles (finally diagnosed as Asperger syndrome). DSS intervention came too late to repair Abby's strained marriage or to address her husband's entrenched denial—and sadly, too late to repair her daughter's educational prospects. But Abby explained that she was deeply grateful for the six months of required supervision and counseling: rather than finding herself under surveillance and threatened with child removal, as a Black or low-income single mother would likely face, Abby found positive support for her divorce and for her mothering.[50] Moreover, school officials might have been mollified to learn that Abby was soon actively encouraging Matt's gender-normative enthusiasm for rock-climbing lessons.

Molly Greer, also a married, white mother of two, had evidently never faced intrusion by child protective services and seemed to have a more supportive husband than did Abby Martin. But she described similar experiences rearing a typically developing son and a daughter diagnosed with dyslexia and ADD. Molly compared her dealings with schools on behalf of each, particularly noting, like Abby, that it was a son's "more visible" behavior that had garnered school attention: "Yeah, not so much with Andrea [daughter Andi]. It was more Nicholas's behavior, because Nicholas's behavior was more *visible*. Where Andi was just Andi, and where *he . . . he* was ditching school or wouldn't work. Or, you know, the school was *constantly* calling me."

According to Molly, Nicholas had struggled through adolescence, primarily because he had had difficulty negotiating a nonnormative sexual orientation: "My son is also gay, so he was dealing with that." She observed that Nicholas was doing well in his early twenties (when Molly and I met), yet it is striking that in school he had been so overvisible compared to a daughter who tended to internalize her troubles in gender-normative fashion: "Nobody would know in school that she [Andi] has any problem . . . they don't even notice that she has ADD!" This had real consequences, though it may have also protected Andi from punitive sanctions: Andi received only minimal special-ed services, though Molly had struggled mightily to obtain them. Molly supplemented those services herself, putting in hours reviewing schoolwork with her daughter each evening. She also sought out private summer programs and reading tutors, using her earnings as a self-employed housecleaner and her husband's from long hours managing rental units and selling real estate. Molly claimed, "We were lucky that we could pay the $10,000 to [the highly regarded summer reading program]. I mean, as I said, I know people that mortgaged a house [for it]!" Nonetheless, because Molly hoped to have twelve-year-old Andi's dual diagnosis better recognized by their urban school district well before the girl entered high school, she explained she was investing more. For the next IEP meeting, she announced, she had hired both an educational attorney and an advocate.

Without such financial resources, low-income single mother Rhonda Salter emphasized the same near-impossibility of getting school personnel to acknowledge a daughter's (Rachael) learning issues against the relative ease of validating a boy's issues. Rather than comparing her own son and daughter, Rhonda compared her experience with Rachael to the fast attention a friend's son had received. She recounted that, unlike Abby Martin's and Molly Greer's typically developing sons, her friend's son was "a special needs child, too":

> But see, her son, it was the behavior, while Rachael's was not really so much behavior. It was her passiveness: it was an act of defiance. OK? But it wasn't such an act that they [school personnel] considered it defiant because she was quiet. She didn't speak out, or kick, or scream . . . But her very passivity was Rachael's act of defiance. She *refused* to pick up a pencil and do the work. And *they refused* to see that as a problem.

Thus to Rhonda, a daughter's feminine "passivity," her internalizing rather than externalizing "behavior," posed a bigger maternal challenge than a boy's active disruptions. A boy might rudely "speak out" or more aggressively "kick or scream" and the school would simply be unable to ignore him. Rhonda, in night school studying for her high-school equivalency exam, observed that, in contrast to her friend, she had few fans among school personnel: "As a parent, if you argue, then OK, you're the Uncooperative Parent! I've actually had that written on reports, yeah, 'uncooperative' . . . I went through six years of what I just thought were *sheer school hell* with Rachael. You know, she hated it, she didn't want to go. She hated her teachers, she hated her class, she hated everything, everybody."

Other mothers of daughters I spoke with did not make such direct comparisons between sons and daughters or boys and girls. Nonetheless, they shared accounts confirming the difficulties of gaining services or assistance when daughters caused so few outward problems at school. This lack of recognition in the daily life of mothers' routine engagement with schools may have increased their need for support and validation from family members, particularly from partners. Such a recognition deficit was certainly emphasized by Abby Martin in the breakdown of her marriage, and it may have contributed to the three other midlife divorces among the mothers of vulnerable daughters—a group which also included Rhonda Salter and Donna Simon.[51] Donna—raising three daughters, two with ADD and emotional issues—complained of this lack of recognition explicitly. She reported that the schools simply had *not* believed girls could have ADD when her oldest, Lynn, had started first grade (Lynn was twenty when I met Donna): "The school didn't recognize the ADD . . . the family [in-laws] didn't recognize it either. ADD back then was, especially in girls, was almost unheard of . . . It was a long wait, about six or seven years, maybe even longer, maybe even ten years before they really recognized it in girls." Donna gained initial recognition from medical providers: "She [Lynn] was probably one of the first [girls] in this area to be diagnosed!" Yet this had surprisingly little impact when the local schools, the site of children's and mothers' daily lives, ignored it. And Donna received little support from her husband, Lynn's stepfather: "It made it very difficult because she's not his biological daughter. . . . We got married when she was four. So with a child like that not being your own, it's difficult . . . so that's probably one of the reasons why we separated."

Painfully, Donna repeated much of the process with her second daughter, Ann—also a child from a previous relationship—sealing the demise of her marriage: "I said, 'God, just shoot me'!" With middle daughter Ann struggling in high school at the time of our conversation, Donna relied on an implicitly gendered binary to compare her two vulnerable girls, somewhat reminiscent of the comparisons Abby, Molly, and Rhonda had made between sons and daughters. Donna described her eldest, Lynn, in more masculine terms: Lynn was a "tough kid," one who "every time you turned around, she was doing something!" But importantly, her greater worries were over middle daughter Ann, whom she described in feminine terms: "[Ann] more or less drew it inward . . . she was very quiet, what you would call the compliant child . . . she was so inward, she was like *invisible*!"

Kelly Carothers, a Euro-American working-class mother, had also experienced serious marital strain from a husband's denial of a daughter's issues and was in the midst of a divorce when I met her. Similarly, Kelly had struggled with schools on a daughter's behalf: "Academically everything fell into place," so her issues were seen as "nothing that constituted special ed," with "really nothing they could do." Kelly, however, reported years of her daughter Stacey's "horrible, horrible school" isolation, teasing, and harassment, with "major, major meltdowns at very unexpected times" outside of school. Kelly, a high-school graduate, had responded protectively by making herself a vigilant presence in Stacey's schools, over the years combining volunteer and paid aide and monitor positions. Members of her close extended family, however, were not very supportive: "They kind of laugh off my concerns. [They said] I was too sensitive to certain things . . . Still, all the while, I felt like the most important person that I should communicate with would have been my husband. But that *wasn't* happening. So that added a lot of stress to the situation, too."

Kelly's long vigilante efforts within the educational system's dense bureaucracy were made easier by her daily presence as employee and volunteer, and eventually resulted in important alliances with skilled, "compassionate" teachers and specialists. The latter, in turn, facilitated Kelly's efforts to gain a more accurate evaluation for Stacey. After the "horrible, horrible" years, a meaningful label brought a sense of *"great relief"* and much-needed visibility: "[Finally] . . . going into the sixth grade, we had the diagnosis that made a whole lot of sense [Asperger syndrome]. And I had things to share with the teachers, guidelines, and I think it helped. I think us just *being visible* . . . gave her and us more consideration."

The greater invisibility of vulnerable daughters created added challenges for their mothers in obtaining institutional and familial support, but a possible benefit to mothers of such daughters, in addition to lessened fear of punitive school sanctions, was suggested by those with whom I spoke. Compared to mothers of troubled sons, the mothers of focal girls reported receiving little direct, primary mother-blame. None reported blame for being too close, too attached, or for sexualizing their attachment, the accusations that could be so hurtful to mothers of troubled sons. Psychologists might add—again building from

Chodorow's psychoanalytic theory[52]—that this difference has little to do with disability. It might simply reflect that our culture never requires daughters to separate as fully, rigidly, and traumatically from mothers because of their shared gender.[53] But complaints, self-criticism, and proximate blame were frequently reported by mothers rearing vulnerable daughters—and this was not so different from accounts of mothers of disordered sons. Daughters and sons were also depicted with much individual specificity and variation; and while mothers often drew on gender-dichotomized terms to describe them, children and their experiences of course did not just fall neatly into overdrawn categories of gender difference.

Donna Simon, for example, had depicted her oldest, Lynn, in terms more similar to boys, as "acting out" rather than turning "inward." Not surprisingly, Donna also told of an ex-husband, Lynn's stepfather, who berated her lax disciplining of this behavior, a complaint much like the proximate blame received by many mothers of sons to be tougher, to "crack down." Donna remained keenly aware, however, that Lynn's gender trumped her behavior at school, as personnel continued to ignore her diagnosis. In contrast, Kelly Caruthers, whose husband remained "in *big* denial," berated herself for being too tough and misunderstanding her daughter's more inward, feminine-typed struggles. Kelly described that only in the past two years, since obtaining Stacey's diagnosis on the autism spectrum, had she accepted her daughter's differences and stopped attempting to change her "bad behavior": "I would do *a lot* of incentives and punishments and takeaways. And I can see major mistakes that I made early on. *Major* mistakes." Yet, if daughter Stacey's invisibility at school was gender-appropriate, Kelly, at some length and wholly unprompted, depicted the girl's lack of gender conformity from an early age as a part of her disorder:

> I took her out [of the dance class] and I remembered just feeling—I think I cried for about a week . . . I felt like a complete failure, that something was wrong with me, something was wrong with her. . . . She has a cousin the same age. They were just born a couple of months apart, lived in the same town, and we [Kelly and her sister] were kind of trying to keep abreast of all the same activities . . . And there was such a stark difference between the two girls! . . . We started giving her like a Little Tikes

[brand] kitchen and a table. . . . She didn't go near it. And I thought she'd have been thrilled. . . . She had baby dolls, but never played with them. A couple of Barbie dolls, never played with them!

In many ways Kelly's depiction of daughter Stacey, with "major meltdowns" at home, invisibility and intelligence at school, reminded me of affluent Judith Lowenthal's depiction of struggling son Allan. Kelly's and Judith's narratives underscore that across gender lines there can be many similarities in children's troubles. Both mothers also confronted extended diagnostic uncertainty, with daughter Stacey's issues tentatively thought of as ADHD or possibly bipolar before being reframed as Asperger's at age eleven; and Allan's diagnosis moving from separation anxiety to dyslexia, and next to dyslexia with bipolar disorder at age ten. Such "exceptionally long" struggles to find an accurate diagnosis, according to an Australian in-depth study of parents of children with high-functioning autism, had very negative consequences to mothers, particularly in exposing them (far more than fathers) to "charges of parental incompetence" from healthcare providers, spouses, and kin.[54] To the extent that my research suggests this is more likely to be the experience of those raising troubled daughters, it raises the level of challenge compared to raising disordered sons.

Mothers of sons and daughters, however, were more alike than different in their shared exasperation with contradictory criticism and advice. Rhonda Salter, mother of a struggling daughter Rachael, sounded remarkably similar to the mothers of more visibly troubled sons as she railed, only half sarcastically, "What did I do wrong? . . . Did I smoke too many cigarettes? Was I away too much [when employed]? Was I there too much [when unemployed]? Did I nag her enough? Did I *not* nag her enough? I mean, I have torn myself up, down, sideways, and slantways."

Another similarity in mothers' accounts across gender lines might lie in the extent to which verbal teasing and harassment of girls was similar to the physical (as well as verbal) threatening and bullying of boys. Three of the ten mothers mentioned that daughters had been victimized. Kelly Carothers, for example, had sadly noted at two different points in her narrative the teasing her daughter Stacey had endured at school—yet at the time I was preoccupied with Kelly's qualms about additional medications and failed to probe further into this victimization:

"When she was in third grade and all the trouble of the teasing and the reactions were going on, we got her seeing a licensed social worker, who put us in touch with one of their own psychiatrists, who wanted to prescribe a different kind of medications." At another point, Kelly went on to link this third-grade "teasing" to the more serious term "bullying": "I think part of the problem too was that no one [in the school] knew how to deal with it, the *bullying and the teasing* and the whole thing. A lot of crying went on at that time" (my emphasis).

In retrospect, I cannot know what the content of this *bullying and teasing* was that Kelly suggested pervaded daughter Stacey's most difficult school years. And without knowing if the bullying involved gay taunts or physical aggression, we cannot fully understand the sense in which Kelly drew the two terms, typically held apart by gender and degree of harm, as similar or synonymous. (Leiter similarly reported a gender divide, with the disabled young men in her study more likely bullied, and the young women, socially isolated.)[55] Happily for Kelly and daughter Stacey, at the time of our interview the "horrible, horrible" years seemed over. Kelly was some months into a better full-time classroom-aide position in a nearby town, comfortable that her daily vigilante presence in Stacey's school was no longer necessary.

Sadly, in the other two instances in which mothers mentioned the teasing of vulnerable daughters, the behavior had more serious, lasting consequences and was far more gendered, targeting girls in early adolescence in sexualized terms. Donna Simon only alluded to the sexualized nature of the incessant teasing of her middle, internalizing daughter, Ann, when emphasizing that it had jeopardized her "safety" at school and led to a "traumatic" end in a sexual assault. First, the "constant teasing" triggered or exacerbated serious depression on top of Ann's learning disorders:

> This was in a drama class, they were acting out. And these kids, oh God, I guess they harassed her daily, were constantly teasing her. You know? [Like] some of the shows you'd see on *Oprah* [laughs], if you know what I mean.[56] I mean these kids were *unmerciful*. So ah, they didn't feel that she needed to be hospitalized when I took her to [a consulting psychiatrist]. But they did set me up with a psychiatrist that she saw on a weekly basis. He also dealt with her ADD and put her on Ritalin[57] . . . Ah, and Prozac.

But mother and daughter soon learned that Prozac alone could not lift Ann's depression when kids continued "just taunting her unmercifully every day." At that point, Donna fought the school system for an out-of-district placement: "I told them because of the peers, and the way the things were, they couldn't provide her safety." But the school change intended to provide safety instead left Ann vulnerable to a sexual assault, tragically, by the driver of the "special needs van": "She was twelve when it happened . . . it was pretty, pretty traumatic." Five years later when I met Donna, the family had begun to emerge after much intensive psychiatric treatment, with Ann in a private therapeutic day school: "She's, she's maturing very well. She really is. She's doing so much better."

Another who emphasized that her daughter faced more difficult consequences from peer teasing was Vivian Kotler, who had been so articulate about her experiences as a single mother. Vivian reported that the "harass[ment]" of twelve-year-old Isabel by kids in the neighborhood continued although she had been in an out-of-district placement for nearly a year at the time of our meeting. Without prompting Vivian bared the ugly content, her speech becoming more broken as she became more upset.

> I mean even though she's been out of the public school system for a long time, she's been like harassed even today . . . We can be standing in front of the bus right here and people will call out her name, "Isabel," ten times . . . and so I made a game out of it. I said, "Let's count how many times they say your name." "Oh that's ten times, that's ten times you had ignored." You know, [I] tried to see the positive . . . And still when we come down, I can be with her even, when they're disrespecting her, even coming to our home. "Isabel['s] a whore," "whore!" and all this kind of stuff. And she's not *a whore* at all, you know. So just, just even she's been, like she hasn't seen anybody from any of the schools for almost a year now. And they're still, it's still backlashing on her. It's still bad.

Vivian did not explicitly link this "backlashing on" Isabel to her recent escalation of challenging, oppositional behavior; however, I knew that the past year had been particularly hard, with Isabel more aggressive and irritable at home. Indeed, Vivian reported that she was considering a "suggested" diagnosis of bipolar disorder and a turn to antidepressant medications.[58] Though the harassment may have been only a partial or contributing cause to Isabel's aggression at home, sociologists Nikki Jones and Laurie Schaffner have each shown that much of the aggression of at-risk girls may result from having endured persistent sexualized hectoring and harassment. The aggression can represent girls' attempts to regain control after victimization. Schaffner, in fact, has maintained that the nation's zero-tolerance policies aimed to prevent male school violence ought to be redirected against the sexual harassment of girls, with the latter posing the far larger, routine event making schools unsafe.[59]

The troubling accounts of Vivian Kotler and Donna Simon illustrate a conclusion shared by sociologists Jones and Schaffner and suggested by Pascoe: girls are most likely to be bullied, teased, and harassed in hyper-heterosexualized terms as "sluts" and "whores" rather than to be taunted as gay like boys. And though no young women are completely safe, this hyper-sexualized harassment may be amplified when girls lack class or race privilege.[60] White Euro-American Donna Simon was a home owner living with her daughters and a very cute puppy in a pleasant lower-middle-class suburb, but this had not protected middle daughter Ann from sexual assault. Vivian, also a white single mother, lived with daughter Isabel, in contrast, in a project in the midst of a diverse, rapidly gentrifying community. Vivian described Isabel's harassment as a reaction by peers to "her special needs and her issues." But this was likely intertwined with peers' awareness of Isabel as biracial and a public housing resident, with "whore" a condemnation, a "disrespecting" that may go beyond "sped." Vivian, who was prone to statements of color-blindness whenever I came close to asking about Isabel's racial identity, did admit that Isabel might face "disrespect" from both white peers and peers of colors: "I think the people that are Haitian, Black American, any of that, they, they make fun of her *more.*"

Conclusion: Policing the Gender Binary

In the next chapter, I return to the mothers like Vivian raising sons and daughters of color and of mixed race. But before turning to this longer discussion of how race may intersect with gender (and social class) to change the meaning and experience of children's invisible disorders and of the accompanying challenges for mothers, what can I suggest from the above accounts about the gendered dimensions on their own? It does seem as if vulnerabilities to peers differ, or at least that mothers perceive differences that are aligned with findings from other research. Their narratives suggest that the bullying and teasing pervading schools, and disproportionately targeting those with vulnerabilities, may target the smaller numbers of disordered girls differently from the ways similarly vulnerable boys or young men are targeted. The content of the harassment tends to be overly heterosexualized in the case of girls and tends toward gay-baiting or gender policing in the case of boys. In a sense this poses a reversal, with too much womanliness in troubled girls, yet too little manliness in disordered boys—though no doubt, either way, this causes kids and their families distress and emotional pain.[61]

Similar cultural logics in how we all understand gender shape the perceptions of adults as well as peers, creating different challenges for mothers of sons and daughters, who themselves live with and draw from these same normative gender relations. Mothers recounted a range of strategies to invest troubled boys with greater masculine body capital and the physical self-assurance to confront peer taunting. And this could be a challenging responsibility taken on in vigilante fashion when fathers largely withdrew. Other research suggests that such building up of masculine embodiment is typically a father's contribution, but with vulnerable boys the inability to conform more closely to normative expectations may signal a more feminized child still needing maternal protection. Mothers similarly drew from normative gendered understandings to describe troubled daughters, their passivity and internalizing of distress. My findings suggest that whichever side of the binary mothers drew from to describe their troubled daughters—even if daughters were, like Donna Simon's eldest, Lynn, closer to masculine externalizing of their issues—they still encountered greater layers of invisibility and denial in gaining recognition and appropriate services for troubled girls. And overextended schools may have little choice, as Rhonda Salter came close to acknowledging, but to prioritize containing disruptive kids rather than attending to the individual needs of nondisruptive girls or boys.

Mothers of both sons and of daughters reported similar distress on one score: the victimization of their kids, seemingly happening under the radar of school personnel, other parents, neighbors, and responsible adults. In contrast, when troubled kids lashed out to compensate for or retaliate against such victimization, this was, according to mothers, what came through "on the radar" and received institutional attention. Yet, despite these important similarities, embodied brain disorder remains an overwhelmingly masculine category capturing disproportionately larger numbers of boys along with the mothers who rear them. Underlying this anxious response, however, seemed to be particular fears and (rather contradictory) beliefs attached disproportionately to boys, to their strength, physicality, and aggression. Such cultural logics led mothers to worry over the criticism surrounding them of being too soft, too lax, too coddling, too attached with sons who might switch violently, unpredictably, from far-too-little to far-too-much masculinity. While these concerns in some ways echo the criticisms of children's medicalization by conservatives anxious about a future with less solid manly authority, biomedicine may be just as preoccupied with masculinity, or at least its hormonal components, as a possible major cause of burgeoning brain problems. In its most extreme and now discredited form this led to the unfortunate (and expensive) use of Lupron, a chemically castrating drug shutting down the production of testosterone, to purportedly cure boys and young men with autism.[62] But research continues to explore "the extreme male brain hypothesis" linking higher rates of fetal exposure to testosterone to the disproportionate numbers of boys diagnosed with invisible disabilities—and perhaps some such research is credible.[63]

Surely the whole story of invisible disabilities is multiple and interactive, including layers of "nature," neurochemistry, hormones, and inherited genetic tendencies, with layers of "nurture," complex family dynamics, and social environments. Yet invisible disabilities also represent and reinforce gendered norms for mothers and for their sons and daughters. With the overwhelming preponderance of sons diagnosed, these disorders are surely enmeshed with heightened fears of failed masculinity. For mothers of the smaller number of similarly struggling girls, the challenges differ, as "neurodiverse" girls tend to be erased from the picture or, as cultural studies scholars conclude, they are rendered "culturally unintelligible" when we are so preoccupied with maintaining the gender binary of strict masculine and feminine difference.[64] Perhaps in this sense, we fear even greater competition for the limited opportunities facing the next generation of productive citizens entering the

New Economy, and we may wonder who will be future family providers with such imperiled paths to meaningful, sustaining adult work. But as researcher Ilina Singh concluded in an in-depth analysis of mothers raising boys with ADHD, "Mothers' struggles to satisfy cultural ideals of successful boys are supported and complicated by their struggles to satisfy cultural ideals of good mothers."[65]

Next I continue to explore the ways gender and the disproportionate number of boys and young men diagnosed with invisible disorders intersect with racial and class divides to shape and reshape the gendered meanings by which we think about such burdensome or precarious children. I will suggest that women raising children of color may draw selectively on medicalization with even greater ambivalence than those raising white children, to protect their vulnerable children from a persisting legacy of negative racialized sorting within the educational system. While the medical system and the discourse of neuroscience may hold authority over labeling, categorizing, and treating their children's troubles, schools remain the site organizing daily life, engaging mothers' work, and shaping children's futures.[66]

6

"A Strange Coincidence"

Race-ing Disordered Children

I felt, "OK, you can't deal with the Black *male'* . . . You can't deal with the Black male, give him a nice little tranquilizer. . . . That's a way of saying, "You shut up, sit over there, take your medication." . . . It's hard to put it exactly into words because you don't want to make it look like this big huge racial-type thing. But my children definitely felt the difference; they definitely felt the tension. . . . It's always most of the Black kids are special ed. It never fails . . . It's such a strange coincidence.
—"Rosa Branca," interview, June 2004

Historically shaped binaries, often drawn on ethnoracial lines, have long measured mothers in the United States, dividing the respectable from the disreputable, the fit from the unfit, the selflessly devoted from those ostensibly too lazy, neglectful, or immoral to raise healthy children.[1] And the children of the disreputable, likely to inherit their mothers' degeneracy whether through "nature" or "nurture," were suspect as potentially polluting and costly to the nation.[2] A century ago, eugenics movements provided the first "scientific" legitimation for such racist beliefs through the fixation on ostensibly biological, evolutionary hierarchies among ethnic, racial, and religious groups, with those least "fit" supposedly behind urban unrest, adult criminality, and juvenile delinquency. Educators, in response, adopted the first large-scale testing and sorting of children in schools, capturing many young children of color, especially boys, within categories of heritable brain deficiency or degeneracy.[3]

Current national research finds that this link between race and perceptions of organic deficiency persists. Children of color, particularly boys, continue to be overrepresented among those labeled with the "high incidence" educational categories of emotional and behavioral disorder and assigned to special ed—and this overrepresentation by race occurs across levels of social class, with little progress despite monitoring by the civil rights community.[4] In addition, the mid-twentieth-century categories of "minimal" or "educable" mental retardation still include disproportionate numbers of children of color.[5] Such children of color, particularly the boys and young men, are then overrepresented among those suspended and expelled, with this pipeline leading to higher rates of school failure, dropout, unemployment, and involvement in the criminal justice system.[6] Indeed, when federal disability legislation was being drafted in 1990 determining eligibility for special ed, the National Association for the Advancement of Colored People (NAACP) fought vigorously *against* including ADHD, fearing the label might be "applied excessively to African-American children," "especially black males," and exacerbate these disparities.[7]

Paradoxically, if medicalization were to recast their deviance or deficiency as treatable illness—as it generally does for white Euro-American boys—parents of children of color might more readily embrace it to foreclose the serious risks of entering this pipeline. Yet, contrary to the NAACP's concerns, children of color are significantly *less* likely to be given the most prevalent biomedical diagnosis, ADHD, and are significantly *less* likely to be treated with the psychoactive medications whose use is soaring among white children.[8] The reasons for this puzzling and perhaps lamentable "undertreatment" are unclear and have received relatively little attention. Epidemiologists suspect that "cultural differences" and lack of access to mental healthcare play the largest part.[9] Undoubtedly these factors, particularly the latter, do contribute;[10] but the situation is also more complex. It involves both the educational and medical systems, institutions in which race continues to shape everyday interactions and major life chances, independently of as well as in concert with class location.[11] While professional researchers tend to study the two systems separately, each with distinct categories and labels, mothers with vulnerable children have no choice but to engage with both.

Moreover, the statistical relationships in medicalization patterns are themselves complex and sometimes appear contradictory. Epidemiologists report, for example, that poverty and Medicaid use increase children's likelihood of treatment with second-line antipsychotic medications. But the prevalence of such medications is still low, and even among this small proportion of children, white kids are *more* likely to be medicated.[12] Social scientists and feminist scholars studying children's medicalization have been largely silent on such racial patterns, perhaps because they are so puzzling, even as they have analyzed the stigma attached to children, their families, and their mothers.[13]

In this chapter, I make a modest start at addressing this silence by hearing from the sixteen mothers raising children of color and wrestling with labels, school services, medications, and stigma. These mothers articulated an ambivalence toward medicalization that was more complex, more initially distrustful than mothers raising white children, freighted with the awareness that race continues to influence everyday interactions and major life chances. They had to balance the hope that medication might lessen their children's risk of school failure with the danger of reinforcing entrenched and resilient images of "badness." What seem to be "cultural differences," then, may in fact refer to rational responses to life in a still racialized society more than to beliefs and values inherently outside the American mainstream.

These sixteen mothers raising children of color described four focal daughters and sixteen focal sons labeled invisibly disabled, with another twelve sons and daughters considered typically developing (see table 6.1 detailing these families). Ten of these mothers seriously questioned whether race alone and particularly being Black—a term many supplied— had negatively affected their child's categorization or access to school services. The others worried about pervasive inequality in the U.S. healthcare system, questioning if it was due to economic disadvantage or to racial discrimination. This included Lucy Nguyen, whose biracial son was fair skinned but had been taunted as a "chink." Patricia Gwarten, who had worried about bullying, also recounted her earliest questions about services for preschoolers offered through schools but requiring medical diagnoses:

> I would say that, with the first doctor, a lot of his patients were African American, or Hispanic, or low-income Caucasians. Not only was my doctor telling me about my son, "Oh, he's developing OK," [but] I found out [from] other parents that [this] doctor said the same thing about their [similar] children. And my mom said that the clinic is now under investigation! And I don't want to say it was because I was Black. But I

TABLE 6.1. Mothers Raising Children of Color: By Income (Most to Least), Included in Chapter 6

Income	Interviewee	Marital Status	Focal Child
High	Virginia Caldwell-Starret	Married	Henry
	Gabriella Ramos-Garza	Married	Diego
Middle	Cara Withers	Divorced	Michael
	Dory Buchanan*	Never married	Khari
	Hermalina Riega	Married	Mateo
	May Royce	Divorced	Robert
	Lucy Nguyen*	Married	Ken
	Marika Booth	Never married	Geneva
Low	Rosa Branca	Married	Frank, stepson Justin
	Mildred Andujar	Divorced	Gil
	Lucia Santos	Married	Carlos (Eduardo, Grace**)
	Patricia Gwarten	Divorced	Jacob
	Vivian Kotler*	Never married	Isabel
	Caron Ross	Divorced	Rashaun
	Leesha Baker	Never married	Dion
	Joann MoGinnis*	Never married	Thomas

Note: * = white women raising children of color; ** = mistakenly categorized as special ed.

think when you're low-income, people say, "Oh, low-income get the same health services as higher income." But I don't see that.

Sadly, research points to a double disadvantage, but one in which being Black regardless of income level shapes nearly all routine medical interactions.[14]

I will focus on the stories of five mothers, with glimpses of the others in supporting roles. I begin with Rosa Branca's narrative, treating it in the greatest depth. With sons nearly grown, Rosa offered her own greater sense of outcomes than those with younger sons whose stories were still in progress. But with younger sons, I profile Cara Withers, Dory Buchanan, Mildred Andujar, and Virginia Caldwell-Starret, each with her own wonderful perspectives to offer. These five women capture the range of household arrangements, and cultural and economic resources, among those who shared the rearing of vulnerable children lacking race privilege.

Rosa Branca, Mother of Frank, Stepmother of Justin

Rosa Branca supplied a particularly vivid, instructive account of serious questioning about the difference race might have made for nearly grown son Frank and stepson Justin. Rosa was a full-time homemaker who described herself as "Black Honduran"; she lived with her large, blended family in an appealing townhouse within a largely white suburb. In the household were her second husband, stably employed in appliance repairs, and their six kids—two from Rosa's previous marriage, two from her husband's first marriage, and the youngest from their remarriage. Rosa explained that worries about special needs first arose with Frank, the oldest child from her first marriage. It was initially very confusing, she offered, when the suburban, white school system suggested the ADD label for Frank, at the time in sixth grade. The family had only recently moved from an urban, diverse district, in large part for the quality of the suburban schools. Wholly unprompted, Rosa emphasized how jarring the move had been because of the family's race: "I'm from Central America, but African American [in the suburb] was like a bigger adjustment." Before I had the chance to ask how or why a "Black Honduran" or "Central America[n]" identity became "African American" in the suburbs, Rosa's next observations indirectly explained: "The schools in this town were only about 1 percent Black," or "maybe," she corrected, "5 [percent] *at the most.*" In contrast, in their urban school, "We weren't minorities because most of the people where we lived were Black." Indeed, according to state figures, their urban district was 75 percent Black and Hispanic, their suburb just 4.8 percent Black and another 6 to 7 percent Hispanic.

Over several visits, Rosa explained a sequence of negotiations with the school over Frank's ADD categorization. Initially, when his middle-school teachers encouraged Rosa to seek an evaluation, she struggled with contradictory reactions, both acquiescent and resistive to the medicalization of Frank's "behavioral problems," his "disturbing the class," "not following directions," and being "very, very social." While most of the women raising white children who shared their stories with me described initial trust in school personnel—even if later that trust was broken—Rosa was skeptical. Yet she also described herself as a mother "in denial" who required long months to admit that her son had an innate neurological problem. Rosa recounted how she first began to accede to the suburban school's interpretation:

> The kids in [the city], to us it was normal to see a kid run around, jump, hop, or be happy. . . . Basically the kids in [the urban school], a lot of them were rowdy, loud, you know? It looks normal to just see that type of behavior. But coming here and noticing the difference, with children a little, maybe you can say quieter or calmer—you know, it started really shouting out there to see the difference with Frank.

Rosa described initially questioning whether his physicality—being "rowdy, loud"—was disability or just "showing off," as she compared Frank to her other kids. Frank was always taking apart the vacuum cleaner and the radio for the challenge of putting them back together, but he was never one who "tried to climb the wall or knock pictures down" and rarely a child who "needed discipline." Yet, as sociologist Ann Arnett Ferguson discovered, school personnel often "decipher" the meaning of children's physicality, their bodily "demeanor, posture, proper gesture," through racialized norms, expecting Black children to enact deference through quiet, stilled bodies.[15] I was struck when Rosa again moved race to central focus when I merely asked if she agreed with suggestions for a medical evaluation. "I was in denial for awhile. I *was* in denial. *Why?* The reason I was in denial is because I knew another parent [a neighbor] who, they [the schools] had the same thing to say about her son. And he was also African American. So she was refusing his medication because she felt like they were just, maybe, in a way, outcasting the few Black children that were there. Like, 'Oh, they're ADD!'"

Notably, Rosa describes her neighbor's son as "*also* African American," again, as in discussing their move to the suburbs, collapsing her family's distinct ethnoracial identity into the hegemonic U.S. Black-white dichotomy.[16] In fact, late in our interview Rosa described a quite specific background with evident pride: "OK, I come from Honduras . . . [but] my mother was this very, very strong-willed Jamaican . . . and my father was from Honduras. [My first husband] was from Honduras, and his family on his mother's side were the indigenous Indians from Salvador. And then her father's side was from Jamaica, so he was part Jamaican."

Next I asked, "So what would you put for your kids on their [school] forms?" and Rosa acknowledged:

> It's weird because I always wrote "Black." And [sometimes] the schools would be like, "No, you can't write Black because it falls under Hispanic." But then I [said], "You know, it doesn't really matter to me, but the color of our skin is considered Black." So I always just write "Black."

Two other women of color, each originally from Jamaica, suggested in contrast that they disliked having their families considered just Black; but all three revealed insightful knowledge of the still dichotomized basis of U.S. racial boundary-making. In this sense, Rosa's seemingly odd statement suggesting that immigrating to the urban United States as a "Central American" was easier than becoming "African American" in the suburb, explained her fearful reaction to a neighbor's assertion that the school was "outcasting" both of their "African American" boys by labeling them with ADD. Even if today the attentional disorders remain disproportionately white,[17] Rosa still had reason to be concerned, as civil rights advocates have long been, with the tendency for special-ed assignment to relegate children of color to lowered expectations and subpar services.[18]

Rosa said (again indicating the specificity of her identity) that her Honduran kin network believed in strict discipline and had no familiarity with notions of invisible disability or ADD: "No one even knew what that [ADD] was." She decided that if this was a brain illness, it made sense to at least consult the family's pediatrician—a reaction at once typical of mainstream American beliefs and indicating that "cultural differences" are not static. The kids' primary-care provider for several years, however, insisted that Frank did not exhibit the disorder's traits. Without blood tests or other biological markers, ADD and ADHD are ambiguous, though healthcare providers would more often look to teachers' assessments rather than exclude them.[19] Rosa mimicked watching a tennis game, swinging her gaze back and forth to illustrate her experience of being caught between opposed sources of professional authority: "Doctor—teacher. Doctor—teacher. Doctor—teacher."

Rosa then redeployed the phrase "I was in denial" to signal that her initial resistance had been misguided: "I was in denial for a very long time." Frank's ADD, she explained, had been "really, really hidden"; with "attention deficit disorder, *not* hyperactive disorder, his was the sneakier type of ADD. . . . They [the personnel at the suburban school] kind of opened my eyes to this ADD thing." Strikingly, in these comments Rosa implied eventually moving to full agreement with the school: they "opened [her] eyes" to a neurochemical problem. Immediately after this acquiescent account, however, Rosa suggested that relenting had been her only option. Had she continued to reject putting Frank on stimulants, she explained, she would have risked his education—the outcome befalling her African American neighbor's son: "The boy ended up getting thrown out of the high school because she [his mother] just didn't follow [the school's recommendations]." "At first, yes, I disagreed, [but] I just basically aim for my children getting a high-school diploma. It was like, 'OK, *whatever* we have to do, we have to do.'" "I just gave in. I threw the towel in and said, 'Well, maybe he is ADD.' And they gave him Ritalin."

The phrase "threw the towel in" stands against the phrase "opened my eyes," sounding as if Rosa had never truly accepted that Frank's behavior reflected an invisible disability. To throw in the towel instead connotes surrender, forfeiting the game, quitting the contest over the ADD label. A moment later, she reiterated this point: "Either way [whether she resisted or not], they ended up winning because he still got put on medication." This statement, in the context of her other remarks and the cautionary tale of the neighbor's son, indicates that Rosa experienced the choice to medicate Frank largely in racial terms.

Though mothers of white children hardly confront such school recommendations easily, they at least confront them without institutional "rules of the game" already, according to sociologists Annette Lareau and Erin Horvat, "built on race-specific interactions" and "socioemotional style[s]."[20] Schools, Lareau and Horvat found in a broader study of parent involvement, expect parents to be "positive and supportive" with initial trust and calm, uncritical responses to professional assessments; and yet, "many Black parents, given the historical legacy of racial discrimination," find it difficult to comply regardless of class resources or even shared cultural capital.[21] Although I have argued that raising a costly, invisibly disabled child places mothers at a disadvantage within institutions that largely fail them, raising a child of color contributes another distinct layer of difficulty; this interacts with the other resources, cultural and economic, which mothers marshal for the task. Indeed, as

Lareau and Horvat wrote of parents' school negotiations, in many contexts, "being white becomes a type of cultural capital."[22]

When Rosa Branca and I met a week later, I jumped back in, referring again to her striking cautionary tale about race: "Did you end up feeling that you kind of agreed with her [the neighbor]? Do you think they target African American kids?" She responded thoughtfully:

> I don't want to sound as strong as to say, "Yes, they are *targeting* African Americans." But I really don't feel they get an equal chance at all. . . . It's already a thing, like, "OK, they're Black—boom!" You know, it's already that thing. It's hard to put it exactly into words because you don't want to make it look like this big huge racial-type thing. But my children definitely felt the difference; they definitely felt the tension. . . . It's always most of the Black kids are special ed. It never fails . . . It's such a strange coincidence. Like most of the Black kids I know . . . either it's a behavioral problem or there is ADD. So there is special ed. . . . OK, wait a minute. Is it that they can't deal with children of color?

Research on schools confirms the "strange coincidence" Rosa noted. The greatest overrepresentation of nonwhite kids in special education actually does occur in whiter, more affluent districts like the Brancas'.[23] In contrast to her neighbor's blunt accusation of intentional "outcasting," Rosa's perceptions of school staff are similar to sociological notions of the "racism without racists" predominant in the post–Civil Rights era.[24] Her well-chosen words, "[not] a big huge racial-type thing, but . . . ," similarly exemplify Lareau and Horvat's focus on the interaction styles and institutional "rules of the game" which unwittingly normalize white privilege, particularly when over "ninety percent of teachers of grades K–12 are of white, European descent."[25] Put differently, "race and culture [are] inextricably woven into the fabric of the school contexts" such that well-intentioned, even selflessly committed personnel are "cultural hegemonists" rather than explicitly prejudiced.[26]

Rosa offered further evidence of such cultural hegemony through the experience of her stepson Justin, in the ninth grade when Rosa and his father were married:

Once I married my husband, you know, we got [custody of] the [his] two kids . . . Justin [his oldest] was not considered special-ed. Everything was fine [in his K–8 school]. And as time went by, you know, meetings and meetings. Then it was the special-ed thing. . . . He got to [the suburban high school], the first two years I guess he slid by. And then the last two years of high school it was like, "No, he's special-ed."

Despite the seeming antagonism to suburban school personnel and other professionals in these stories, Rosa, like several others raising children of color, expressed sympathy for teachers and healthcare providers. Perhaps sociologist Claudia Malacrida would find this surprising; she indicated, in a study of Canadian and British mothers of children with ADHD, that mothers regardless of race and class location were primarily antagonistic toward "normalizing" professionals pushing medicalization.[27] However, Rosa's account suggested she had been confounded instead by differences among professional authorities and thought about these carefully: "I understand the struggle that teachers may go through, you know, through the day. So . . . I was never against the school per se. . . . I, at first, yes, disagreed [with the ADD diagnosis]. I said, 'OK, I want to check into this' . . . I asked the doctor . . . [But] of course, the doctor only gets to see him fifteen to twenty minutes, versus the schools have the child for six hours."

Moreover, Rosa's ambivalence toward school authorities may be better understood by the race differences that divide her from the majority of mothers I spoke with—as from the majority in Malacrida's research, also a predominantly white group. To protect her child from greater harms, Rosa, like many U.S. mothers raising children of color, ultimately had to do whatever was required for him to remain in school: "I finally threw in the towel. You know, if it took that [ADD diagnosis and medications] for them to keep him in school . . . then I said, 'Fine.' . . . Did I agree 100 percent with everything they said? Under *no* condition, I *never did*." Thus she concluded her narrative by describing a reluctant and somewhat temporary acquiescence, almost boasting that after four years (at age sixteen) Frank had taken himself off Ritalin. While he had graduated high school and had just begun attending a community college at the time we met, Rosa sadly recalled how much the two had fought over his medications—and how ironic it was that she had enforced a practice she so seriously questioned.

Other parents with sons of color, along with educators of color, face similar dilemmas over schools' behavioral standards. Researchers contend that many capitulate to unfair, overly harsh and punishing standards in order to inculcate necessary adult survival skills.[28] Relenting to medication, as Rosa suggested, might now represent a part of this unfair necessity—Frank, after all, had graduated and represented a school success. Among the sixteen mothers rearing children of color, a majority had relented to medications at some point, with mothers recounting that ten of the sixteen focal sons of color, including Frank and his stepbrother, and three of the four focal daughters of color, were medicated for some school years.

Cara Withers, Mother of Michael

Divorced Afro-Caribbean mother Cara Withers made race less explicit than Rosa Branca and was more outspoken about her efforts to inculcate a sense of masculine embodiment in struggling, "extremely sensitive" young son Michael. Cara shared Rosa's working-class origins; but unlike Rosa, Cara was upwardly mobile, a college-educated businesswoman and successful breadwinner, whose own mother lived in the household sharing childcare and providing much-needed domestic labor. Cara accepted a neuroscientific diagnosis for her son more readily than Rosa had, perhaps because Michael's vulnerabilities, diagnosed as learning and emotional disorders, seemed genuinely more pronounced than those of Rosa's son Frank. Yet Cara shared a very similar resistance to medication: "I'm still a parent struggling with the medication portion of it. I just don't like the idea of it. . . . I would *not* administer it. I would only allow it to be administered at the school . . . I was omitting the dosage at home . . . so I would only allow the medication to be administered then [at school], just at the lowest dosage."

Cara had reluctantly agreed to this "lowest dosage" of a stimulant to treat Michael's learning disorder only when Michael became very distressed at being held back in school—but she had rejected additional mood-stabilizing medication for his emotional disorder.[29] She also shared this cautionary tale of two nephews: Both of these "good kids" were given medication to improve school behavior. But when coming off doses led to the common "crashing" and "violent, extreme hot temper[s]," their mother appealed to the prescribing physician. The boys' doctor just "kept increasing the dosage," finally "sedating [them into] a zombie state." Cara thus emphasized her partial resistance in insisting that her son Michael's dosage remain low. And, like Rosa, she depicted her acquiescence to such medicalization as only partial: "I'm only willing to let him take the meds for academic reasons. . . . I'm just saying, 'Oh OK, fine. If that's what it takes for him to function in this environment . . . I'm giving you permission.' I'm giving permission for someone else to administer, to take that responsibility. I don't want it."

Although Cara made race less central to her narrative than Rosa had, she was, at the same time, more critical of the contemporary educational "environment" within which the kids had to "function." Cara explained the burgeoning medicalization of childhood through a sociological lens, pointing to several major facets of social change, but also expressing sympathy for teachers:

I know a lot of ADD adults [laughing] . . . but there was no meds behind it [back then]. Parents and friends and neighbors probably said, "Oh my God, you were the worst child of the block!" . . . I just find in today's world it's so easy to sedate a child just so the teachers can get their job done. . . . The demands on them [teachers], I have to admit . . . they're expected to do a lot more with a lot less!

In other remarks, while emphasizing her similarity to any parent facing this dilemma, Cara briefly pointed to a possible ethnoracial difference:

It's hard for *any* parent to see that we have to give our child drugs just to have them function . . . but unfortunately, when we have to take our child to a [stressful] learning environment so they can eventually be productive citizens in society, I'm sorry, [but] now society has it where, yeah, in order for these kids to function, we will have to medicate them. We are, a lot of us, initially, when you try to introduce medication to modify behavior to *any* minority, we're very apprehensive. . . . We were taught . . . that it takes an entire neighborhood to raise a child. And we don't do that anymore. . . . You are kind of compelled to go with what's there so your kids can somehow fit into that environment.

Within this explanation, Cara underscored awareness of the account-ability pressures schools confront as they attempt to turn out "pro-ductive citizens." Her complex ambivalence or even antipathy toward medication, evident in terms like "it's so easy to sedate" or her nephews' "zombie state," was here suggested by the phrase "to modify behavior" with its hint of Pavlovian conditioning, dog training, and blind ma-nipulation.[30] Such ominous words stand in marked contrast to the flat, technical terms usually employed by proponents of medicating kids.[31] But several white Euro-American mothers had made similarly ominous allusions to "zombies" and the like—for example, Judith Lowenthal, who had referred to the child psychiatrist encouraging drug combina-tions as "the Witch Doctor." Cara's emphatic mention of an extra layer of "apprehensi[on]," however, for "*any* minority" is distinct, alluding to the long American legacy of (quite intentional) racism and perhaps specifi-cally to the medical exploitation and experimentation it justified.[32] The remark that follows, "It takes an entire neighborhood to raise a child," evokes shared community parenting norms which stand in contrast to the neoliberal motherhood and vigilante heroics examined in this book. But the remark possibly contains another glancing reference to ethnora-cial difference, especially since it is preceded by the phrase "we were taught." "We" might refer to the earlier "*any* parent," rather than to those raising children of color, and, in this sense, it might point simply to gen-erational change. Black feminist scholars, however, argue that women's kin networks have specific historical roots in communities of color,[33] and the proverb "It takes a village" popularized by Hillary Rodham Clin-ton has been widely touted as being of African origin.[34] Perhaps Cara referred to these layered meanings, as she linked her apprehensions both to the words "*any* parent" and to "*any* minority"; yet it seems likely her worries were more particular, given her attunement to social factors, fearing what it would take for Michael, a young Black male labeled with a disorder, to "eventually" be among the "productive citizens in society."

Mildred Andujar, Mother of Gil, with Lucia Santos, Mother of Carlos, and Hermalina Riega, Mother of Mateo

Mildred Andujar, a divorced Dominican mother of two, illus-trated another variation on the theme of complex ambivalence to medicalization.[35] One of the mothers most distrustful of school authorities—more so than either Rosa Branca or Cara Withers—Mildred was among those who most strongly resisted medicating a young son. She described school pressure to do so beginning when Gil was just six years old. Mildred recounted finally relenting when he was seven, but only to a brief trial that she ended after four months. She concluded, after discussions with their family provider, that each of the three stimulants tried brought on too much of the "crashing" to which Cara had referred, the excessive irritability as each dose wears off.

Although Mildred evidently trusted her family's primary-care physician in a local clinic, she was more antagonistic toward school staff. School personnel, in Mildred's account, had become increasingly hostile since she had rejected medication, even referring to her as "crazy." More upsetting was the manner in which they targeted Gil, suspending him from school on two occasions for minor offenses, with Mildred alleging one teacher had also been physically abusive. Mildred had not relented but had joined a local Latino community organization for assistance in filing complaints against the school.[36] Though I cannot judge the veracity of her account, Mildred was palpably shaken recalling these events. As well, her narrative exemplifies larger, troubling patterns: according to government data, students of color are far more likely to be suspended for minor, nonviolent misconduct, with disability labels seeming to offer less protection than families might expect. Moreover, Black and Hispanic students with disabilities are more likely to be physically restrained in school—and such racialized patterns seem to have been only amplified or exacerbated by the post-Columbine, zero-tolerance climate (though in actuality, nearly all the school shooters have been young white men).[37]

Mildred's narrative also suggests that language difference and anti-immigrant sentiment may contribute to such racially disparate patterns. According to Mildred, the family was "looked down upon" because they were "Black Latino immigrants" with Spanish their primary language. Another Black Latina immigrant, Lucia Santos, a married Puerto Rican mother active in the community organization with Mildred, similarly complained that one of her sons, Eduardo, had been mistakenly labeled learning disabled, an error taking several years to rectify: "It's the same discrimination from the barrier about the language. A barrier . . . because we had accent[s]!" Researchers in California, a state with a large immigrant population, have argued that stories like Mildred and Lucia's deserve more attention: "Although considerable efforts have been devoted to understanding African American placement in high-incidence disabilities, we know significantly less about ELL [English-language learners'] representation in these [special-ed] programs."[38] Their study of urban California school districts found that Latinos without English proficiency were significantly overrepresented from fifth grade on.[39]

The NAACP has repeatedly spoken out against racial disparities in relegation to special ed (as in their 1990 opposition to including ADHD in federal disability legislation), though without reference to language or immigration issues. My analysis of the NAACP newspaper *The Crisis* confirmed this pattern, revealing that between 1998 and 2008, some twenty-six articles called for action on racial disparities in school disciplining and special-ed assignment without mention of non-English speakers. The NAACP, however, supported legislation that might have assisted Mildred, aiming to prohibit schools from insisting that a child take psychiatric medication (a stance that found the civil rights group oddly allied with conservatives). Such measures were eventually enacted by some U.S. states but were rejected on the federal level for fear of inhibiting open communication between schools and families.[40]

To be fair, although several mothers spoke, like Mildred, of feeling pressured by schools to medicate their children, none recounted receiving any ultimatum. In my fieldwork at special-ed parent advisory council meetings, I did observe two mothers who seemed to be at the meeting in a diverse urban district together, each angrily claiming that school officials had threatened to file for protective service intervention if they did not medicate their (respective) sons.[41] Each appeared to be white Euro-American, but because I did not interview them, I cannot be sure, nor can I know if either boy was bi- or multiracial. This was, however, the only such incident I observed in the dozen parent special-ed meetings I attended. At all others, parents (overwhelmingly mothers) praised at least some school personnel, and such selective praise was offered by many of those I interviewed as well. Among the sixteen mothers raising children of color, Lucia Santos and Hermalina Riega found allies in their children's teachers, who helped them resist overmedicating young sons.

Hermalina Riega, however, also revealed anger at the local schools, sounding more like Mildred. Hermalina thoughtfully detailed the complexities of her husband and three children's ethnoracial identification after speaking of the humiliation of her own treatment upon immigrating in high school: "[My daughter] she just says, 'I'm American.' 'Cause she was born here. Yeah, so she identifies more with that. But I tell her all the time, I said, 'No, you're not. You're *not.*' I say, 'You are a Black woman, Latino woman, Jamaican, Costa Rican, Honduran-Black woman.'" As I followed up, "Do you ever feel that being a Black Latino woman, and your kids being Latino, has [still] affected . . . ?" Hermalina interrupted energetically, "Of course they're stigmatized!" She continued, "I think if, for instance, me waiting since October to June for a core evaluation [to evaluate son Mateo's need for special ed]—and they're giving me all these excuses. I'm sure if Mateo was a different race he would have been seen right away." Hermalina, who had consulted attorneys through a local office of the NAACP before finally obtaining her son's evaluation, concluded that "the public system doesn't work, at least for me. It doesn't work for my children."

Two additional points stand out from the narratives offered by Mildred, Lucia, and Hermalina of rearing young sons of color: first, unlike Rosa Branca or Cara Withers, none of the three was strictly opposed to psychiatric medications. Lucia felt that both she and an adolescent daughter had benefited from treatment with an antidepressant, a treatment Mildred was considering for herself after receiving a recent diagnosis for depression; and Hermalina continued to administer an antiseizure medication in low dosages to her son Mateo. But second, Mildred, Lucia, and Hermalina may offer a glimpse of what a "village" might resemble among mothers, evoking something of the neighborhood support that Cara Withers recalled from her youth. Beyond the neoliberal version of social support which had to be individually hunted down, patched together, and paid for, the three explained that through the Latino community organization they supported one another. Along with several others whom I was unable to meet, they coached one another for the team meetings surrounding a child's individualized education plan, helped one another with letters of response, and tried to attend together as well. In contrast to the special-ed parents advisory councils which I had observed, these mothers identified more oppositionally as ethnoracial, immigrant outsiders linked in a network of reciprocity, as Mildred explained: "It's very hard fighting the system by yourself. They say a lot of bad things, and the language, they have problems with it . . . they blame the parent. And you have no witness to prove that they say that. In the school, [it's] better [if] the parents [are] more together. It's better like that than [if] we go alone to the school." Lucia's involvement had begun similarly, when she was encouraged by a teacher to learn her rights: "One of the teachers call me ... she call me [to] say, 'I want to tell this to you. I'm very angry because of the way they treat you ... You've got rights!'"

Yet each of the three mothers and the organization itself seemed stretched thin by larger New Economy–neoliberal conditions. Lucia's involvement and volunteer hours depended on receiving a small stipend from uncertain public funds, while the stipend and a husband's earnings still left the family in poverty. Mildred, also living in poverty, worked the night shift cleaning offices, and as a single parent had little extra time or energy. Hermalina, in contrast, enjoyed a healthy household income, with a full-time and a part-time job as a health aide–dietician; but two jobs, three kids, and a husband in trucking often on the road limited her involvement: "We're [each] into our own problems, you know? So there's not like social kind of thing ... I do what I can." Mildred had separately conveyed similar thoughts: "The support that I get from the mothers sometimes is very important, but you don't want to tire them with your problems too. You know, like everyone has their own problems."

Dory Buchanan, Mother of Khari

Dory Buchanan offered another slant on complex ambivalence as the white adoptive mother of a young boy of color and a teacher in a relatively under-resourced high school. Dory, a single mother, had an older (biological) daughter who was white and a younger adopted African American son, Khari. Khari was in a prekindergarten program when we met and had already been diagnosed with multiple issues: developmental delays as well as sensory integration, behavioral, and attentional issues. Dory, who had adopted Khari at a year old from the foster care system, had sought repeated evaluations and a variety of early intervention services; but she had been taken aback when specialists "recommended drugs for when he goes to school": "It was a big reality check, 'cause I had been very hopeful that he'd be OK." Yet she also laughed slyly when explaining that, as a teacher, "I would love to hand them out at the door. ... But you're not using my name, right?"

For Dory, being a lesbian single mother put her well "outside the norm," but she admitted that as a member of the white middle-class, she had not sufficiently questioned racial dynamics prior to adopting Khari. She raised two troubling incidents, yet cautioned that "I don't know truthfully [if race mattered], I really don't know what to believe." The first was ambiguous: a speech therapist reported in her documentation that Khari was "oppositional," "a very strong word. And I was like, 'He's being a kid; he's just being a kid. He's not trying to—he's not a bad kid.'" While it might be overinterpreting, as Dory acknowledged, the incident nonetheless parallels Ferguson's finding that schools tend to interpret African American boys' misbehavior as "willfully bad" compared to that of white boys, while also expecting greater deference. And at just under five years of age, Dory suggested it was much too early to label Khari with something like oppositional defiant disorder, though Ferguson also argued that Black boys are often "adultified" as well.[42]

Dory's second example was clearer, following the findings of civil rights research on disparities in special-ed services.[43] After losing the fight for more extensive services from Khari's school, Dory had enlisted a professional advocate and gone to mediation at the district level. After losing again, Latino and Black colleagues told her, "If he wasn't Black, you would get what you need!" Indeed, according to Dory, the mediation itself seemed unfair because school officials had concluded that Khari, again just shy of five years old, had limited potential. Dory instead blamed a special-ed program which "doesn't have very high expectations of the kids." Dory concluded by reflecting on her own seeming loss of privilege as the mother of a burdensome young boy of color: "I don't know that it's any better in any other community, but as a parent who works in a school system, a *middle-class white* parent, I feel like, incredibly frustrated . . . I feel humiliated. I ha[d] an advocate, we went to mediation, and it's just like . . . unbelievable!"

Race, Gender, Ritalin?

Only a few of the mothers raising children of color explicitly added an intersectional dimension to their accounts of invisible disability, with most, like Dory, raising concerns about race alone. The NAACP discussions evidenced a similar pattern, with more attention paid to race than to intersections of race and gender: stereotypes of dangerous Black masculinity possibly behind school racial disparities were mentioned in only three of the twenty-six relevant articles.[44] Yet, as the previous chapter emphasized, in the United States invisible disabilities and special-ed referrals are both gendered and racialized: according to one large-scale study, Black boys are 5.5 times more likely, and white boys 3.8 times more likely to be referred to special education than white girls.[45]

Black Honduran homemaker Rosa Branca was one who did articulate an intersectional analysis: "I felt [like], 'OK, you can't deal with the Black *male*,' because . . . for some reason, the *Black female* is never a threat. Why? I don't know. Why wasn't *my daughter* ADD? Why my son? . . . You can't deal with the Black male, give him a nice little tranquilizer. . . . That's a way of saying, 'You shut up, sit over there, take your medication.'"

Rosa's contention that masculine racial ideology gives a different meaning to the medicalization of sons of color makes particularly vivid the statistical findings on school disparities. At the same time, it parallels research on employer discrimination, police profiling, and differential incarceration rates, all of which target Black men over white men and over Black women.[46] Moreover, research on school disparity, while ignoring medicalization, suggests that disability labels for young men of color may do more harm than good. Rather than enabling such kids to receive helpful services, labels increase the odds of school failure and of being removed for "dangerousness."[47] With few young women of color typed by such masculine "dangerousness," Rosa's acerbic comment, "Give him a nice little tranquilizer," aptly captures one mother's resentment.[48] Despite the fact that her strategy may have temporarily shielded a son and stepson from school sanctions, Rosa seemed aware that medicalization unwittingly reinforced larger cultural images of Black male badness at the same time.

Virginia Caldwell-Starret, Mother of Henry

Virginia Caldwell-Starret, a married African American mother and high-earning professional, offered another explicitly intersectional analysis. Her narrative points to how deeply class location reshapes racialized and gendered meanings of invisible disability, suggesting that medicalization may be more readily embraced and may work better to protect boys of color in highly privileged class contexts—perhaps because their participation in such contexts already challenges the way that the ideology of Black masculine badness rests on lower-class identification.

Virginia, the mother of one young son, Henry, was worried for him, but little of her concern centered on medicalization: "Certainly, when I was coming through there was the expectation that the Black kids are going to do lesser than, or not as well as, or very much behind the other kids. And *males*, doubly so!" Virginia had been raised by a single mother, an office worker, scrambling to get by. She and her sisters, however, obtained scholarships to the elite K–8 private school where their mother worked, setting them on high-achievement trajectories to attend equally elite high schools, colleges, and professional schools. Virginia reported being repeatedly struck: "There were almost no Black males *in any* of these schools."

Virginia brought up race issues early in our conversation to describe the "crisis" Henry experienced just the previous year in kindergarten, at the private school that was her alma mater. Now a full-tuition-paying parent and trustee, Virginia had addressed Henry's crisis by working with the school and a highly respected child psychiatrist to secure the ADHD diagnosis earlier offered by his pediatrician. Provoking the crisis was teachers' concern that kids were starting to "shun" Henry because of his "exuberance":

> Understand that I'm just about six feet [tall]. My husband is six foot three. My son is in the ninety-ninth percentile for height, and he's a head-plus taller than the tallest kid in his class and the other [age-level] class. Then, it's a predominantly white school. He's probably one of the two or three—no, let me see, *five* Black kids out of both classes [about thirty kids]. And one of *two* Black *males*. So, my point being that he's different than what a lot of the kids are used to. And bigger. And then on top of that, [he's] all over the place and hyper. . . . [When] I went through there were *no* people of color. That was *hard*. [But] to add hyperactivity on top of it!

Here, Virginia specifically linked perceptions of Henry's Blackness with imposing male bodies, adding, "I've read it's the whole threat factor." Though Henry, similarly to Dory Buchanan's Khari, might seem young for such stereotyping, sociologist Ferguson argued that boys of color tend to be "adultified" in schools in just this manner.[49] Virginia further differentiated Black masculinity by setting aside the Black girls in the age cohort from the boys' "different," "bigger" bodies. She and her husband were relieved and thankful that stimulant drugs immediately contained Henry's physicality—his racing around the playground, his jostling, bumping, and jumping in the classroom.

However, medication was less successful in improving Henry's academic performance, also part of Virginia's crisis. School personnel questioned whether Henry was ready for a challenging first-grade curriculum: "That teacher that I love . . . she pulled me aside because she was concerned that we have an unusually *gifted* class of students." In itself, this reference to "gifted students" is intriguing as it may be a category bounded by white privilege: national data show that whites are strongly overrepresented and students of color significantly underrepresented among those labeled "gifted and talented."[50]

While Virginia may not have heard this or been aware of these additional racialized trends, her account suggested a sense of urgency that drove her to quickly secure costly private services: a daily reading tutor, a special summer camp, a behavioral therapist, and increased visits to the psychiatrist. Virginia recounted that the latter suggested upping Henry's stimulant dosage, but the ambivalence and objections so central to the other mothers were largely absent from her narrative. Instead—and understandably so—Virginia seemed intent that Henry benefit from her dramatic upward mobility. And like the affluent white mothers featured earlier, she seemed to prioritize the transmission of her hard-earned cultural capital—the tacit skills in bodily deportment, language use, wielding of "good taste," and the sense of entitled self-assurance—to succeed in elite social networks.[51] Virginia thus spoke emphatically of being "proactive," fearing that school personnel would slip into an assumption that "it's because of his *race* that he's behind" rather than because of his "learning disability."

Being "proactive" and closely monitoring Henry's progress required Virginia to scale back her career. Yet with the privilege of flexible hours, Virginia sacrificed only plum assignments, extracurricular civic engagement, and the hope of ever getting a full night's sleep. Because she had a well-established career with high earnings, a supportive spouse, and a nearby kin network, Virginia navigated the intensified work-family conflict a needy child brings better than most, if also admitting to exhaustion and being overstressed. However, her narrative also poignantly represents a mother's awareness of the extraordinary vulnerability of a young Black son. In this sense, Virginia may amplify Lareau's argument that if both Black and white affluent parents engage in "concerted cultivation," mothers of Black children must go further to maximize their children's opportunities, ever "vigilant" for possible racial exclusion or insensitivity.[52]

Several school ethnographies supply more evidence of the role class resources might play in mitigating the challenges Henry faced. Such in-depth research demonstrates that schools do tend to assume that racial otherness and cultural difference are responsible for the badness of boys of color—but only because of entrenched stereotypes that all have deeply dysfunctional, impoverished, father-absent families.[53] Virginia, in contrast, signaled repeatedly the importance she attached to legal marriage and family respectability. For example, she confided that Henry had been conceived on her honeymoon, at a late age (thirty-five) because she had waited for a strong and appropriate partner. Moreover, Virginia seemed to recognize a need to display this family respectability, as she kept Henry medicated on weekends and school breaks specifically to join in school-related gatherings—many, in her words, in "structured," high-status venues. Similarly, she spoke of having her husband, a musician with an erratic schedule, more visible at school by bringing Henry most mornings. And she signaled their financial status by hosting or sponsoring several class events.

In short, with considerable resources, Virginia employed a range of strategies to protect her young Black son. Though long-run outcomes for six-year-old Henry were unknowable, Virginia exuded confidence that her maternal work would succeed. Not coincidentally, among the group raising children of color she was the least hesitant to use psychoactive drugs. Intriguingly, though, Virginia alluded to a need for constant vigilance near the end of our long conversation over dinner: "Even now they have an issue with retention of Black males at the school," she whispered. "A couple of the teachers [were] telling me" that, just prior to Henry's enrollment, "two young Black boys . . . I don't think they were even in the first-grade yet . . . both were asked to leave the school."

Class, Race, and Gender?

Cara Withers placed neither race nor intersections of race and gender as explicitly at the forefront of her narrative as Virginia had—yet she, too, suggested the importance of class context to the meaning of boys' medicalization. In contrast to Virginia, Cara pointed to a working-class masculinity, underscoring her more tentative upward mobility. Cara was much less comfortable medicating her young son than was Virginia. Cara's middle-class moorings were insecure, as she alone among her extended family had earned a college degree. Her narrative illustrated life on the cusp between social classes, having enjoyable workplace perks, gym membership, and catered lunches, but also facing tough times after her divorce, fostering her sister's kids, and moving her mother into the household. Moreover, while Michael's father lived in the same city and visited regularly, as a single mother Cara could not demonstrate the same family respectability as married Virginia; neither could she, on one income, provide elite schooling.

Cara had also invoked a working-class context in comparing Michael to his younger sister Delia, worrying that they were nearly gender-reversed. She described Delia as "streetwise," with Michael the one unable to cope with life "in the city." Her language codes an urban, working-class manliness defined by self-control and muscular physicality, as well as, for some scholars, connoting Blackness.[54] Cara's words were perhaps more ambiguous about the racial context than about the classed, gendered context: "[Michael] tends to get upset about everything and he cries. And the hardest thing is we live in the city. You *can't afford* to cry, not often, not as much . . . So it's very, very, very, very hard!" Cara also listed her objectives for their early morning gym workouts—without Delia—with notably gendered imagery: to toughen Michael's "overly sensitive" nature, his "overreacting to any little, slight pain," his getting "embarrassed very easily." Michael must move out of his "cocoon" and "get the harsh reality of what life really is like." Perhaps in her ability to shield a neurochemically vulnerable son, Cara, like all the mothers in this group (except perhaps for Virginia, though it may be too early to judge), is caught in the more entrapping racialized meanings of medicalization.

Working-class Rosa Branca, who was perhaps the least inhibited in discussing the pejorative meanings attached to disordered boys of color, could not protect her kids with middle-class cultural or economic resources, though she and her blue-collar (second) husband had managed to move their large blended household to the edge of an affluent white suburb with highly ranked schools. Rosa detailed near the end of our conversations the following scenario of escalating stigmatization, conveying what might have befallen son Frank without her vigilant but selective use of medicalization. With fears centered on the label of inherent mental deficiency and mental retardation, Rosa underscored the persisting weight of historical legacies of scientific racism and eugenic movements on poor and working-class boys and young men of color:

> That's why I agreed for him to take the pills because I didn't want it to be like after ADD, all of a sudden then he would be *retarded*. So no, let's leave it at that point. And also they offered me that Social Security, SSI I guess, like the government would give him money. And I said, "Wait a minute! NO!" This is too much of a label on my son. OK, one minute ADD, and the next minute we qualify for SSI? And then the next minute, he would be staying for life [in an institution]? So I said, "*no thank you!*"

In fact, research on mental retardation indicates that Rosa's fears are realistic. Rather than diminishing, large racial discrepancies have persisted since the Civil Rights era in categories of such inherent brain deficiency, with African Americans more than twice as likely as whites to be categorized as mentally retarded.[55] White boys tend to be more concentrated in categories like ADHD denoting greater cognitive *potential* despite low school achievement. "Minimal" or "educable mental retardation," in contrast, defines young boys of color as low achievers with *inherently limited* cognitive potential, with this conclusion largely based on culturally biased IQ testing.[56] None of the thirty-two mothers of white sons or daughters mentioned the mental retardation label at all, in any context—though many worried about academic problems and poor school performance. In contrast, four mothers of Black sons—Rosa Branca, Mildred Andujar, Lucia Santos, and Dory Buchanan—raised the issue without my prompting. I learned that Mildred's son Gil, Dory's son Khari, and Lucia's Eduardo, had been threatened with the "minimally" retarded label that Rosa only feared laid in wait for Frank if he sought public disability assistance. Each impressed me with their understanding, on some level, of the historical weight of this category and its association with racial otherness. Lucia was perhaps the most outraged and might have spoken also for those like Dory and Rosa, whose sons had no accents but whose skin was dark: "[You] think we [are all] *retarded* because we have accent[s]. That's not true. We are the same human beings as other people. Because we [do] no[t] have the perfect English . . . that [does] no[t] mean we [are] retarded!"

Rosa's rejection of a government handout, though some might applaud it as an act of personal responsibility, might actually signal something more. Of course Rosa wished to see Frank become self-sufficient; but the receipt of SSI can be demonized as "the Other Welfare" and stamp an already-at-risk young man and his mother as scheming welfare cheats. It also involves demonstrating that a youth's functional limitations are "marked and severe."

Conclusion: Listening to Mothers

The narratives of the women here richly depict the distinct maternal work involved when children of color are labeled with em-brained issues, becoming part of Rosa Branca's "strange coincidence" of persisting, unintended racial sorting in schools. The mothers expressed complex ambivalence toward the medicalization that, in the age of neuroscience, now accompanies most such school sorting. They demonstrated a greater initial wariness to any label than did white mothers, who often found relief and recognition in gaining a diagnosis; and they were torn differently over whether to comply with or challenge recommendations to administer psychoactive drugs. Both reactions emerge precisely from their awareness that racial exclusion and insensitivity persist in U.S. institutional life.[57]

I suggest, then, that mothers raising children of color are not inherently different from other mothers and are not carriers of unchanging cultural difference. Those I spoke with simply knew that they must be doubly vigilant to protect sons of color, who even if not actually neurologically vulnerable, already faced more precarious life chances. Medicalized disabilities like ADHD more associated with white youths thus seem to offer a bit of white privilege, and at least partial protection against academic failure or exclusion, compared to "Blacker" labels of irreparable organic deficiencies. Yet at the same time, the mothers raising vulnerable sons of color sensed that disability labels might also pose risks, inviting

as much as protecting against the harsh, unfair framing of any disruptive behaviors. Listening closely to mothers' narratives and the discourses
they invoked, I suggest they may, like Cara Withers, feel "compelled to
go with what's there." They thus accede to psychoactive medications to
ease sons' ability to comply with such harsh behavioral standards as well
as our era's strictly standardized academic markers. Even in a time of
"racism without racists,"[58] the full stigma attached to Black masculine
dangerousness may be held in abeyance if a mother relents—though as
Rosa Branca sensed, this protection of an individual child's education
may unwittingly reinforce or perpetuate the larger stereotype. That is,
what does it tell us when Frank Branca, or Michael Withers, or Mateo
Riega, or Henry Caldwell-Starret needs to be "tranquilized"?

Importantly, the mothers raising children of color did not condemn
school personnel despite the pervasive racialized frames which made
their sons appear more willful and "adultified" than white sons as well
as, at times, less intelligent. Well-meaning school personnel, already
pressed by tight budgets and high-stakes testing, may believe that special-ed designation will bring helpful early intervention, or generous
academic support and mental health services, unaware that children
of color tend to find instead more restrictive settings, lowered expectations, and less rigorous curricula. Still, most of the mothers had found
at least a few allies in the schools and, like Cara Withers, were at least
partially sympathetic to the institutional pressures teachers experienced.
(And Dory Buchanan reminds that some teachers live with both sides of
these issues, as she was fast disillusioned with early intervention.) Even
Rosa Branca had significantly corrected any notion that she saw intentional targeting of "African American" sons in her thoughtful declaration
that the "strange coincidence" is not "this big huge racial-type thing"—
though she was emphatic that we see the disparities nonetheless.

Listening to the narratives of such mothers may also help us think
more carefully about the limited suggestions offered in the research as
to why nonwhite sons are less likely to receive psychopharmaceutical
treatments. In addition to the relatively ill-defined suggestion of cultural differences and the very real problems of access and affordabil-
ity, epidemiologists seldom consider the full picture surrounding such
"undertreatment." Mothers struggling with a limited set of choices may
not perfectly articulate their suspicions of disparate treatment, but it is

reasonable for them to approach the healthcare system with as much distrust as they do the educational system. As Black feminist scholar Dorothy Roberts concluded after reviewing the evidence on health inequities, inequities which continue even where access has been ensured, "Blacks are less likely to get desirable medical interventions and more likely to get undesirable interventions."[59]

Although the mothers were clearly most concerned with protecting vulnerable children of color from institutional disparities, they may rightly want to protect themselves as well. In the United States we continue to demonize racially other mothers, made monstrous to cover over larger cultural anxieties about growing economic inequality, the erosion of decent jobs, and gendered family changes, as sociologists studying neoliberal welfare reform have detailed.[60] Thus mothers like those featured here may be right to fear being considered ill informed in rejecting psychoactive drugs—and just as insightful to fear being considered a new kind of "calculating parasite" if they turn to medications.[61] Certainly their odds of raising normatively gendered, yet less threatening, more compliant young men of color are severely constrained by America's transformed opportunity structure. With or without psychopharmaceutical help, mothers like Cara Withers—or Leesha Baker—walk a very fine line rearing sons who can move with agility and assurance between the "street" and the institutions of a shrinking white middle class. It may be that only extraordinary individual and extended-family upward mobility, like that of Virginia Caldwell-Starret, brings less risk to mothers and sons of color when selectively drawing on white medicalization.

I do not mean, however, to overstate the difference race makes in rearing kids with invisible special needs: among all those I interviewed, only *one* multiply privileged mother, Colleen Janeway, had spoken enthusiastically about psychopharmaceuticals—and she had not been without initial reservations. Moreover, no mother can fully escape the double-edged stigma surrounding medicating children—all are in some way "damned if they do, damned if they don't." Mildred Andujar was certainly not alone in receiving harsh judgments of her maternal valor for refusing to medicate a struggling child or for challenging school authorities. Yet ethnoracial and class location, along with a child's gender, may shift the meaning of children's invisible em-brained troubles from reparable to irreparable, and of mothers' actions from selfish to monstrous.

Mothers, Children, and Families in a Precarious Time

When I undertook this study of mothers raising kids with invisible, em-brained disabilities, I suspected it would be a complicated story, involving issues of gender, social class, and race, and of educational, medical, and social policy. Still, through long years of research and analysis, I kept realizing even more was involved, most notably the precarious futures for both adults and children in New Economy labor markets, the influence of neoliberal values embracing private market-based solutions to these perils, and the diffusion of neuroscience through our popular culture, reframing our public discourse. The mothers I interviewed were all struggling to do what was best for their children while entangled in the web of these larger sociological forces. As I listened, I became increasingly convinced that for all their often heroic efforts, solutions to the challenges their children pose, to themselves, their families, their schools and the larger society, are ultimately a public, not a private matter.

As a feminist sociologist, I place mothers center stage in this story. The full story involves many individual and institutional players, all with their own experiences, interests, and stories to tell. Fathers, partners, other family members and devoted caregivers, as well as most importantly, kids themselves, all deserve to voice their own perspectives.[1] Moreover, there are many professionals—teachers and educational specialists; psychiatrists, therapists, and other psy-sector workers within and outside state social services, as well as alternative service providers, some carving out new markets—who are also devoted to children. Many of these professional workers, especially in the female-dominated "semi-professions," have chosen relatively under-rewarded, over-burdened fields to serve diverse children and surely deserve books of their own.[2]

I would argue, however, that mother-blame and the tensions within current gender relations which this represents are among the most significant and under-studied aspects of this multifaceted tale. U.S. families are changing, with men and women on more equal footing now that most mothers are also employed outside the home and many live outside of nuclear-family households. But norms of womanhood are still tied to care and nurture, to the practical and symbolic responsibility for the nation's children and its future. Mothers whose children are uncommonly needy pose a most troubling case, illuminating how little the United States does as a nation to protect reconfigured families from harsh postindustrial capitalism, to press for workplace change and against an ADD-ogenic pace of life. And in this "end of men" era, with widespread concern for the future of men's breadwinning and a sharpening gulf between winners and losers, mothers become responsible for shoring up the shaky masculinity, and the shaky gender divide itself, represented by burgeoning numbers of vulnerable, feminized boys.

This central responsibility of normative mothers for their children's development is vividly portrayed in best-selling essayist Ayelet Waldman's *Bad Mother* and "commercial fiction" writer Jodi Picoult's *House Rules*.[3] With self-deprecating humor, Waldman defends her decisions raising a son with ADHD amid suburban nuclear-family affluence, a context much like that of the affluent mothers featured here. Picoult weaves a more earnest fictional account of the divorced character Emma Hunt raising a son diagnosed with Asperger syndrome. Like the real-life single mothers I interviewed, Picoult's Emma has hard-earned expertise in disability rights and special-education laws, gluten- and casein-free diets, psychoactive medications, autism specialists and tutors of various persuasions, and behavior modification and psychodynamic therapies. To avoid losing a key audience, Picoult even has her protagonist give a respectful nod to the discredited vaccine theory for rising autism rates and its zealous advocates among mothers.

At the other extreme, the acclaimed 2011 film *We Need to Talk about Kevin*, based on a prize-winning 2003 British novel and its 2008 BBC radio serialization, presents a nightmarish cautionary tale of an affluent married mother, her sociopathic son, and the school massacre that he ultimately commits. The film's elliptical portrayal of Kevin and his mother, Eva, played to fears of the violence lurking within a normal-looking son and of the disorder that could befall us if mothers fail to be selflessly and relentlessly attentive to their children's neurobiological development. In an online film forum, one lay reviewer asked, "Anyone else think the movie actually implicated [sic] that it was the mom's fault?" A spate of responses precisely articulated how older tropes of mother-blame have been revised by the age of neuroscience: "Eva was a terrible mother. How can people not see this! It doesn't excuse everything Kevin did, but holy *bleep* man she did nothing to stop it when SO MANY signs were there."[4] Where were all the experts relentlessly pursued and researched, the services and treatments relentlessly advocated for by Waldman, by Picoult's Emma Hunt, and by nearly all of the forty-eight mothers who shared their stories with me? As cultural theorist Murray emphasized, our cultural representations of child disorder nearly all center on such individual mothers, fit mothers who bring healing and hope, or those unfit mothers like Eva who bring tragedy.[5]

Mothers as Vigilantes

Yet as I interviewed real mothers, it was a different image from popular culture that kept coming to mind, that of the lone warrior struggling for justice against an indifferent or hostile world with whatever tools and tactics are available, like the vigilante heroes in many of Clint Eastwood's films. As in those iconic stories, a mother's unyielding watchfulness and advocacy for her child took on the imperative of a lone moral quest. Indeed, sociologist Amy Sousa referred to similar mothers of autistic children as isolated "warrior-heroes" reinventing a masculine archetype.[6] And Valerie Leiter, in her study of disabled youths' transitions to adulthood, similarly discovered that mothers practiced an "advocacy imperative" whose "moral framing is quite powerful," dividing good mothers from bad.[7]

Admittedly the metaphor of the vigilante is imperfect, most associated with violence and actions outside the law. Yet there is also the sense of one who acts on her own, in pursuit of justice for a family wronged.[8] And there is the adversarial dimension, the seizing of authority, taking the "law" into one's own hands in a system where information and expertise are difficult to locate, fragmented among many narrow specializations, or "secret" within constrained and opaque bureaucratic offices. Leiter again had similar findings, with mothers reporting that the budget pressures in educational and social service agencies inadvertently pressed staff to conceal resources and treat them with a policy of "if you don't ask, you're not told."[9] Faith Prenniker captured this sense of a lone quest in her efforts to gain a better diagnosis for son Miller: "Sometimes *I* just will get this fear, like there's something else. And *nobody else* is going to find it, and *I* don't know what it is." Faith, and many others, brought out files, logs, and notebooks, showing me meticulous records of their "battles" with schools and special-education procedures, health-care systems and insurance firms, psy-sector and state social services on behalf of children innately vulnerable, but also wronged by a precarious, uncaring social context.

Some mothers did find allies—usually teachers—among the educational, medical, and social service personnel with whom they dealt. At least three mothers echoed Patricia Gwarten's complaint that "everything is a *secret*"—though they variously referred to getting physical therapy, an outside evaluation, more hours with a reading tutor, or summertime services included in a child's IEP. In each case, it was a sympathetic teacher who finally clued them in. Yet the distinct, adversarial institutional level was highlighted—and thus mothers' critical perspectives— when each reported these teacher-allies vigorously advising, "But you didn't hear it from me!" or "Don't say I told you!"[10]

Mother-Blame in the Age of Neuroscience

A core finding in this book is the extent to which mother-blame has become so expansive, yet so indirect. Few of the mothers encountered such direct indictment of their emotional or sexual character, of their psychological capacity for care, as with the infamous "refrigerator mothers" blamed for their children's autism in the twentieth century—and few blamed themselves as the underlying, root, or whole cause for a child's struggles either. Yet they described being surrounded with proximal blame from many sides, but now couched in the language of postindustrial management—as at a public school special-ed parent meeting I attended where we were exhorted to "raise the bar on being a parent professional" and more expertly manage a child's "executive function."

Though valorous mothers have been charged to turn to medical guidance and practice "scientific motherhood" for a century or more,[11] twenty-first-century engagement must be with the most advanced sciences; and as feminist scholar Joan Wolf emphasized, it must be "total," with greater maternal responsibility for self-taught expertise to individually assess risk and optimize every possible opportunity for a child's embodied and em-brained advantage.[12] The evident commitment to this normative standard is clearly what is most admirable in Picoult's fictional Emma Hunt as in Waldman's self-deprecatory confessional essays—and its absence is what is perhaps most disturbing about Eva in *We Need to Talk about Kevin*.

A striking aspect of mothering in the early twenty-first-century United States is the widespread diffusion of the language and ideas of neuroscience. This trend, so pervasive we might well refer to our era as the age of neuroscience, is said to date just since the 1990s with the proliferating use of brain-imaging technologies and, most important in the case of invisible disabilities, brain-altering psychopharmaceuticals. Some suggest it goes even further, representing a major "paradigm shift" in understanding what it is to be human, to believing we *are* our embodied brains, so that our health and well-being and that of our children depend on optimizing our (and their) neurochemical-electrical hardwiring.[13] Amid political discord and economic weakness, even President Obama sought to capitalize on the popularity of neuroscience, in his 2013 State of the Union address proposing the launch of the BRAIN Initiative. Modeled on the European Union's Human Brain Project and the public-private collaboration in the Human Genome Project, it is intended to "develop technologies to track the electrical activity of every neuron [some one hundred billion] in the brain."[14]

In the United Kingdom, the center-right government has taken up new parent-education campaigns promoting the privatized "development of early brain architecture" as a major route to "increasing social mobility." Employing the seeming neutrality and objectivity of neuroscience, the campaign exhorts parents to become "brain architects" implementing "Home Learning Environment[s]" to stimulate and maximize brain development in children's early years. This program not only masks the gendered imperative in such early "parenting," but also the need for political action to stem rising inequality and create actual opportunities for increased mobility. A more caring public might also affirm the value of nurture and familial intimacy for their own sake rather than in the instrumental language of optimizing cognitive stimulation.[15]

Similar if less centralized campaigns have emerged in the United States, like the Massachusetts public awareness program "Brain Building in Progress," its logo a yellow highway sign making early optimized brain development the figurative road to "our future economic prosperity" and "productive, responsible citizenship." The Massachusetts campaign's website and videos feature attractive, racially diverse men and women engaged in such traditional activities as reading to toddlers, but alongside dramatic neuroscientific discoveries: "Young children's brains develop 700 synapses (neural connections that transmit information) every second."[16] While broadly invoking the responsibility of other community members, the campaign primarily depicts feminized teachers, day-care providers, and other underpaid, mother-like care-workers. And the most important responsibility in this largely unfunded mandate is relegated to families, and thus once more, to mothers.[17]

No doubt this focus on the physical brain, and the accompanying rise in those deemed non-neurotypical, has been promoted and encouraged by Big Pharma, a significant New Economy knowledge-based industry: in the United States Big Pharma pours billions of dollars into direct-to-consumer advertising of psychoactive drugs and many billions more into promoting them to healthcare providers.[18] Yet as communication studies scholar Thornton argues, pharmaceutical companies are not the sole or perhaps even the major contributing cause of our "cultural saturation" with "brain-based ways of thinking and acting."[19] Indeed, to both Thornton and sociologist Pitts-Taylor, extending the work of Nikolas Rose, neuroscience finds its purchase precisely because of its "affinity" with the privatizing values of neoliberalism so convenient for postindustrial firms in the face of global competition.[20] And I agree that it is largely this "convergence of interests," this minimizing of public obligations, which gives neuroscience its more ominous edge.

The neuroscientific paradigm reshapes mothers' accountability for children's troubles, making it in some sense more palatable, less overtly misogynistic than the Freudian-inflected blame of earlier eras. But it does nothing to alleviate a mother's individual responsibility and often reinforces such privatized views. Commercial enterprises cashing in on our age of neuroscience like the online game site Lumosity.com, "trusted by over 35 million users," offer to "harness your brain's neuroplasticity and train your way to a brighter future,"[21] suggesting that a "normal" brain is simply not good enough in the global economy.[22] At the same time, other popular voices affirm the central gendered responsibilities of individual mothers, rather than larger publics, for children's brighter futures. Like the popular advice books, news media discussions sort good mothers from bad, assessing just who is individually fit to manage vulnerable children or to make truly responsible decisions regarding psychiatric medications.[23]

Against such repeated affirmations of the solely private basis of family life and children's development, a feminist sociological lens reminds us that childrearing always occurs in a social context—or as a colleague put it, in frustration over our students' individualistic brain-centered explanations for every social ill, "brains always move around in space, *social space*." The rise of invisible childhood disability is a multifaceted "dialectic of biology and culture," in which children's less perceptible quirks or differences become formally recognized only in a particular time and place.[24] But if mothers accept their individual responsibility for their children's' optimal neurological development, effectively raising the bar on themselves, does this contradict the feminist assumption that women are active, critical subjects? I hope I have demonstrated that their words and accounts reflect both acquiescence *and* critical recognition of institutional failings—indeed, their narratives might be seen as attempts to work out just what portion of such private blame ought to be placed back on public shoulders. This was strikingly evident in the special-ed parent meeting when parents, mainly mothers, repeatedly rejected the guest speaker's chiding to "take the olive branch, acknowledge we're part of the problem."

Finally, a feminist sociological lens, treating women as active, thoughtful subjects, illustrates that mothers are not simply duped by Big Pharma or biomedical authority. As social actors crafting individual narratives, the women who shared their stories with me selectively and sometimes critically drew on dominant discourses and were far from passive recipients of our cultural paradigm shift. They did remain, however, ultimately dependent on institutional and professional resources to help their struggling children. Their perspectives were also shaped by intersectional locations, how their relative lack of social power as women with burdensome, not-normal children also varied by their access to class resources, white ethnoracial advantage, and more surprisingly, to heterosexual-marital privilege. Feminist sociological lenses help explain their more critical perspectives on social power and cultural authority as partly a consequence of their lived experiences of marginality.[25] Such marginality is a fact of life for all mothers raising non-neurotypical kids, but those outside ethnoracial or hetero-marital privileges seemed to develop more critical insights because they perceived processes of institutional sorting which those with more privilege could afford to overlook.

Mothers and Inequality, Unequal Mothers

The differences and inequalities among mothers raising invisibly disabled children in this age of neuroscience are therefore as central to my argument as their commonalities. It is not a simple argument: I found no obvious differences in the accounts of mothers of divergent ethnoracial, marital, or class location as they struggled to understand and ameliorate their children's troubles. Even the most privileged mothers, for example, could not escape stigma and spoiled identities. And I did not find less privileged women significantly less engaged in vigilante efforts to navigate educational and medical systems.[26] Moreover, nearly all described decisions about administering psychopharmaceutical drugs as among the most difficult they faced—and, with great, vigorous detail, they demonstrated that managing the medications was anything but a quick fix.

Still, single mothers and those raising children of color experienced a higher level of mother-blame, describing greater dangers and suspicion of their fitness because of their social location. They also described encountering negative institutional sorting along lines that recapitulate persistent inequalities in the United States, perceiving differential risks for their stigmatized children depending on intersecting lines of race, gender, and class. I discovered that those most critical or with the most complex ambivalence toward childhood medicalization were those raising sons of color.

Mothers' experiences also differed according to the package of economic and cultural resources, of tangible and intangible assets, they could marshal to rear their neurodiverse kids. Yet those assets matter in rather surprising or paradoxical ways. A high income allows one to purchase services, to have more choice of providers, and to seek out more and better forms of commodified support—but these privileges come with costs seldom examined in either scholarly or popular discussion. Also, the presence of a husband may still be a crucial cultural resource, a form of cultural capital despite women's gains and our more varied, postmodern households.[27] Although even married women perceived the disadvantage beginning when husbands were not in the room at the school IEP meeting or the psychiatrist's office, the absence of a husband loomed far larger in the accounts of the mothers who were single, whether divorced or never married. Each of these important dimensions, money and men, interacted with other advantages—educational attainment, fit bodies and self-assured demeanor, and most importantly, white ethnoracial privilege—in how mothers experienced bureaucratic gatekeeping within the educational and medical systems and within state social services.

The narratives of the advantaged mothers who could afford to raise "multimillion-dollar" children were replete with private schools and tutors, educational advocates and attorneys, family therapists, homeopathic practitioners, and pediatric psychiatrists, neurologists, and psychopharmacologists. But children's volatility and disruptions threatened class transmission and mothers' efforts to inculcate the cultural and body capital, the internalized sense of entitlement, verbal skills and demeanor, superior tastes, and sense of distinction sociologists find crucial to interacting successfully in upper-middle-class and elite environments. Because class transmission of such intangible assets is not automatic, but requires familial effort primarily assigned to women, I heard stories of arduous maternal efforts to carry on with high-brow outings and activities despite youths' anxieties, tantrums or meltdowns, or to keep challenging, unruly children in carefully chosen school environments.

In addition, while living in a community with well-educated neighbors and just the right schools would seem to maximize opportunities for class transmission, along with improving children's well-being, women's stories of painful rejection suggested that it may also increase the stigma of "not-normal" kids and their mothers. In an anxious, competitive context, less perceptible but burdensome impairments can disturb neighbors and school personnel who have their own investments in class transmission and community standing to protect. Further, the stealth quality of invisible disabilities, the sense that they may strike or invade anywhere, may make them more disturbing than clearly marked physical impairments. But affluent mothers' painful stories involved more than difficulties protecting vulnerable children and maximizing their cultural capital: they involved mothers' own lack of social support and their exclusion from practical and emotional relations of care and reciprocity among neighbors, friends, sometimes even kin. Whereas other researchers emphasize the positive exchanges and networks between middle- or upper-middle-class mothers,[28] I found that affluent mothers raising vulnerable kids were more likely to describe communities drawn up against them. Such mothers turned to the credentialed psy-sector professionals they had laboriously located as individually patched-together substitutes for this missing community support. Purchasing such private services (or employing private health insurance to do so), however, creates a commodified, asymmetric transaction despite the compassion of practitioners. Even when on a first-name basis, like Judith Lowenthal's relationship with her son's "brilliant" pediatric psychopharmacologist, such hollow substitutes are thus another paradoxical consequence of social privilege.

I learned from the affluent mothers' narratives that marriage also often posed a key paradox: while heterosexual marriage still confers important cultural and economic resources and of course can be an important source of intimacy and care, husbands' emotional and practical support for rearing troubled children was often described as sorely lacking. There were exceptions, such as Judith Lowenthal's account of a genuinely companionable marriage, but more affluent mothers endured inequitable, even strained relationships in exchange for at least some respite from stigma and recognition of their vigilante efforts and daily challenges. In contrast, single mothers voiced some unexpected advantage in their ability to organize day-to-day life around the needs of unruly children without enduring a husband's criticism, his expectations for family order, and what Hochschild might term an unfair "economy of gratitude."[29]

Many colleagues and students with whom I've discussed this work wonder whether the concerted class transmission practices of such affluent married mothers lend credence to the image of intrusive "helicopter" moms medicating normal but unruly kids because they mar otherwise orderly upper-middle-class lives, underperform in school, and frustrate class transmission if they do not gain entrance to selective universities. In our college classrooms we see the growing number of students with invisible disabilities, for whom campuses are legally obligated to provide accommodations just as they are for those requiring wheelchair ramps or American Sign Language interpreters.[30] No doubt some few families may unfairly take advantage of these supports, just as they may use psychiatric medications as academic performance-enhancing drugs. I suspect, however, that such images are overstated caricatures. Disability services on many, if not most, college campuses are far from generous[31]—and this is little different from the strapped special-education programs in many K–12 schools.[32] Also, the extent of palpable pain I encountered in my interviews makes me skeptical that many would actually subject their children (or themselves) to the stigma of such labels—or especially to the rigors of daily life with the idiosyncratic effects and side effects of medications—without serious cause. Abby Martin, a mother with both undergraduate and graduate degrees from elite universities, expressed this most bluntly: "Medications, they are no panacea!"

Other investigations, in fact, suggest that the parents and compassionate professionals likeliest to use psychoactive medications to turn around kids' school performance are those more precariously located and hardly looking for perfect, displayable children. Sociologist Regina Smardon uncovered the highest rates of Ritalin usage in declining white working-class communities, among those families hardest hit by the waning of U.S. industries and decent jobs.[33] Admittedly, I did not study college youth or their parents—or those living in former factory towns. And my methods of recruiting mothers at multiple sites may have tapped only those with more serious concerns—those who felt some desire for greater engagement, some need to "out" themselves as Brooke Donnelly put it, poignantly explaining why she had responded to my newsletter ad.[34] I am torn myself, thinking of mothers like Judith Lowenthal, knowing that their actions to protect sensitive, highly reactive children also reaffirm unfair boundaries of privilege. Still, Judith, Abby, and others who may seem to be "helicopter" moms make convenient targets without being major causes for rising inequality or economic precariousness.

Another paradoxical disadvantage faced by privileged mothers emerged when they spoke self-critically of their initial "naive" trust in educational and medical professionals. As Theresa Kelleher explained, "I thought all these people are taking care of my child, that's *their job*.... [But] I was so naive and idealistic ... I never thought people would put cost over children's needs." Mothers raising children of color and many of the single mothers, particularly those who had never married, were not handicapped by such excessive trust in the system.

I had not originally thought of the single mothers as a distinct group, since their divisions along class and ethnoracial lines seemed so much greater than any commonality. Their narratives taken together, however—filled with their self-identification as single parents "having to advocate five thousand times harder"—prompted me to suggest that women raising burdensome, unruly children in "fatherless" homes may heighten the discomfort many Americans already feel with fast-rising rates of single motherhood. Once only associated with poor minority communities, over a quarter of U.S. households with children under eighteen are now headed by single mothers. Yet they are nearly invisible in the best-selling parenting books I analyzed. And the lone mothers whom I met, white and nonwhite, with good earnings and without, nearly all described encountering continuing suspicion of their fitness, feeling compelled to defend their "broken," morally questionable homes to educational and medical professionals and social service providers.

A Quick Fix?

Single mothers across divides of income and education were little different from married mothers in reporting how difficult it was to make decisions to administer psychoactive drugs to their children. Single mothers may be perceived quite differently, however, as when they are portrayed at all in public media it is with few strengths, in "broken homes," where it is suggested they medicate difficult children all too quickly.[35] Lone mothers' detailed narratives, however, suggest an alternative explanation: negative cultural imagery of morally questionable, fatherless homes may influence harried professionals, wittingly or unwittingly, to press more quickly for medications. Certainly this is a more plausible explanation for aggregate disparities when we consider what nearly every one of the forty-two mothers, married and single, who reported turning to medications for a precarious child described:

medications are simply not a quick fix, but instead, their limited benefits require extensive maternal management.

Much of this vigilante effort in managing medications is missed if we focus on medications as a one-time either/or decision and count only whether children are or are not medicated. Rather, my research suggests we might respect mothers' ongoing work to monitor the number and type of drugs prescribed, the daily and weekly effects, at what dosages and with what side effects. I discovered, as well, that mothers often do this with little professional guidance, with psychiatrists and psychopharmacologists only reimbursed by insurance for intermittent fifteen-minute appointments.[36] Instead of mothers duped by Big Pharma and biomedical authority—or mothers flatly rejecting or resisting both—I found mothers actively negotiating with and selectively drawing from such medicalization. But for mothers lacking the cultural capital or legitimation of a father in the home, these interactions with the medical system on behalf of a burdensome child may carry different meanings or prove more fraught.

Gender and Race in the Institutional Sorting of Precarious Children

The stigma or threat posed by disordered or needy children is inseparable from a long history in the United States of sorting those wanted for the nation's future from those unwanted, expendable children, originally along eugenic lines of ethnoracial otherness. These lines were also gendered, demarcating different threats to the nation from lawless or feeble-minded boys and girls. In the present social context, the sorting of normal from not-normal children is more fine-grained and individual, and arguably more accurate—but it is still influenced by gendered and racialized processes that disproportionately cast boys and young men and children of color as having deficient brains. The gender dimension or the targeting of boys, much noticed by conservative pundits, also reveals tensions provoked by New Economy transformation and threats to men's continued social advantage.

Destabilizing men's advantage also threatens the strict maintenance of the gender binary of masculine and feminine difference, and mothers of vulnerable boys expressed responsibility for shoring it up anew. Surrounded by proximal blame from kin and professionals for boys' shaky masculine development—and a larger culture that, according to sociologist Michael Kimmel, "vilifie[s] mothers as feminizing their boys"[37]—it is not surprising that mothers spoke in detail of their strategies to instill greater embodied self-assurance, to "build up muscles" and physical strength in boys seen as too weird, too soft, or too sensitive. They also worried a great deal that they had been too coddling or too attached, spoiling rather than toughening young sons. Such concerns were rarely voiced by the mothers of disordered girls, whose normative attachment to mothers, "inwardness," or "passivity" are culturally expected or encouraged. Each mother may be acting to protect her own child from stigma, the harsh treatment of peers, and an overly precarious future, yet in aggregate their actions and attitudes sadly reinforce normative gender relations.

Mothers reflected national patterns, and the dialectic interaction of biology and culture, in identifying far more focal boys than girls among their children and in speaking of both differences and similarities between them. Mothers of vulnerable sons and daughters recounted similar issues of peer victimization, bullying, serious teasing, and harassment. Mothers of sons, however, suggested that too little manliness invited harsh treatment and gay-taunting from other boys, whereas the few daughters were targeted for too much femininity or were overly (hetero)sexualized. Troubled girls were also more often isolated or verbally teased rather than subjected to the physical aggression vulnerable boys received.[38] Yet girls' internalizing posed great obstacles for mothers negotiating on their daughters' behalf—with the gender norms that mask girls' issues in public spaces unwittingly reinforced by tight budgets and harried school personnel. Conversely, sons who lashed out against bullying, even in relatively minor ways, suffered from over-visibility and fears of male violence. Recent zero-tolerance policies greatly exacerbated the tendency toward harsh punishment of initially victimized boys.

Such multiply layered cultural anxieties surrounding masculinity are no doubt on high alert in the United States today. But for those with burdensome, vulnerable boys, these anxieties are two-sided, signaling both the peril and the promise of the New Economy. The United States, in this time of high-stakes global competition, wishes to capitalize on unconventional forms of male giftedness. Dreaming of the next Steve

Jobs, Bill Gates, or Mark Zuckerberg potentially creates space to appreciate neurodiversity. Yet alongside such entrepreneurs and innovators, New Economy firms need large supplies of cheap, contingent labor. Affluent Colleen Janeway aptly captured both edges of the sword: "My son will either end up at MIT or working at Blockbuster!" Mothers walked a fine line between pushing boys to separate and stand up for themselves in training for such competitive opportunities, but without pushing too fast or too hard for boys already exquisitely sensitive. As Colleen observed of twelve-year-old James, "My God, he's so sweet. He's so happy. He's *so dependent* on us. How independent is he going to be?"

Mothers of troubled daughters drew on the same cultural logics of gender, worrying, from the other side of the gender divide, over daughters' silences and gender conformity, but with little of the preoccupation with separation expressed by mothers of boys. Nonetheless, it was Vivian Kotler, mother of Isabel, who expressed the strongest sense of what might be at stake for vulnerable girls and boys in the postindustrial United States: "I need to bring her up to speed as far as her education is concerned because, as you know, this world, it's *very* competitive. And if you don't have the edge in some way, and if *I* don't do all that I can for my daughter, you know she's going to lose out. And I don't want her to lose out, you know, just because she has all these issues. That's no excuse."

Changing School Cultures?

Clearly the narratives of mothers point to the need to change school climates in the United States and to transform such harshly competitive peer cultures. While a good deal of attention is now being paid by educators and school systems to school-wide anti-bullying and social-emotional learning programs, the formulaic approaches being widely used may only paper over serious problems.[39] Genuine public investment might recognize as well that bullying and peer harassment are also problems of gender and sexuality. Some of the worst harms may come in gendered and sexualized forms through the gay-baiting of boys, as Michael Kimmel has argued, and following Laurie Schaffner, in the (hetero)sexualized harassment of girls.[40] In the long run, changing school cultures may lead to savings in special-education costs while improving outcomes for neurotypical children, who also suffer in schools with widespread harassment and gay-taunting. Several mothers in my group felt that their children might have functioned well, without costly out-of-district placements to private schools, had such respectful environments, along with skilled classroom teachers, inclusion specialists, and smaller class sizes been in place in local public schools—particularly if the repeated incidents that "scarred" already needy kids or induced their "school phobia" had been prevented.

The narratives of the sixteen mothers raising children of color made it clear that centuries-old perceptions of organic deficiencies among racial others persist in today's United States, leading to the racialized sorting of vulnerable children in schools. Boys and young men of color remain overrepresented in school categories of emotional and behavioral disorder, and the mothers of children of color I spoke with, far more than those raising white children, distrusted educational and medical professionals—they were sharply, painfully torn about labels and medications precisely because of their awareness that race continues to influence everyday interactions and major life chances within U.S. institutions. Their reflections on the distinct maternal work involved in raising children of color, and of the "strange coincidence" of largely unintended yet persistent racial sorting, shed light on paradoxical statistical findings: although overrepresented in categories relegated to special education and at higher risk for school failure, children of color are *underrepresented* in the most prevalent medicalized diagnosis category, ADHD, and in the numbers treated with psychoactive medications.

White mothers raising white children often described finding relief and recognition in initially gaining a diagnosis, though this reaction might be tempered with sadness and evolve over time to frustration with inadequate or inaccurate services.[41] The mothers raising children of color, however, knew they must be doubly on guard to protect their sons, who, whether neurologically vulnerable or not, already faced more precarious life chances. The medicalized labels and medications associated with whiteness might offer protection against school failure, the harsher, "adultified" framing of their disruptive behavior, and ultimately the racialized pipeline that siphons large and disproportionate numbers of young Black men from school failure to unemployment, the streets, and incarceration. In addition, I was surprised to learn, mothers saw the medical diagnoses as protection against the far more damaging labels of minimal or educable retardation. Fear and anger over those labels, which cast disproportionate numbers of Black youths with irreparable brain deficiency, arose without my prompting in four of the sixteen interviews with mothers raising children of color—yet labels of retardation were never mentioned by the thirty-two white mothers raising white children.

On the other hand, weighing against such protections, mothers raising children of color suspected that medicalized labels and pharmaceutical treatments carried different meanings for their nonwhite children. They suggested that pervasive cultural imagery of Black masculine dangerousness might only be reinforced by labels and medication, conveying the message that young Black men, inherently "bad," need to be neurochemically contained, "sedated," or "tranquilized." Nonetheless, ten of the sixteen sons of color—and three of four focal daughters of color—were medicated for at least some period, with mothers describing painful, selective decisions to relent in order to protect their children from school failure and its potentially devastating consequences.

Private Costs, Public Benefits

Large-scale studies find that many mothers with disabled children in the United States either cut back or withdraw completely from the paid workforce, a worrisome trend considering the numbers of single mothers this must include and the need for two incomes even in many two-parent families.[42] The narratives in this book capture the complex and varied ways that mothers cope with the strain on family resources of raising a needy child in a nation that largely lacks family-friendly workplaces or public family supports.[43] Only two mothers with high-earning husbands, Colleen Janeway and Judith Lowenthal, had happily chosen full-time homemaking well before their troubled children were born. Three others reported being content as homemakers, but while Lucy Nguyen's husband worked lots of overtime and brought in a decent income, Rosa Branca and Heather Dunn relied on husbands with low and, in Heather's case, less stable earnings. An exceptional few were lucky to have enough stable family support to continue working full-time. Others patched together private care arrangements or sacrificed sleep to remain in valued jobs, or worked part-time and suffered the financial consequences. At the other end were mothers who reported unhappily that they had been compelled to withdraw from the world of work. While the loss of sociability and adult identity was painful to all of them, single mothers certainly faced the most serious financial consequences.

Several, like Vivian Kotler, were compelled to turn to the state and negotiate for meager public resources to care for vulnerable kids. But in a nation still clinging to a married-couple norm and demonizing public dependence, accessing benefits through Medicaid for health coverage, Section 8 for public housing and rent subsidies, the reformed welfare system for time-limited cash assistance, or the most convoluted, Supplemental Security Income for low-income families with disabled children, requires tremendous vigilante efforts and brings a degree of surveillance in exchange for paltry assistance—surveillance that was strikingly more intrusive and threatening for the single mothers and women of color. Ironically, however, state programs—when they worked—also offered genuinely helpful programs, particularly in child mental health services, services largely unavailable or difficult to obtain privately.

This helpful impact of public psy-sector professionals like social workers and community mental health, crisis intervention, and family counselors, would be greatly enhanced if their employment conditions fully recognized feminine-typed skills and training, implemented reasonable case loads, and offered security rather than threatened austerity cuts. The same might equally well be said for educational-system personnel. It is possible that with enriched, respectful regular-education classrooms and a commitment to public neuroscience that encouraged less high-stakes standardized testing and more respect for the training and skills of feminine- or maternal-typed professionals, fewer children would be pushed over the threshold into special education to begin with or might require only limited support in mainstream classrooms.[44]

Here we do not need to reinvent the wheel or wait for further advances in neuroscience to assist more families, but to simply find the political will to expand public provisions. Well-publicized sliding-scale packages in community settings linked to schools might be made available to provide the multimodal or wraparound treatment that research has shown to be most effective. For example, though at present "unrealistic" for many families, researchers found seven-to-nine-year-olds with ADHD in a fourteen-month randomized clinical trial did best with medication and "expensive and intensive behavioral treatments" compared to those treated by either pharmacological or therapeutic treatment alone.[45] The package of costly psychosocial-behavioral supports, which included group and individual counseling for parents, summer interventions for kids in camp-like settings, extra trained aides, daily messages to parents via "report cards," and biweekly teacher consultations at schools, led to substantial improvement in behavior problems at significantly lower doses of medication than those treated with medication alone.[46] Such neuro-developmental services also reduced parents' stress, perhaps simply because each mother was not, as Vivian Kotler had so vividly explained, left to be "a team of one." If regularized, even if in somewhat less intensive forms, and if welcoming to diverse families and households rather than coming with punitive surveillance, this experimental treatment might model a truly public neuroscience.

Greater public provisions such as these would also allow women to turn away from private dependence on abusive or exploitive partners, a cost of our neoliberal conditions that also risks harm to already precarious children. Fleeing an abusive marriage, Beverly Peterson was unable to obtain SSI coverage for a troubled daughter; and while employed, she had earned too much for welfare assistance, but too little to attend to her daughter's needs. In Bev's account, this led to disastrous dependence on an exploitive boyfriend with whom she had another child, and finally, may have pushed her into a second marriage.

As I write this in fall 2013, with the federal government shut down and the country flirting with defaulting on its debts, it is difficult to be optimistic that the United States will move in the direction of greater public support in these areas. Calls for belt-tightening continue to undermine public support for the education, healthcare, and social services that all children and families need. In the United States, billions of dollars have been cut from mental health[47] and preschool early intervention programs, while federal funds for K–12 special-education programs remain inadequate.[48] The slow recovery from the 2008–9 recession, which itself stemmed directly from the neoliberal embrace of deregulated markets, continues to spark anxiety about the growing U.S. class divide and diminished prospects for youth—though we are increasingly polarized about what to do.[49] Meaningful public investments in living wages and job growth firmly located in decent, family-friendly workplaces seem a distant dream.

Yet perhaps the age of neuroscience offers more than just another way to blame mothers and enrich the large pharmaceutical companies. Rather than continuing to expect mothers to act alone, each managing her child's unique brain development, we might better use neuroscience to reinspire or reinvigorate a genuinely inclusive sense of public responsibility for children—an inclusion that does not simply relocate deficiency in ethnoracial others. Perhaps reconceptualizing children's unique hard-wiring as a critical national resource could reinvigorate a more inclusive sense of public responsibility. Rather than using new brain research to tell mothers over and over just how much depends on them, it could stimulate support for public investment in brain building and family well-being in general. As Vivian Kotler ruminated:

> How can we as a society make a good brain? Well that doesn't sound right, but you know. Because the medications are given to correct the brain, but how can we start out with a good brain in the beginning so that—the impact of these kinds of kids on society is monetarily tremendous. Not just my kid, but other kids like, like my next-door neighbor has a severely autistic kid . . . I mean that's gotta have a drain on society, not that I'm saying there's something horrible in doing that, but let's try to prevent it in the first place. Let's study the mind. Let's put our resources, a lot of resources there, so that we can have the society, you know, with upward mobility.

Here even Vivian is caught within neoliberal values, wrestling with the "drain on society" posed by burdensome children, though she comes out firmly on the side of a public neuroscience. I would urge that we make it even more public by addressing more directly our nation's contracting opportunity structure. The enemy, then, is neither neuroscience nor even Big Pharma, but each of these only when coupled with political views that deny public accountability, efface the social body, and invite the oh-so-easy targeting of "unfit" mothers.

NOTES

CHAPTER 1. MOTHER-CHILD TROUBLES, PAST AND PRESENT

1. I use the term "race" following critical race theorists to include the historical and political construction of difference, power, and inequality on the lines of ostensibly biological group differences. I thus use "race" to signal, in Brodkin's terms, ethnoracial identity and assignment (Brodkin 1998; also Omi and Winant 1994; Roberts 2011). I do not mean to suggest that understandings of ethnicity can be simply collapsed into one construct.

2. Pascoe 2007.

3. I considered both tangible and intangible economic resources, which were not always distributed consistently. Following feminist sociologists like Judith Stacey (1990) and Karen Hansen (2005), who considered New Economy restructuring and household diversity, tangible class resources included, most notably, women's household income (summarized in table 2.1), but also their education, occupation, and work history, and major assets like home ownership, family-household arrangements, and partner's (or ex-partner's) resources. In terms of intangible class resources, I primarily considered cultural capital, a concept from sociologist Pierre Bourdieu (1984) explored at length in chapters 3 and 4.

4. Mother-blame refers precisely to our tendency to hold mothers responsible for children's troubles and thus for the larger social ills ostensibly stemming from them. See, among many, Ladd-Taylor and Umansky 1998; Singh 2004.

5. Karp 2001; Malacrida 2003; Singh 2004.

6. See, among many, Murray 2008; Nadesan 2005.

7. In this sense, my argument is indebted to scholars who find mother-blame "reconstitute[d]" rather than "pierce[d]" by "brain-blame" (Singh 2004: 1193), although they do not characterize the form of this reconstitution or its intersectional dimensions.

8. Pitts-Taylor 2010.

9. CDC 2010a, 2010b; King and Bearman 2011; U.S. Department of Health and Human Services 2008.

10. Rafalovich 2005.

11. My research design aimed to capture only "mild to moderate" levels because these are the most invisible, uncertain, and, importantly, the most prevalent. I thus excluded those with children diagnosed with full-spectrum autism, only including those whose kids were considered higher functioning. I also excluded

any whose focal children were not currently living in their home. For more on my sample, see chapter 2 and tables 2.1 and 2.2.

12. See Blum 1999: 204–5; Blum and Press 2002; Malacrida 2003: 44–64.

13. Nadesan 2005: 9.

14. Big Pharma is widely used to refer to the large, multinational pharmaceutical firms and is often employed to call attention to their less scrupulous, profit-driven actions (see, e.g., Warner 2010).

15. David Armstrong in Malacrida 2003: 19.

16. See Thornton 2011: 2, 10; also Dumit 2004.

17. This extensive interdisciplinary literature is insightfully reviewed by Doucet 2006.

18. Lareau 2000b: 425, 430, 428.

19. Summarized in Home 2002; also Gray 2003; Hogan 2012; Scott 2010.

20. Wolf 2011.

21. See ibid.; also Blum 1999; Saguy 2013.

22. Murray 2008: 161.

23. This historical summary relies heavily on Apple 2006; Jones 1998; Litt 2000; Rafalovich 2001; and Rose 1998. For similar developments in France, see Donzelot (1977) 1999.

24. Written with Nathan Glazer and Reuel Denney, *The Lonely Crowd* was first published in 1948, aiming to explain how, why, and with what consequences "one kind of social character, which dominated America in the nineteenth century, [wa]s gradually being replaced by a social character of quite a different sort" ([1948] 1989: 3). Riesman put somewhat less weight on potentials for mass conformity in this shift than did his contemporaries in the Frankfurt School, but the title itself signaled some loss of individual moral autonomy (see also the 1961 preface).

25. On children of color and heritable deficiency, Harry and Klingner 2006; also Carey 2013. On the history of disability and immigration policy, Baynton (2001) demonstrates that fear of nationalities who would "handicap" the nation justified the earliest exclusionary immigration policies.

26. The helpful term "psy sector" is taken from Robert Castel, as used by Canadian sociologist Claudia Malacrida, and is informed by Foucault's emphasis on modern subjects constituted through the normalizing institutions of psychiatry, psychology, and social work (Malacrida 2003: 24, 50). It is similar to Jacques Donzelot's term "the tutelary complex" ([1977] 1997: 96).

27. For the U.S. child guidance movement see Jones 1998: 100; for "dangerous children" see Donzelot (1977) 1997: 96.

28. Tone 2008.

29. Searching http://time.com/ (July 27, 2013) with the term "human brain" revealed 2,061 articles since 1994. There have been at least eight brain cover stories with dramatic imagery since 1997 in the U.S. edition (with most also in *Time Europe* and several in *Time Asia*), including the iconic February 3, 1997, "How a Child's Brain Develops and What It Means for Childcare and Welfare Reform" story.

More cover stories emerge with search terms for specific disorders or medications (e.g., November 30, 1998: "The Latest on Ritalin"; May 6, 2002: "Inside the World of Autism"). For detailed analysis, see Thornton 2011: 92–110.

30. The term is from Judith Stacey (1990). Married-couple households made up 48 percent of American households in 2010, but 78 percent in 1950; those married couples with children under eighteen made up 20 percent of households in 2010, but 43 percent in 1950. At the same time, dual-income marriages, the largest group of those married with children in 2011 at nearly 60 percent, were just under 25 percent fifty years earlier (U.S. Census Bureau in Tavernise 2011; and Wang, Parker, and Taylor 2013).

31. Griffith and Smith 2005.

32. Nordal 2010.

33. See, among many, Furedi 2008; Nelson 2010.

34. From Blum and Stracuzzi 2004. See also Thornton 2011.

35. Mayes, Bagwell, and Erkulwater (2009) address important policy changes in the 1990s provoking greater diagnoses of ADHD, yet they assume the neuroscientific, biomedical paradigm.

36. "Cultural capital" refers to that set of intangible assets in presentation of self enriched by the right schools and summer camps, but primarily conveyed by family background, that allow one to successfully navigate professional environments, and on a larger scale, naturalize social inequality (Bourdieu 1984). This issue is explored in depth in chapter 3.

37. Eberstadt has commented that she also blames career-driven and divorced fathers (1999, 2004); a *New York Times* columnist pointed out, however, that she dispensed advice from her own life of part-time writing and featured on the front cover of her book the figure in a skirt, pumps, and briefcase, with child clutching at the ankles, while relegating the father figure to the back (Wyatt 2004).

38. Huffington 1997.

39. Conrad 1976, 2005; Conrad and Potter 2000.

40. Peter Conrad clarifies that the "engines" of medicalization have changed, with corporate profit-seeking overtaking the earlier expansion of medical authority (2005). By contrast, the greater regulation of this profit-seeking outside the United States seems to account for less medicalization of child troubles, though trends point to global increases (e.g., Zito et al. 2008; also Malacrida 2003, Watters 2010).

41. Many feminist sociologists have revised and extended medicalization perspectives by including the complexity of women's lived experiences of premenstrual syndrome (Markens 1996), childbirth (Riessman 1983), postpartum depression (Taylor 1996), and elective hysterectomy (Elson 2004), among many.

42. Conrad 1976.

43. Singh 2004: 1193.

44. Litt 2004.

45. Malacrida 2003: 136–37.

46. Each is sensitive to some intersectional dimensions. Litt (2004) attended to the particular context faced by low-income mothers from a larger study of welfare reform. Malacrida (2003) suggested many important links to class and cultural capital, but her primary focus remained the cross-national comparison. And Singh (2004, 2005), the only one to consider the masculine gender of most children, largely ignored the social privilege of her research group.

47. Warner 2010: 3, 197, 28–30.

48. Warner 2005; and 2010: 15–16.

49. Mayes, Bagwell, and Erkulwater 2009.

50. From *the Boston Globe*, Allen 2007; and Wen 2007.

51. See the websites of the National Alliance on Mental Illness, under "About Medications," http://www.nami.org/template.cfm?section=about_medications (accessed June 9, 2014); and of the National Institute of Mental Health, under "Medications," http://www.nimh.nih.gov/health/publications/mental-health-medications/index.shtml (accessed June 9, 2014).

52. See http://www.indigochild.com/ (accessed July 15, 2011).

53. Brown et al. 2004.

54. Harmon 2004; http://www.neurodiversity.com/ (accessed June 10, 2012); Solomon 2008.

55. See, among many, Harmon 2013; Padden and Humphries 2009.

56. Murray 2008.

57. Goffman (1963) 1986: 1.

58. Ibid.: 42.

59. Ibid.: 16, 19, 62, 74.

60. Murray 2008: 8.

61. Garland-Thompson 2002, 2005.

62. Leiter 2012: 20–26.

63. For collections, see Davis 2012; on passing, see Brune and Wiilson 2013: 5.

64. Leiter 2012.

65. Massachusetts state law requires school districts to have parent advisory groups of those utilizing special-education services. Such groups bring together families and mothers with a wide range of traditional and invisible disabilities, as I discuss further in the next chapter.

66. Hogan 2012; Shandra, Spearin, and Hogan 2008; Hogan, Shandra, and Msall 2007. The survey drew on an elaborated model of disability from the World Health Organization focused on degree and domain of impairment (Shandra, Spearin, and Hogan 2008: 364).

67. Also cited by Scott 2010.

68. U.S. Department of Health and Human Services 2008.

69. CDC 2012. The CDC cautions that their multisite, longitudinal surveillance method, while more accurate on each case included, is neither regionally nor nationally representative.

70. CDC 2010b. These are based on surveys of parents.

71. Carey 2005a.

72. Because of public concern with increases in autism, the CDC attempts to combine multiple data sources, including educational and health system reports, in each surveillance site for tracking autism spectrum disorders (ibid.: n. 69); but more often surveys gauging prevalence rely solely on parent reports.

73. See, for example, Akinbami et al. 2011: 5.

74. APA 1994, 2013; for criticism of the fifth, 2013 edition, see, among many, Carey 2012; and Harmon 2012.

75. Questionnaire items during the time of my research included nine impulsive-hyperactive and nine inattentive behavioral symptoms (APA 1994). On diagnostic/clinical uncertainty, see Carey 2005b, 2007; Conrad 1976; Rafalovich 2005. On seeking diagnostic technologies, Ellison 2010.

76. Diller 1998: 315.

77. "ADHD" 2007. See also Malacrida 2003; Zito et al. 2008.

78. Ritalin history, Conrad 1976: 13; in 1990s, Diller 1998: 34; with antidepressants, Zito et al. 2002; first- and second-line psychoactives, Zito et al. 2003; concomitant use, Safer, Zito, and dosReis 2003; and Harris 2006. Prozac was approved for use in children as young as seven in 2002 ("U.S. Approves Prozac for Treating Children" 2002).

79. See, among many, Bloom 2000; Schwartz 2012.

80. For more on these mothers and how I elicited volunteers, see chapter 2 and in particular the summary in tables 2.1 and 2.2.

81. Sociologists Joseph Howell (1973) and Judith Stacey (1990) use the term "hard living" to distinguish those smaller numbers of working-class families with instability, strife, and alcohol and drug problems from the large majority of "settled living" families with no greater levels of income or education (see chapter 4).

82. See Allen 2007; Carey 2007; Lavoie 2007; Murphy 2008; Reinert 2007; Wen 2007, 2010a.

83. SSI began in the 1970s for low-income families with disabled members unable to qualify for the larger, contribution-based Social Security Disability Insurance benefits (see chapter 4).

84. Wen 2010b.

85. See Bousquet 2008; also Schwarz 2012a.

86. Riesman, Glazer, and Denney admitted as much (e.g., [1948] 1989: 41).

87. Jones 1998.

88. CDC 2010b; Zuvekas and Vitiello 2012.

89. CDC 2010a.

90. "U.S. Approves Prozac for Treating Children" 2002; Guevara et al. 2002; Safer and Malever 2000; Zito et al. 2003, 2002. See also Pratt, Brody, and Gu 2011; Zuvekas and Vitiello 2012.

91. On men, masculinity, and disability history, see Hickel 2001; and Williams-Searle 2001; on women's worthiness for assistance, see, among many, Hays 2003.

92. Even with visible disabilities, U.S. policies were not need based (as in Europe) and required medical proof years after the fact, thus inviting the reinforcement of ethnoracial prejudice (Hickel 2001; Williams-Searle 2001).

93. Hickel 2001: 250.

94. Contention over the prevalence of posttraumatic stress syndrome among veterans continues however (Smith 2006).

95. Rosin 2010, 2012.

96. Rosin 2010. The dominance of biologism was also evident in her mention of testosterone as perhaps being responsible for Wall Street brokers taking on such "excessive risk" (7).

97. Kimmel 2008: 17.

98. Mishel, Bernstein, and Allegretto 2007. From the same source, prerecession income growth (between 1979 and 2000) was very unevenly distributed. Fully 77 percent of income growth went to the top fifth of Americans (see also Wilson 1998). Since 2000, this trend has only picked up. For further sociological analysis, see Smith 2001.

99. Kimmel 2008.

100. See, for example, the *PBS NewsHour* June 27, 2012, discussion of the future of public universities, especially the closing comment of George Cohen (http://www.pbs.org/newshour/bb/education-jan-june12-uva_06–27/, accessed July 1, 2012).

101. See Diller 1998: esp. 96; also DeGrandpre 2000; Hallowell and Ratey 1995; Hallowell 2006. Some brain scientists do also see causality moving in two directions—that rather than neurochemistry as destiny, psychosocial environments can modify neurochemistry (e.g., Kramer 1993).

102. While Judith Warner emphasized the importance of European work-family policies to prevention of the *Perfect Madness* (2005) of mothering in the United States, this insight was lost in her discussion of childhood medicalization (2010). See also Gornick and Meyers 2005; Mishel, Bernstein, and Allegretto 2007.

103. Cherlin 2005; Hochschild 2009; but myriad differences, in educational systems, in religious attitudes, in tighter pharmaceutical regulation and restricted advertising, may also contribute to our nation's lead in the medicalization of childhood.

104. Kimmel gets the trend right though he exaggerates the extent of the gender gap in ADHD rates (2008: 54).

105. See, for example, Warner 2010; Mayes, Bagwell, and Erkulwater 2009

106. CDC 2010b; Liu, King, and Bearman 2010

107. Murray 2008: 139–42; Nadesan 2005: 3, 129.

108. See, for example, Mullard 2009; and discussion in chapter 5. For larger critiques of neuroscience on hardwired gender differences, see Fine 2010; Jordan-Young 2010.

109. Nadesan 2005: 129; also Murray 2008: 155.

110. Nadesan 2005: 9, 128, 130.

111. Nadesan 2005: 130, my emphasis.

112. Kimmel 2008: 54; Murray 2008: 153–54.

113. Nadesan 2005: 128–34; Murray 2008: 140, 160–65. See also Bazelon 2007.

114. Discussed in Fumento 2003; also Fukuyama 2002; Will 1998.
115. Cited in Mayes, Bagwell, and Erkulwater 2009: 166, from Sowell 2001. See also Eberstadt 2004; Hart 2006; Limbaugh in Fumento 2003.
116. Steinberg 2008.
117. Thirteen of forty-eight were without paid work (a few were among the "hard-living" or were dealing with their own disabilities, as I discuss in chapter 4).
118. It was no coincidence that the 1996 legislative act ending six decades of guaranteed assistance to low-income families was titled the Personal Responsibility and Work Opportunity Reconciliation Act (Hays 2003).
119. Wolf 2011: 67; also Rose 2007.
120. Pitts-Taylor 2010; Thornton 2011.
121. Sunderland 2006: 20.
122. Shelov and Altman 2009: 156.
123. Medina 2010: 64, 6.
124. Martin et al. 2007.
125. Cheaper, quick-fix, profitable, see Harris 2011; Nordal 2010. Multimodal approaches, see Carey 2006b; Mayes, Bagwell, and Erkulwater 2009; and chapter 7.
126. Parker-Pope 2008.
127. Singh 2004, 2005.
128. Blum 2011.
129. Ferguson 2000.

CHAPTER 2. "WELCOME TO YOUR CHILD'S BRAIN"
1. Ratey 2002.
2. Aamodt and Wang 2011.
3. The research was conducted in two New England states.
4. See table 2.1.
5. Names and identifying circumstances have been changed to protect interviewees' confidentiality (also see table 2.2).
6. The psy sector, as in chapter 1, usefully refers to the range of credentialed professionals who deliver mental healthcare (Malacrida 2003); while most are located in the healthcare system, some smaller number work within the educational system.
7. Karp 2001: 222–23, 191. Karp's research focused on mental illness among adult or child family members rather than invisible disability among kids and thus did not include navigating the educational system.
8. Gabriella went through a lengthy appeal process with the insurance firm: "In the end, I had gone through their little hoops. So in the end they paid for it."
9. This particular meeting was in a largely white, middle- to upper-middle-class suburb.
10. The Supreme Court's decision of June 2012 on the Patient Protection and Affordable Care Act of 2010 left key problems unresolved. For example, access to public coverage through Medicaid for low-income Americans varies by state, with

individual states able to opt out of expansion. The Mental Health Parity and Addiction Equity Act of 2008, with added "Obamacare" provisions, should improve access; however, shortages of primary and community care providers and child psychiatrists remain unaddressed (Pear 2012; Lowrey and Pear 2012).

11. Attendance varied at the twelve PAC meetings I observed, ranging from about one dozen to several dozen.

12. The number nationwide receiving public funds for private education is often overblown by those attacking special-education budgets (UCP 2008; Winters and Greene 2007).

13. At minimum, quarterly progress reports, annual reviews, and three-year reevaluations are required (Federation for Children with Special Needs 2003).

14. Park 2003.

15. A 2005 Supreme Court decision shifting the burden of proof from schools to parents if parents contest the adequacy of special-ed services intensifies the adversarial nature of team meetings and mothers' need for legal expertise (Greenhouse 2005).

16. See, for example, the website of the largest autism advocacy organization, Autism Speaks: http://www.autismspeaks.org/what-autism/treatment/applied-behavior-analysis-aba (accessed October 3, 2010).

17. There are remarkable parallels in this exchange to corporate rhetoric and the management "retraining" meant to inspire active compliance with downsizing (Smith 1990).

18. From the Massachusetts Association of Special Education Parent Advisory Council, n.d., obtained at a local district PAC meeting in 2004.

19. The mechanistic, dehumanized talk, which I found somewhat off-putting, is simply dominant in brain research (Pitts-Taylor 2010).

20. Litt 2004.

21. The term "vigilante" in the United States spans a wide array of characters. My Google and Wikipedia search found roughly equivalent positive cultural icons (from Robin Hood to anti-whaling activists) as negative (from Ku Klux Klan lynchings to George Zimmerman's 2012 shooting of Florida teen Trayvon Martin) (also Blum 2007).

22. Merriam-Webster Online, accessed July 14, 2013.

23. Sousa 2011: 234, 236.

24. Warner 2010: 17.

25. McLeod et al. 2004: 62.

26. Stracuzzi 2005: 82.

27. This tended to be less true for those raising children of color; see chapter 6.

28. See, for example, Scheff (1966) 1999; Szasz 1974.

29. See, for example, Markens 1996; Taylor 1996.

30. On psychiatric diagnosis as a more continuous, reflexive process, see Jutel 2009; Rosenberg 2002, 2006; also Brown 1995. On the importance of naming distressing experiences, see Thoits 1985.

31. Multiple studies have found either *no* link to later drug abuse or that treated children are *less* likely to abuse drugs; see Mayes, Bagwell, and Erkulwater 2009; "Study Finds No Ritalin Link to Later Drug Abuse" 2003. *The Valley of the Dolls*, a steamy Hollywood best seller by Jacqueline Susann (1966), became a hit movie, mythologizing the eventual ruin resulting from the abuse of "dolls," "downers" or barbiturates.

32. Of the monthly meetings I was unable to attend that year (2003–4), some focused squarely on educational issues such as assistive reading and writing technologies or college advice. But others focused on recreational opportunities or sibling issues, indicating that PACs provide information on noneducational issues *other* than medications.

33. I observed seven monthly meetings in the affluent district and only five in the two diverse, less affluent districts. I attempted to compensate with phone and e-mail exchanges with two of the urban group's volunteer leaders, one of whom then joined my interview group. I also purposefully kept the in-depth interview group better balanced.

34. NIH 2011.

35. Litt 2004; Loe and Cuttino 2008; Malacrida 2002; Mayes, Bagwell, and Erkulwater 2009; Rafalovich 2005; Singh 2003, 2004, 2005.

36. Harris 2006 (also see n. 37). With thirty-two of forty-eight mothers (67 percent) administering or having administered some psychoactive drug combination, I do have a disproportionate number. Whether they are on the leading edge of this trend or represent a group whose kids were genuinely more disordered is hard to disentangle. I tend to suspect the former because of my location in New England, a highly medicalized region. Self-selection might also weigh in this direction, with many mothers I met in the field unable to meet for an in-depth interview because of their child's latest crisis.

37. For trends regarding the increasing use of these drugs among children, see Safer, Zito, and dosReis 2003; Zito et al. 2002, 2003, 2008. See also Harris 2011, 2006.

38. Psychiatrists disagree on the prevalence of such disorders in kids and on the ability to diagnose accurately at young ages, with estimates of oppositional defiant disorder ranging from 2 to 16 percent of school-aged kids, but bipolar just 0 to 1 percent (Carey 2006a).

39. My graduate research assistant and I looked for research to substantiate Rosemary's account of an eventual tolerance for ADHD medications cutting into their effectiveness. Two experts explained (in personal communications) that regardless of whether talking about stimulants, antidepressants, or antipsychotics, there is no evidence of tolerance; parents simply do not want to increase doses to handle children's physical growth or increased pathology (see, e.g., Walkup and Labellarte 2001); however, Sroufe (2012) cites at least one randomized, longitudinal study that found treatment effects of stimulant medication fading after three years.

40. Fildes 1986.

41. Goffman (1963) 1986.
42. Martin et al. 2007: 62.
43. Bellafante 2012.
44. Murray 2008: 148.
45. Jared Dunn had initially been diagnosed with pervasive development delay, an autism spectrum disorder lower functioning than Asperger. But Heather questioned this when discovering that Jared's IQ score was high. Later he was diagnosed with depression or possible bipolar disorder.
46. Garland-Thompson 2002, 2005.
47. Goffman (1963) 1986: 42, 74.
48. Allen 2007; Carey 2006a; Goldberg 2007.
49. Expert debate over *DSM*-5 centers on whether the changes are cosmetic, remaining descriptive of "constellations of symptoms" (Tanner 2012) rather than creating a "new paradigm" to press "biology, genetics, and neuroscience" to unravel causality in "the labyrinth of the brain" (Belluck and Carey 2013). Parents may be more concerned with losing insurance coverage or school services, though advocacy organizations like Autism Speaks suggest that changes are not intended to restrict access (Gorenstein 2013; Pearson 2013).
50. Carey 2005b.
51. Carey 2005a.
52. See, for example, Martin et al. 2007.
53. MAPPS 2002.
54. Martin et al. 2007: 55–56.
55. While the Amazon list is recomputed hourly, my graduate assistant and I relied on repeated checking across the latter six months of 2011.
56. Aamodt and Wang 2011.
57. Siegel and Bryson 2011.
58. Medina 2010.
59. Shelov and Altman 2009: 156, my emphasis.
60. Siegel and Hartzell 2004, my emphasis.
61. See, among many, Apple 2006; Litt 2000.
62. Hays 1996.
63. See, for example, Siegel and Hartzell 2004.
64. Sears and Sears 2003: 14.
65. Ibid.: 43.
66. Bronson and Merryman 2009: 27.
67. Pitts-Taylor 2010; Wall 2004, 2010.
68. Koplewicz 1997.
69. On the brain connectivity hypothesis see, for example, ABC NewsRadio 2012.
70. *Driven to Distraction*, by psychiatrists Hallowell and Ratey (1995), argued that ADD represents a biomedically real brain difference bringing both limitations and gifts.
71. Wymbs et al. 2008: 741.

72. Strohschein 2007.
73. Cosh 2007.
74. Wymbs et al. (2008) cautioned, however, that their measure of paternal disability was questionable, with many cases relying on the assessments of ex-wives.
75. Cosh 2007.
76. Medina 2010: 58–59, 46.
77. Ibid.: 69–70.
78. On the effects of divorce on children see McLanahan 2004; also Cherlin 2005; Rutter 2009.
79. See, for example, "Living with Autism" 2008.
80. Bolman 2006; Gray 2003; Gray and Holden 1992; Siegel 1997.
81. This literature is usefully summarized in Home 2002; see also Cohen and Petrescu-Prahova 2006; Hogan 2012; Leiter et al. 2004; McKeever and Miller 2004; Scott 2010.
82. Hochschild 1989.
83. On the relation between men's unemployment, the adult disability rolls, and the recession see Leonhart 2011; Rich 2011; Porter 2012.
84. See, for example, Legerski and Cornwall 2010.
85. Nineteen of the twenty-one turning to a psychiatric drug turned to an antidepressant, though two used antidepressants in combination with another psychoactive. On debates about the proliferation of antidepressants, see Mukherjee 2012.
86. Pratt, Brody, and Gu 2011.
87. Comparison to Valium, Koerner 1999; also Metzl 2003. For other quotes, see Blum and Stracuzzi 2004.
88. Conrad and Potter 2000; Diller 1998.
89. Singh 2004, 2005.
90. Ratey 2002.
91. Crohn's is an inflammatory bowel disease, but as Angie added, it can be triggered by stress.
92. Explicitly in Hart 2006. Suggested by the findings on stigma of the Indiana University group (McLeod et al. 2004; Pescosolido et al. 2007a, 2007b), and the conservative pundits discussed in chapter 1.
93. Kureishi 2012.
94. Ibid.
95. See http://www.shutupabout.com/ (accessed October 1, 2013).
96. Murray 2008; Nadesan 2005; Osteen 2008.
97. This dialectical notion goes beyond the social-political model that insists our notions of the body and ability are socially constructed (see, among many, Berger 2013). Instead, the dialectical model finds biology itself shaped by history, social location, and cultural practice. Disability scholars increasingly acknowledge the invisible "neuro" disabilities, though attention to what may make them distinctive yet also "disabilities" remains limited (e.g., Berger 2013; Davis 2012; Leiter 2012).

CHAPTER 3. "THE MULTIMILLION-DOLLAR CHILD"

1. On workplace inflexibility and affluent married women, see Stone 2007. On the decline of the manly industrial economy, see, among many, Rosin 2010, 2012.

2. All ten with high household incomes were married when I met them—though one, as I discuss below, subsequently divorced her husband.

3. Of the twenty-one middle-income mothers with household incomes between $30,000 and $70,000 per year, just two were full-time homemakers, six were employed part-time or intermittently, and thirteen worked outside the home full-time. I also interviewed seventeen low-income mothers, nine of whom were out of the paid labor force.

4. Cotter, England, and Hermsen 2010.

5. Malacrida 2003.

6. Ong-Dean 2009; Malacrida 2003.

7. Bourdieu 1984: 56.

8. Ibid.: 152.

9. Ibid.

10. Lareau 2003.

11. Bourdieu 1984: 186.

12. See, for example, Hays 1996. In her influential 2003 book, Lareau ignores such work (but see 2000b).

13. Lareau 2003: 180.

14. In fact, as Karen Hansen demonstrated in *Not-So-Nuclear Families* (2005), in our culture of "personal responsibility" we often overlook that parents with typically developing children also strive to create such non-commodified "networks of care."

15. Lareau (2000a), however, did point to the heavy symbolic weight accorded to upper-middle-class fathers' (infrequent) involvement with their children's schools.

16. Jacobs and Gerson 2004; Hochschild 1997; Schor 1999.

17. Giddens 1991.

18. Lareau 2003; Lareau and Horvat 1999: 42.

19. Bourdieu 1984: 215.

20. Ibid.

21. To Bourdieu (ibid.: 211–18), this is a dynamic process: elites respond to populist trends by creating renewed distinctions such as between learning a sport through early private training rather than through a school club. Such "bourgeois" athleticism also disguises class dominance as naturally occurring individual talent.

22. Ibid.: 218.

23. Styles of embodiment, in addition to being class-based, are importantly gendered and racialized, as I explore in chapters 5 and 6. On neoliberal risk culture and medicine, see, among several, Pitts-Taylor 2010; Wolf 2011.

24. The first SSRI, Prozac received approval in the United States to treat youths as young as seven in 2002 ("U.S. Approves Prozac for Treating Children" 2002); but

in 2005 the U.S. Food and Drug Administration added a label warning about the risk of suicidal thoughts and actions in some children (Harris 2006; Rose 2007). My conversations with Judith occurred in fall 2003, as the issue had begun to receive attention (e.g., Friedman 2003; Goode 2003; Harris 2003).

25. Hochschild 1989.

26. Lareau 2003: 245, 124–27.

27. See, for example, DeVault 1991.

28. Saguy 2013; Wolf 2011.

29. Swarns 2012, my emphasis. In a feminist Goffmanian sense, such initial visibility also prevents discrediting the mother if passing fails.

30. See NIMH 2012.

31. Others were also concerned with their sons' embodied fitness and the weight gain from atypical antipsychotics; see chapter 5.

32. Bourdieu (1984) noted that such foods convey particularly high status.

33. Bourdieu (ibid.: 192, 199, 201–11) might see some rejection of the "elective asceticism" required of elite women, though Judith compensated in her devotion to exercise and health foods.

34. The coincidence struck both of us that I might easily have interviewed her for my previous book, on ideologies and practices of breastfeeding (Blum 1999). While this forged a bond, Judith alluded to looking up my work and disagreeing with some of its arguments.

35. See "Munchausen Syndrome by Proxy" 2010. Among the ten affluent mothers, Gabriella Ramos-Garza made a similar quip about her struggle to gain a diagnosis for her son Diego.

36. See Ahmed 2011. For non-U.S. readers, CVS is a retail pharmacy chain; MIT, the prestigious Massachusetts Institute of Technology; and Blockbuster (was) a retail DVD chain.

37. Much research on families with disabled children confirms that mothers rather than fathers tend to cut back or quit paid work (see chapter 2, n. 81).

38. Theresa also acknowledged sadness about gaining extra pounds and sacrificing the professional wardrobe, the lunchtime gym workouts, and the manicures which represented investment in her own body capital. Privileged women's work in the New Economy does involve skilled deployment of feminine display containing pleasurable, empowering aspects (Adkins 2001; McDowell 1997).

39. According to Swedish sociologist Kitty Lassinanti, such long-term leave was relied on by the mothers she studied whose children were diagnosed with ADHD (personal communication, Uppsala University, Sweden, October 2012).

40. Another affluent married mother, Gabriella Ramos-Garza, also claimed work was a much-needed respite from a young son's volatility. Gabriella reported heavy reliance on a generously paid nanny.

41. Ong-Dean 2009, 10.

42. The Indiana University group studies stigma and children's disorders within the field of mental health and illness rather than disability as such. Thus they

compare ADHD and depression with chronic illness (asthma) and "normal troubles" (Martin et al. 2007), rather than with visible physical impairment as mothers did, detailed in the previous chapter.

43. McLeod et al. 2004.

44. Martin et al. 2007: 59, 62.

45. Nedelsky 1999: 326; also Hansen 2005.

46. Lareau 2003: 187.

47. Oakley (1974) 2005. Neither Lareau or Nedelsky consider these negative possibilities.

48. Sterzing et al. 2012.

49. Griffith and Smith 2005: 24, my emphasis.

50. Ibid.: 29.

51. Virginia also suspected there were subtle racial biases involved, and I take this up in chapter 6 (see also Blum 2011).

52. According to disability rights law, public funds should support "out-of-district" placements if an eligible student's instructional needs cannot be met in the public setting. The numbers nationwide receiving public funds for private education are quite small, however (UCP 2008: 34; Winters and Greene 2007). My interviewees include a disproportionate number with such out-of-district placements, due both to my difficulties recruiting mothers through other means and to the fact that such placements are more common in the New England states where I conducted the research.

53. The cost of hiring an attorney or educational advocate can be substantial, as discussed in the previous chapter (see also Ong-Dean 2009).

54. Park 2003.

55. Moreover, like Judith and the astute mother I observed at a special-ed parents meeting (described in chapter 2), Theresa, Colleen, and Angie each had typically developing kids in regular ed in addition to their children with special needs.

56. Ong-Dean 2009: 160. Admittedly, however, his data are limited. Also, because he considered only a large California district, he seems to put aside the impact of residential segregation and the ability of privileged parents to live in better-resourced districts where they compete primarily against one another.

57. Ong-Dean (ibid.), however, ignores the gendered dimensions of "parenting" and thus misses the multiple paradoxes confronting affluent mothers for whom privilege may make managing a disordered child both better and worse than for mothers less pressed to transmit class advantage and to confront affluent communities of negative judgment.

58. A term from Ong-Dean (ibid.: 43); and Lareau 2003.

59. Bundeson (1950) 1998: 268. Indeed, from such a Freudian perspective, Judith's extended breastfeeding might be seen as related, a symptom of maternal overinvolvement, with overinvolved mothers metaphorically described as unwilling to "wean" even adult sons (e.g., Rascoe [1938] 1998: 266–67).

60. See chapter 2 for discussion of neuropsychological assessment, originally developed to gauge brain injuries, and of dyslexia, a non-medicalized diagnosis of language-based learning differences.
61. I am cutting short a segment of Judith's narrative in which, in the aftermath of the harsh mother-blame from the public school, she secured admission midyear to a "holistic," "nurturing" private school. The school offered small classes and little academic pressure, yet it had no special-education expertise and also failed to recognize Allan's needs. Thus for several years the Lowenthals paid for a highly trained reading tutor on top of tuition while Allan's emotional turbulence at home continued unabated.
62. Federation for Children with Special Needs 2003.
63. See chapter 2.
64. Elaine offered fascinating observations about a marriage in transition as she sought to change the couple's inequitable gender division. She was clearly complaining, for example, when she said, "We sort of take turns taking Micah to the psychiatrist . . . Actually 'take turns' is the wrong word. Occasionally he will take him." But Elaine was to begin a full-time teaching position soon after I met her, a change she was anticipating happily.
65. The silence about medication issues at the special-ed parent meetings I observed, discussed in chapter 2, also evidences the shamefulness of the issue.
66. See Malacrida 2003 for Canadian and British mothers who turned to such labor-intensive alternative approaches; also Parker-Pope 2008 on growing numbers trying alternative approaches in the United States.
67. On SSRIs' effectiveness for premenstrual syndrome, see Shah et al. 2008. For feminist analysis of the "reality" of PMS, see Markens 1996.
68. Pharmaceutical firms must submit clinical data showing safety and effectiveness for new uses to the federal Food and Drug Administration and wait for approval (see Tone 2008). However, physicians may and routinely do prescribe medications "off-label," for unapproved uses, guided by the needs of their individual patients.
69. These conversations occurred in October 2003. By May 2004 Pfizer had pled guilty and accepted fines of nearly $500 million for unscrupulous marketing of Neurontin (Harris 2004; Kowalczyk 2004). By 2012, British drugmaker GlaxoSmithKline agreed to pay $3 billion and pled guilty to similar charges, marketing antidepressants Paxil and Wellbutrin and antiseizure drug Depakote for unapproved uses (Thomas and Schmidt 2012). Also see the following note, below.
70. Wilson 2010; Carey 2007. A class-action lawsuit was later filed against Eli Lilly, maker of similar drug Zyprexa, charging that Lilly hid knowledge of these common side effects; the firm agreed to settle the following year for fines of $1.4 billion (Harris and Berenson 2009; Walsh 2008). Judith also questioned the practice of prominent child psychiatrists accepting research funds from the

industry for this class of drugs, an issue receiving national attention in a 2008 Senate investigation (Carey and Harris 2008)

71. A study conducted for the *New York Times* estimated that 1.6 million youths were given at least two psychiatric drugs (Harris 2006; also see Safer et al. 2003; and discussion in chapter 1).

72. According to experts, "lithium poisoning occurs frequently" and the drug was banned between the 1940s and 1970 because of such problems (Lee and Gupta 2010; also "Lithium Toxicity" 2008, 2010). Psychiatrists currently acknowledge that some bipolar patients do better with lithium, as the alternative—the atypical antipsychotics—carry their own side effects and are more expensive (Carey and Harris 2008). Judith was well informed on this and another score: since Reagan-era deregulation, lithium falls outside the jurisdiction of the FDA, with no clear protocol to establish the safety and effectiveness of new formulations or to treat youths.

73. If affluent Elaine Irving found solace in administering only lithium to her vulnerable son Micah, less advantaged mother Rosemary Hardesty administered it on top of a drug combination to her son Josh. Working-class Jenny Tedeschi, who had done well managing her son on lithium for "awhile," had seen its scarier side when an effective level suddenly made him "very ill" and she switched to another drug combination.

74. Belkin 2004; Conrad and Potter 2000; Von Bergen 2006.

75. Pearson 2002.

76. Holden 2011.

77. McDowell 1997; also Adkins 2001.

78. Term from Stacey 1990, although she coined it to capture a more positive vision than conservatives find in contemporary family change.

79. Sociological research includes, among many, Jacobs and Gerson 2004; Hochschild 1997, 1989; Stone 2007; and in popular writing, among many, Pearson 2002; Warner 2005.

CHAPTER 4. "I THINK I HAVE TO ADVOCATE *FIVE THOUSAND TIMES HARDER!*"

1. Generous professional staff at three such schools helped me solicit volunteers. I also recruited from special-education parent meetings of three public-school districts (see table 2.2).

2. In addition to Abby Martin, those confessing a separation were Louise Richardson, Jenny Tedeschi, and Kelly Caruthers. From the remarried mothers, I include only Bev Peterson in this chapter because of the long period she had spent as a single parent (see table 2.1).

3. Census bureau data reported in "The Wage Gap over Time," National Committee on Pay Equity (http://www.pay-equity.org/info-time.html, accessed July 11, 2011); also Woolhouse 2011.

4. "Hard living" refers to precarious households with high instability of income and residence, often including substance abuse, family violence, or other traumatic

issues; see Stacey 1990; Howell 1973. Hays (2003) found that only a small minority of low-income single-mothers approximated such negative stereotypes.

5. Malacrida 2002: 377; 2003: 132.

6. Brodkin 1998: 76; also, among many, Collins 2005.

7. According to the U.S. Census Bureau (2012), 10 million of the nation's 37.8 million mothers living with children under eighteen were single in 2011. While divorce rates have been stable, divorce has become more concentrated among less educated Americans (McLanahan 2004); but unmarried motherhood has increased, as in other developed nations, across age and ethnoracial groups (Ventura NCHS 2009; also Cherlin 2005). According to DeParle (2012), motherhood outside marriage "is growing fastest in the lower reaches of the white middle class."

8. At a later point, getting back in touch with never-married Cassie Mueller, she too reported having withdrawn from all paid work to homeschool her troubled son Ned. Married Charlotte Sperling had also homeschooled one of her learning disabled sons for some years.

9. U.S. Department of Health and Human Services 2008; see also Scott 2010.

10. Hogan 2012.

11. This large-scale overhaul of "welfare as we know it" under President Bill Clinton ended federal guarantees of assistance to low-income single mothers and signaled greater national consensus around neoliberal values. TANF, with strict work requirements and lifetime limits of sixty months, is funded through state block grants which reward states for slashing the rolls and making low-income single mothers accept "personal responsibility" for falling into poverty (Hays 2003).

12. I gauged the importance of religion by how much mothers spoke of it unprompted as well as by their responses to questions in my semi-structured interview asking if they went to church, synagogue, or other religious organization, and if so, if they found this to be a support or another place of difficulty with a child's behavior.

13. Gerstel and Sarkisian 2006; McPherson, Smith-Lovin, and Brashears 2006.

14. Formal "team meetings" are mandated by the Individuals with Disabilities Education Act to monitor a student's progress under his/her Individual Education Plan, the yearly written agreement specifying the special-ed services and other accommodations to be received by the eligible child. The team includes teachers, administrators, and other professionals as well as the child's parents (Leiter 2012; Ong-Dean 2009), so the comment suggests that Vivian by herself is more effective than a half dozen professionals.

15. Heimer and Staffen 1995, 1998.

16. Susan could speak with me of the suit to a limited extent only because our lengthy interview was for research purposes and her identity and school district are known only to me.

17. Mayes, Bagwell, and Erkulwater 2009: 26, 30.

18. Perhaps this is because, as Wymbs et al. (2008) suggest, fathers who tend to such disorders themselves have lower odds of marital success, with some single

mothers more likely to regret their relationship choices, or to believe, "I should have known."

19. Medina 2010: x, 46. This advice is cast in the most authoritative terms: "'Brain Rules' are what I call the things we know for sure about how the early-childhood brain works. Each one is quarried from the larger seams of behavioral psychology, cellular biology, and molecular biology" (2).

20. Aamodt and Wang 2012.

21. Brewer 2012: 15.

22. A niche market of targeted advice books has emerged, including, for example, *Single Parenting for Dummies*, which depicts a smiling mom rather than dad on the cover. None of the lone mothers in my research group, however, mentioned consulting such works.

23. DeParle 2012.

24. See feminist columnist Katha Pollitt (2012) for an apt critique.

25. DeParle 2012.

26. Ibid.

27. Ibid.

28. Blum 2007.

29. Lareau 2003: 163, 198–99.

30. Lareau's ethnography did not aim to study children with special needs. It included two focal children, both girls, with some learning issues but no behavioral-emotional or social troubles. Lareau (2003: 209) painted a stark class boundary, however, with the married middle-class mother intrusive and interventionist, but the single (cohabiting) working-class mother, perhaps stereotypically, "content with only a vague notion of her daughter's learning disabilities."

31. Bourdieu 1984.

32. Spitzer et al. 2003.

33. Heimer and Staffen 1995: 646.

34. Stacey 1990: 46; Hansen 2005.

35. Reich 2005: 128.

36. Abramovitz 1988; Mink 1995.

37. Hays 2003.

38. Deborah Becker and Monica Brady-Myerov, WBUR, Boston, "Are the Kids Alright?" January 31–February 4, 2011; also Sasha Pfeiffer, February 2, 2011, http://www.wbur.org/2011/01/31/childrens-mental-health-massachusetts (accessed June 9, 2014).

39. See chapter 2.

40. Note 14 above; and WBUR Radio, Boston, February 2, 2011. Regional and urban-suburban differences, however, may be great: one study of a Chicago suburb found kids on public insurance 1.7 times more likely to be denied an appointment (Bisgaier and Rhodes 2011).

41. Fremstad and Vallas 2012; see also http://www.ssa.gov/ssi.

42. Wen 2011a.

43. Wen 2010c. On the congressional hearings, see Parish and Perrin 2011; Wen 2011a, 2011b, 2011c.
44. Print and online versions open with different shots, but of the same family. Two of the seven women depicted appeared racially ambiguous; however, other visual cues signaled nonwhite ethnoracial assignment, such as foregrounding multiracial children. On the demonizing "welfare queen" stereotype see, among many, Collins 1990, 2005; Lubiano 1992; McCorkel 2004.
45. Wen 2010c.
46. Astrue 2008; http://www.socialsecurity.gov/hearingsbacklog.pdf, 2007 (accessed August 16, 2013). Only some 7.5 percent of poor children receive SSI (cited in Parish and Perrin 2011).
47. Hays 2003: 167.
48. Wen 2010c. The series of four stories, with links to related follow-ups, is posted at http://www.boston.com/news/health/specials/New_Welfare/ (accessed July 20, 2011).
49. Wen 2010c; also Leslie et al. 2003; Zito et al. 2002, 2003.
50. I take up this evidence in chapter 6.
51. Only one other mother, married low-income Lucia Santos, revealed a child being on SSI. Seven mothers, including the four hard-living women whom I soon get to, received disability assistance for their own conditions. These included MS, heart disease, debilitating back injury, PTSD, depression, and bipolar disorder.
52. A large literature demonstrates this social devaluation of care, but on the devaluation of forms of paid in-home care see, among many, Hondagneu-Sotelo 2001; Stacey 2011.
53. "Disturbing cycles" in Wen 2011c. Hays (2003: 199, 212, 166) reports that only some 10 to 15 percent of those on welfare have addiction problems, but at least 15 percent have physical disabilities, and as many as 60 percent may be survivors of violence and trauma. Yet, prior to the 1996 turn to strict time limits, few remained in long-run dependency, with half off welfare in under two years (ibid: 35–36).
54. Following my research design, I excluded those whose focal child or teen was not living in the home. I met two of the four with disorganized, dysfunctional lives through a small public-school intervention program for at-risk teens and the other two through a private special-needs day school.
55. Roberts 2002.
56. I use "DSS" because this was typically the shorthand term supplied by the women themselves.
57. Cases then go to a family court, and if not resolved in court-mandated time periods, parental rights are terminated and children are placed for adoption (Reich 2005).
58. Ibid.: 177–84.
59. National patterns reported in Reich 2005; Roberts 2002.
60. I have here grouped together the single mothers with those few in the process of separation and divorce, because of the timing of state investigation amid marital breakup in the two relevant cases with DSS involvement.

61. Roberts 2002.
62. Of course, my interpretation might be off-base if Marika, more or less consciously, shaded or omitted relevant details to portray herself in a better light. I rely on the rapport evident by the amount of frank detail she did choose to share.
63. Nadesan 2005.
64. Murkoff, Eisenberg, and Hathaway 2008: 224.
65. See Reich 2005.
66. Nora recounted that when her ex-husband had finally racked up $34,000 in unpaid child support, she returned to court and gained sole ownership of the two-family property.
67. "Attachment parenting" centers on long-term breastfeeding and is most popularly advocated by Dr. William Sears and his wife and coauthor, Martha Sears, in multiple best-selling advice books (e.g., 2003).
68. See Blum 1999, chapter 4, for a comparative cautionary tale of a single mother charged with child sexual abuse who lost custody of her child for a year for attachment parenting similar to Judith's.
69. According to Kay, this was badly misconstrued from earlier comments of a private psychotherapist she and David had worked with, made to David's IEP team (Blum 2007: 219).
70. Reich 2005.
71. This became problematic when Marika had her own health scare and required surgery.
72. Malacrida 2003.
73. Roberts 1997: 8, 17.

CHAPTER 5. EN-GENDERING THE MEDICALIZED CHILD

1. On boys versus girls treated for ADHD, see Zuvekas and Vitiello 2012: 162; comparisons including stimulants and antidepressants by gender, see Zito et al. 2003, 2002, 2008; also Guevara et al. 2002; Pratt, Brody, and Gu 2011.
2. CDC 2010a, 2010b, 2012.
3. Conrad 2005; also Breggin 2001; DeGrandpre 2000.
4. See, for example, Litt 2004; Loe and Cuttino 2008; Malacrida 2003. Leiter and Rieker (2012: 1075, 1079) examine multicausal explanations for this gender gap in invisible disabilities in national survey data, concluding that too little is known about the brain or about families' "imbedded gendered expectations" to fully account for it.
5. Singh 2005, 2003.
6. Blum 2007, 2011.
7. Chodorow (1978) argued that in highly gendered cultures in which women are responsible for most early, intimate care, boys must develop greater ego boundaries than girls, renouncing identification with the mother in the individuation process to develop a masculine identity. Connell's (1995) influential work on masculinities explicitly builds on Chodorow.

8. Pollack 1998.

9. Hart 2006: 139; Fukuyama 2002.

10. Hart 2006: 154.

11. See the discussion of this issue in chapter 1.

12. See, for example, Jones 1998.

13. Freud (1930) 1961: 77n2.

14. Lareau 2000b: 426.

15. Messner 2000: 779.

16. Lareau 2000b.

17. Martin 1994.

18. Blum and Stracuzzi 2004.

19. Some frustrated mothers observed that their sons were slower to develop gross motor skills, suggesting that this might be a related neurological aspect of invisible disability.

20. Renee's story of son Bobby exemplifies C. J. Pascoe's (2007) theory of "compulsive masculinity." Pascoe importantly demonstrates that masculinity is a set of practices that demand repetition, that following Judith Butler's theory of performativity, never become one's essential identity but must be continually performed.

21. Cara Withers, while praising her ex-husband, still explained that his lack of support in dealing with their son's issues had contributed to their divorce. Caron Ross similarly complained, "You know, their Daddy, they treasure him: Daddy can do no wrong. He only comes in for the glory part—not the hard work part!"

22. Suggested by Adkins 2001; McDowell 1997.

23. As mentioned in chapter 3, there is growing legal action against pharmaceutical makers of atypical antipsychotics for promoting use among kids and adolescents while making light of such risks (Thomas and Schmidt 2012).

24. Silverman 2012.

25. Cara, from a working-class Afro-Caribbean immigrant background, had achieved a good amount of upward mobility. On the way, she had evidently developed both streetwise and professional vocabularies and hoped to pass such fluencies on to her children.

26. In the previous chapter I explained that Patricia emphasized physical modalities, diet and exercise, to prevent or forestall the need for medications. But to address lagging gross motor skills, she had also been "increasing his exercise" while struggling to have physical therapy included in his IEP for special-ed services.

27. Pope, Phillips, and Olivardio 2000.

28. Many U.S. states have passed legislation mandating anti-bullying school curricula or other related measures, but these remain subject to public debate (e.g., Engel and Sandstrom 2010).

29. Cullen 2010.

30. Kimmel and Mahler 2003: 1450; Kimmel 2008: 80–82.

31. See, for example, Brodkin 1998.

32. Schaffner (2006) finds such gendered stereotypes remarkably persistent.

33. Sterzing et al. 2012; also, a 2005 survey confirmed that kids with nonnormative body types or simply perceived as gay, lesbian, bisexual, or transgender were more likely to be bullied (in Blow 2012).

34. On widespread public perceptions of dangerousness, see Perry et al. 2007; and Pescosolido et al. 2007b. The modest correlation between mental disorders and violence is largely explained by co-occurring substance abuse—and such substance abuse is less likely among those diagnosed and treated as children (Mayes, Bagwell, and Erkulwater 2009; also "Study Finds No Ritalin Link to Later Drug Abuse" 2003; and Warner 2010: 194).

35. Kimmel and Mahler 2003: 1439.

36. Katz 2011; Messner 1992.

37. Kimmel and Mahler 2003: 1445.

38. In retrospect, I realize that my own discomfort with aggression, victimization, and violence make these frank observations from women all the more remarkable. Such comments came up without my prompting and I only truly heard them when reading and rereading transcripts.

39. Kimmel and Mahler 2003: 1448.

40. See, among many, Warner 2010: 13.

41. At Columbine, two students, Eric Harris, age eighteen, and Dylan Klebold, age seventeen, walked into the school and opened fire. In addition to those killed, twenty-three were injured and the school was held under siege (Kimmel and Mahler 2003).

42. Ibid.: 1449; Pascoe 2007. Disability theorist Tobin Siebers (2004) drew an influential parallel to remaining in the closet in his attempts to conceal post-polio syndrome. Such work reminds that there is no homogeneous experience of either visible or invisible disability.

43. Poteat and Espelange 2007; also Kristof 2012.

44. Leiter 2012: 90.

45. Brooke had readily volunteered that she was a single mother by choice, with her son conceived through donor insemination; but she offered no glimpse of past or present partners and nothing of her sexual orientation.

46. Just ten of forty-eight women reported their focal, diagnosed child to be a daughter; but Donna Simon raised three daughters, two with diagnoses and another considered typically developing (see table 2.2).

47. As mentioned in chapter 3, Munchausen syndrome by proxy is a controversial diagnosis, coined in the 1970s by a British pediatric researcher as an extreme version of the psychogenic mother: one who induces her own child's illness, or even death, just to garner attention from professionals ("Munchausen Syndrome by Proxy" 2010).

48. Abby Martin was one of just a few mothers to occasionally recontact me.

49. DSS, the Department of Social Services, investigates complaints of child abuse and neglect.

50. Feminist scholarship has demonstrated that family privacy and protection from state surveillance have long been racial, class, and marital privileges; see Hays 2003; Reich 2005; Roberts 1997, 2002; and discussion in the previous chapter.

51. To clarify, among the ten mothers with disordered daughters, there were four with midlife divorces: Abby Martin and Kelly Carothers were in the midst of the process, while Donna Simon and Rhonda Salter had been divorced for some time.

52. Chodorow 1978.

53. See, for example, Pollack 1998.

54. Gray 2003: 636, 637.

55. Leiter 2012: 90.

56. This phrase "if you know what I mean" may also allude to the sexualized basis of the harassment.

57. Donna and daughter Ann in time discovered that Ritalin was causing "spasticity of the bladder" and had to be discontinued, reconfirming my finding in earlier chapters that psychiatric medications do not work all that well and rarely represent a "quick fix."

58. For Isabel's earlier difficulties with stimulants, see chapter 4.

59. Jones 2010; Schaffner 2006.

60. Jones 2010; Schaffner 2006; Pascoe 2007.

61. Such questions about rampant bullying in schools deserve more attention to also protect transgender-identified kids (e.g., Eckholm 2012).

62. Carey 2013; Shelton 2012.

63. The use of Lupron had little credibility: it was based on the discredited vaccine theory that made thimerosal, a mercury-based vaccine preservative, the cause of autism. Testosterone was implicated only because it was thought to bind mercury to the brain. More recent theories make early testosterone exposure itself causal, though as one expert cautioned, "there is still limited evidence for the 'extreme male brain' hypothesis" (Jabr 2011; also Carey 2013; James 2008; Mullard 2009).

64. Nadesan 2005: 128–34; also Murray 2008: 140, 164–65.

65. Singh 2005: 10.

66. Griffith and Smith 2005.

CHAPTER 6. "A STRANGE COINCIDENCE"

1. See, for example, Ladd-Taylor and Umansky 1998.

2. See, for example, Klaus 1993; Roberts 1997, 2002.

3. Harry and Klingner 2006.

4. Vallas 2009.

5. Ong-Dean 2009: 79.

6. Nationally, African Americans constitute 16 percent of K–12 students but 25 percent of those labeled emotionally or behaviorally disordered in schools. Such students are at least 3 times as likely to be suspended, 2.6 times more likely to be expelled, and have far lower graduation rates than comparably disabled white students (Osher, Woodruff, and Sims 2002; see also Ferguson 2000; Committee

on Minority Representation in Special Education 2002; Losen and Orfield 2002; Rimer 2004; Harry and Klingner 2006; Harry, Klingner, and Cramer 2007; Vallas 2009; Losen and Skiba 2010; Lewin 2012).

7. Diller 1998: 149. Many advocacy groups fought in favor of ADHD's inclusion to increase school services; ultimately they prevailed, though without large gains in funds (Mayes, Bagwell, and Erkulwater 2009).

8. Morgan et al. (2013) drew this conclusion from a large, nationally representative data set which longitudinally tracked children from kindergarten through eighth grade. Safer and Malever (2000) included all Maryland public schools, finding the following ratios in white/black stimulant use: in elementary school, 2 to 1; middle school, 2.6 to 1; and high school, 5.2 to 1. Both studies found similar though smaller disparities between whites and Hispanics, and demonstrated that racial disparities persist across income groups. Zito and her coauthors compared two state Medicaid populations on all psychotropics used by youth, finding similar white/black ratios, though with some convergence over time in one state (Zito et al. 2003; see also Leslie et al. 2003).

9. Morgan et al. 2013. Also see Russell Barkley in Fumento 2003: 21; CHADD 2004; dosReis et al. 2003, 2007; Safer and Malever 2000; also Safer in "Attention Deficit Hyperactivity Disorder" 2000; Zito et al. 2003.

10. See, for example, Roberts 1997, 2011.

11. Researchers tend to focus either on overrepresentation in special ed (as those cited in note 6, above) or on understanding patterns of medical treatment (as in note 8 and 9, above). There are large literatures on the persisting effect of race in each institutional sphere, demonstrating that it is never just a proxy for social class (see, among many, Ferguson 2000; Lareau and Horvat 1999 on schools; Roberts 2011 on medical care; also Bonilla-Silva 2006; Collins 2005).

12. Crystal et al. 2009: 772; also Fitzgerald 2009: 136, 139; Leslie et al. 2003.

13. Social scientific and feminist analysis of childhood medicalization ignoring racial disproportionality in the United States includes Litt 2004; McLeod et al. 2004; Singh 2003, 2004, 2005; Blum 2007; Martin et al. 2007; Loe and Cuttino 2008; Scott 2010. Leiter and Rieker (2012) and Ong-Dean (2009: 75) each touch on the issue, though Ong-Dean with the erroneous assumption that race is only "a proxy for social class."

14. Roberts 2011: 96–97. Gabriella Ramos-Garza, affluent, highly educated mother of young Diego, also emphasized that her ample class resources were sometimes not enough, such as at a consultation with a leading pediatric specialist: "I had a long list of questions [about Diego's behavior]. After two, he stopped me, 'OK, this had better be your last.' This is where I think racism enters."

15. Ferguson 2000: 68, 65.

16. See, among many, Brodkin 1998; Roberts 2011.

17. Morgan et al. 2013.

18. Osher, Woodruff, and Sims 2002; Vallas 2009: 195.

19. Rafalovich 2005.

20. Lareau and Horvat 1999: 42, 49.

21. Ibid.: 43, 42.

22. Ibid.: 42.

23. Harry and Klingner 2006: 48–49, 98; also Safer and Malever 2000; Oswald, Coutinho, and Best 2002; Vallas 2009: 191 n.62.

24. Bonilla-Silva 2006; also Collins 2005.

25. Lareau and Horvat 1999; Vallas 2009: 189.

26. Harry and Klingner 2006: 45, 42; also Ferguson 2000.

27. Malacrida 2003.

28. Ferguson 2000; Harry and Klingner 2006: 97–100.

29. Michael's emotional response to being held back to repeat a grade may not have been unusual. Experts debate the advisability of such policies, with some contending that being held back traumatizes children for only short-run academic gains (Smith 2012).

30. "Pavlov's Dog" 2012.

31. See, for example, Mayes, Bagwell, and Erkulwater 2009.

32. Roberts 2011.

33. Collins 1990.

34. See "Proverb: It Takes a Whole Village to Raise a Child," H-Net, http://www.h-net. org/~africa/threads/village.html (1996, ret. November 19, 2009). Terms like "zombie" and "witch doctor" may also have racialized subtexts resting on African origins; these terms, however, stood in negative contrast to Cara's positive framing of shared childrearing traditions.

35. I interviewed Mildred, Lucia, and Hermalina individually but had been introduced to all three through a helpful staff member at their community organization.

36. Bravo 2004.

37. U.S. Department of Education civil rights data cited in Lewin 2012; also Losen and Orfield 2002; Rimer 2004; Losen and Skiba 2010. On school shootings, see Kimmel and Mahler 2003.

38. Artiles et al. 2002: 121.

39. Ibid.; also Harry, Klingner, and Cramer 2007.

40. Mayes, Bagwell, and Erkulwater 2009: 161–64.

41. That is, school personnel threatened to request that the Department of Social Services investigate the families for child abuse or neglect.

42. Ferguson 2000: 80.

43. Osher, Woodruff, and Sims 2002; Vallas 2009.

44. Smith 2003; Stone 2004; Head 2007.

45. Oswald, Coutinho, and Best 2002.

46. Summarized in Collins 2005.

47. Osher, Woodruff, and Sims 2002: 9; also Lewin 2012.

48. As Vivian's story of a biracial daughter's harassment suggested, Black femininity figures differently, threatening through culturally hegemonic images of

exaggerated heterosexual promiscuity, careless breeding, and public dependency rather than violence (Collins 2005; Schaffner 2006; Jones 2010).

49. Ferguson 2000: 80.

50. Losen and Orfield 2002: xvii; also Baker 2013.

51. Bourdieu 1984; Lareau 2003.

52. Lareau 2003: 180–81.

53. Ferguson 2000; Harry and Klingner 2006; Harry, Klingner, and Cramer 2007.

54. Anderson 1999; Ferguson 2000.

55. Committee on Minority Representation in Special Education 2002; Harry and Klingner 2006: 125; Ong-Dean 2009: 79.

56. Harry and Klingner 2006: 124–26. Litigation challenging such use of IQ testing has met with mixed results (Vallas 2009: 196–97).

57. Lareau 2003; Lareau and Horvat 1999; Ferguson 2000.

58. Bonilla-Silva 2006.

59. Roberts 2011: 102, also 118–26.

60. See, among many, Hays 2003. This was particularly evident in the discussion in chapter 4, above, of the new "welfare queens" trying to gain government disability checks.

61. Roberts 1997: 18.

CHAPTER 7. MOTHERS, CHILDREN, AND FAMILIES IN A PRECARIOUS TIME

1. Several valuable studies do give voice to children and youths with invisible disabilities (Loe and Cuttino 2008; Leiter 2012; Singh 2011, 2013). (Though much of Leiter's study focuses on those with traditional disabilities, she also emphasizes the distinct experiences of those with "hidden" disabilities.)

2. A few can be glimpsed in these pages because, long after choosing such fields, they inadvertently became mothers to troubled children. These include single mothers Brooke Donnelly, Dory Buchanan, Kay Raso, and Shauna Lapine.

3. Waldman 2009; Picoult 2010. On "commercial fiction," see Picoult's website quoting USA Today: "Nobody in commercial fiction cranks the pages more effectively than Jodi Picoult" (http://jodipicoult.com/, accessed May 12, 2013). Also see Murray 2008, chap. 5, on similar popular works in the United Kingdom.

4. http://www.imdb.com/title/tt1242460/, accessed May 4, 2013.

5. Murray 2008: 171.

6. Sousa 2011.

7. Leiter 2012: 69.

8. The film We Need to Talk about Kevin may be so gripping because it also plays on these meanings, taking them to an extreme: Eva, because she was not tirelessly guarding over and seeking treatment for Kevin, became the target of vigilantes, who vandalized her car and home.

9. Leiter 2012: 57.

10. The four in this case were Kelly Caruthers, Heather Dunn, Molly Greer, and Patricia Gwarten.
11. See, for example, Apple 2006; Litt 2000.
12. Wolf 2011.
13. Thornton 2011: 94; also Dumit 2004; Pitts-Taylor 2010; Rose 2007.
14. Requarth 2013.
15. See http://www.centreforum.org/assets/pubs/parenting-matters.pdf (accessed January 7, 2012). This 2011 report was taken up immediately by Sarah Teather, Minister of State for Children and Families in the United Kingdom. See also discussion on http://www.spiked-online.com/index.php/site/article/10968/ and the newsletter of the Centre for Parenting Culture Studies from August 9, 2011, at http://blogs.kent.ac.uk/parentingculturestudies/ (accessed September 2, 2013).
16. See http://www.brainbuildinginprogress.org (accessed May 2, 2013).
17. Thornton (2011) chronicles this "baby-brain movement" and similar state initiatives, yet she ignores their gendered implications.
18. According to the American Psychological Association, in a typical year Big Pharma spent a "whopping $7.2 billion" on promotion of psychoactive drugs to physicians, but also a substantial $4.2 billion on direct-to-consumer advertising of psychoactive medications (Nordal 2010).
19. Thornton 2011: 114.
20. Ibid.: 113, 9; Pitts Taylor 2010; Rose 2007.
21. http://www.lumosity.com (accessed May 1, 2013).
22. See also Thornton 2011: 10.
23. See, for example, deParle 2012; Harris 2006; Schwarz 2012a, 2012b; Wen 2010b.
24. "Brains . . . in space, *social space*," Emily Mann, personal communication March 2013; "Dialectic of biology and culture," Nadesan 2005: 9.
25. This draws heavily from feminist standpoint and multiracial feminist theories (see, among many, Collins 1990, 2005); and also the useful synthesis with feminist poststructural approaches in Malacrida 2003: 44–64 (also Blum and Press 2002).
26. Although this could be explained as a result of my volunteer sample—that is, that more passive mothers would be less likely to come forward—I did make every effort to tap a broader range through diverse school districts and utilizing helpful staff contacts (see tables 2.1 and 2.2). I was also persistent with more than a few who were initially wary and unenthusiastic about participating.
27. Stacey 1990.
28. Hansen 2005; Lareau 2003; Nedelsky 1999.
29. Hochschild 1989.
30. See, for example, Loe and Cuttino 2008.
31. Leiter 2012: 75–95.
32. Marcus 2011; Ong-Dean 2009; Winters and Green 2007.
33. Smardon 2008; also Schwarz 2012b.
34. Most of the forty-eight were recruited with more effort, through multiple calls or contacts. Table 2.2 summarizes this information.

35. A stunning example appeared in the episode "Manic" of the long-running television series *Law & Order: Special Victims Unit* in which a single mother desperate to keep her job and prevent her son's school expulsion gave him a psychoactive she had once taken herself. While laying blame on Big Pharma for its unethical practices, the script implied that a mother's irresponsibility in administering medication without a physician's supervision was also to blame when the son became manic and killed two schoolmates (season 5, episode 2, available at the http://www.tvguide.com/tvshows/law-and-order-special-victims-unit/videos-season-5/100257, accessed June 10, 2014).

36. Harris 2011.

37. Kimmel 2008: 275.

38. See also Leiter 2012: 90–92.

39. Kahn 2013.

40. Kimmel 2008; Schaffner 2006.

41. See also Malacrida 2003.

42. Hogan 2012; U.S. Department of Health and Human Services 2008.

43. See also Scott 2010.

44. Hehir 2012; Marcus 2011.

45. Mayes, Bagwell, and Erkulwater 2009: 38.

46. Mayes, Bagwell, and Erkulwater (ibid.: 40) explain that after the study and intensive therapies ended, most children seen in the follow-ups retained the gains made, but were still below comparable kids without ADHD diagnoses in social and academic functioning.

47. Goode and Healy 2013.

48. For three- to five-year-olds, per-pupil federal contributions declined steadily from a 1992 peak, with the exception of funds allocated under the American Recovery and Reinvestment Act for fiscal year 2009. The number of children served, however, nearly doubled (U.S. Department of Education 2013: 40–41). Federal contributions to K–12 special-education programs dropped from 18 percent of average per-pupil expenditures in 2007 to 16 percent in 2013, with the exception of the 2009 doubling from stimulus funds (ibid.: 25).

49. See, for example, among many, Lowrey 2013.

REFERENCES

Aamodt, Sandra, and Sam Wang. 2012. "Building Self-Control the American Way." *New York Times*. February 19.

———. 2011. *Welcome to Your Child's Brain: How the Mind Grows from Conception to College*. New York: Bloomsbury USA.

ABC NewsRadio. 2012. "EEGs May Someday Be Able to Diagnose Autism." June 26. Accessed June 10, 2014. http://abcnewsradioonline.com/health-news/eegs-may-someday-be-able-to-diagnose-autism.html.

Abramovitz, Mimi. 1988. *Regulating the Lives of Women*. Boston: South End Press.

"ADHD." 2007. *Canberra Times* (Australia). March 27.

Adkins, Lisa. 2001. "Cultural Feminization." *Signs: Journal of Women in Culture and Society* 26 (3): 669–96.

Ahmed, Azam. 2011. "Bankruptcy Judge Approves Sale of Blockbuster." DealBook, *New York Times*. March 10.

Akinbami, L. J., X. Lihu, P. N. Pastor, and C. A. Reuben. 2011. "Attention Deficit Hyperactivity Disorder among Children Aged 5–17 Years in the United States, 1998–2009." *NCHS Data Brief*, no. 70. Hyattsville, MD: National Center for Health Statistics, Centers for Disease Control.

Allen, Scott. 2007. "Backlash on Bipolar Diagnoses in Children." *Boston Globe*. June 17.

Anderson, Elijah. 1999. *Code of the Street: Decency, Violence, and the Moral Life of the Inner City*. New York: Norton.

APA (American Psychiatric Association). 2013. *Diagnostic and Statistical Manual of Mental Disorders*. 5th ed. Washington, DC: American Psychiatric Publishing.

———. 1994. *Diagnostic and Statistical Manual of Mental Disorders*. 4th ed. Washington, DC: American Psychiatric Publishing.

Apple, Rima. 2006. *Perfect Motherhood*. New Brunswick: Rutgers University Press.

Artiles, Alfredo J., Robert Rueda, Jesús José Salazar, and Ignacio Higareda. 2002. "English-Language Learner Representation in Special Education in California Urban School Districts." In *Racial Inequity in Special Education*, edited by Daniel J. Losen and Gary Orfield, 117–36. Cambridge, MA: Harvard Education Press.

Astrue, Michael. 2008. "Disability: Our Most Pressing Challenge." *Belmont Citizen-Herald*. February 21.

"Attention Deficit Hyperactivity Disorder: Ritalin Use in Maryland Schools Lowest for Minorities, Highest for Special Education." 2000. *Health and Medicine Week*. September 18.

Baker, Al. 2013. "Gifted, Talented, and Separated." *New York Times*. January 13.

Baynton, Douglas. 2001. "Disability and the Justification of Inequality in American History." In *The New Disability History*, edited by Paul K. Longmore and Lauri Umansky, 1–57. New York: NYU Press.

Bazelon, Emily. 2007. "What Are Autistic Girls Made Of?" *New York Times Magazine*. August 5: 38–43.

Belkin, Lisa. 2004. "Office Messes." *New York Times Magazine*. July 18: 24–29, 46, 54–55.

Bellafante, Ginia. 2012. "Never Mind the Champagne; Some Workers Can't Buy Groceries." *New York Times*. July 22.

Belluck, Pam, and Benedict Carey. 2013. "Psychiatry's New Guide Falls Short, Experts Say." *New York Times*. May 7.

Berger, Ronald. 2013. *Introducing Disability Studies*. New York: Lynne Rienner.

Bisgaier, Joanna, and Karen Rhodes. 2011. "Auditing Access to Specialty Care for Children with Public Insurance." *New England Journal of Medicine* 364: 2324–33.

Bloom, Amy. 2000. "The Way We Live Now: Generation Rx." *New York Times Magazine*. March 12: 23–24. .

Blow, Charles. 2012. "Real Men and Pink Suits." *New York Times*. February 11.

Blum, Linda M. 2011. "'Not Some Big, Huge, Racial-Type Thing, but': Mothering Children of Color with Invisible Disabilities in the Age of Neuroscience." *Signs: Journal of Women in Culture and Society* 36 (4): 941–67.

——. 2007. "Mother-Blame in the Prozac Nation: Raising Kids with Invisible Disabilities." *Gender & Society* 21 (2): 202–26.

——. 1999. At the Breast: Ideologies of Breastfeeding and Motherhood in the Contemporary United States. Boston: Beacon.

Blum, Linda M., and Andrea L. Press. 2002. "What Can We Hear after Postmodernism? Doing Feminist Field Research in the Age of Cultural Studies." In *American Cultural Studies*, edited by Catherine A. Warren and Mary D. Vavrus, 94–114. Urbana: University of Illinois Press.

Blum, Linda M., and Nena F. Stracuzzi. 2004. "Gender in the Prozac Nation: Popular Discourse and Productive Femininity." *Gender & Society* 18 (3): 269–86.

Bolman, William. 2006. "The Autistic Family Life Cycle: Family Stress and Divorce." Paper presented at the 37th National Conference of the Autism Society of America, Providence, RI. July 15.

Bonilla-Silva, Eduardo. 2006. *Racism without Racists: Color-Blind Racism and the Persistence of Racial Inequality in the United States*. Lanham, MD: Rowman & Littlefield.

Bourdieu, Pierre. 1984. *Distinction: A Social Critique of the Judgement of Taste*. Translated by Richard Nice. Cambridge: Harvard University Press.

Bousquet, Marc. 2008. "Ritalin Generation 1." *Brainstorm: Ideas and Culture* blog, *Chronicle of Higher Education*. September 14. Accessed June 29, 2010. http://chronicle.com/blogPost/Ritalin-Generation-1/6287/.

Bravo, Luis. 2004. "Educacion Especial, En la Escuela William Monroe Trotter" (Special Education, in William Monroe Trotter School). *Perfiles Latino Magazine*. May–June: 11.

Breggin, Peter. 2001. *Talking Back to Ritalin*. Cambridge, MA: Perseus.

Brewer, Kate. 2012. Review of *The Common Sense Guide to Your Child's Special Needs*, by Louis Pellegrino. Federation for Children with Special Needs. *Newsline* 33 (2): 15.

Brodkin, Karen. 1998. *How Jews Became White Folks and What That Says about Race in America*. New Brunswick: Rutgers University Press.

Bronson, Po, and Ashley Merryman. 2009. *NurtureShock: New Thinking about Children*. New York: Twelve.

Brown, Phil. 1995. "Naming and Framing: The Social Construction of Diagnosis and Illness." *Journal of Health and Social Behavior* 11: 385–406.

Brown, Phil, Stephen Zavestoski, Sabrina McCormick, Brian Mayer, Rachel Morello-Frosch, and Rebecca Gasior Altman. 2004. "Embodied Health Movements." *Sociology of Health & Illness* 26 (1): 50–80.

Brune, Jeffrey, and Daniel Wilson, eds. 2013. *Disability and Passing*. Philadelphia: Temple University Press.

Bundeson, Herman N. (1950) 1998. "The Overprotective Mother." In *"Bad" Mothers: The Politics of Blame in Twentieth-Century America*, edited by Molly Ladd-Taylor and Lauri Umansky, 268–70. New York: NYU Press.

Carey, Benedict. 2012. "New Autism Rule Will Exclude Many, Study Suggests." *New York Times*. January 20.

———. 2007. "Charges in Death of a Girl, 4, Raise Issue of Giving Psychiatric Drugs." *New York Times*. February 15.

———. 2006a. "What's Wrong With a Child? Psychiatrists Often Disagree: Overlapping Diagnoses." *New York Times*. November 11.

———. 2006b. "Parenting Therapy for Child's Mental Disorders." *New York Times*. December 22.

———. 2005a. "Most Will Be Mentally Ill at Some Point, Study Says." *New York Times*. June 7.

———. 2005b. "Snake Phobias, Moodiness, and a Battle in Psychiatry." *New York Times*. June 14.

Carey, Benedict, and Gardner Harris. 2008. "Psychiatric Association Faces Senate Scrutiny over Drug Industry Ties." *New York Times*. July 12.

Carey, Matt. 2013. "Mark Geier Loses His Last Medical License." *Left Brain Right Brain: Autism News, Science, and Opinion since 2003*. May 23. Accessed May 30, 2013. http://leftbrainrightbrain.co.uk/2013/05/23/mark-geier-loses-his-last-medical-license/.

CDC (Centers for Disease Control). 2012. "Prevalence of Autism Spectrum Disorders: Autism and Developmental Disabilities Monitoring Network, 14 Sites, United States, 2008." *Morbidity and Mortality Weekly Report* 61 (3): 1–19.

———. 2010a. Data and Statistics, Autism Spectrum Disorders. Last modified May 2010. Accessed March 18, 2012. http://www.cdc.gov/ncbddd/autism/data.html.

———. 2010b. "Increasing Prevalence of Parent-Reported Attention Deficit/Hyperactivity Disorder among Children: United States, 2003 and 2007." *Morbidity and Mortality Weekly Report* 59 (44): 1439–43.

CHADD (Children and Adults with Attention Deficit/Hyperactivity Disorder). 2004. "Experts Assault Undertreatment of AD/HD in African American Youth." *News from CHADD: Children and Adults with Attention Deficit/Hyperactivity Disorder* 4 (8): 1–4.

Cherlin, Andrew. 2005. "American Marriage in the Early Twenty-First Century." *Future Child* 15 (2): 33–55.

Chodorow, Nancy. 1978. *The Reproduction of Mothering*. Berkeley: University of California Press.

Cohen, Philip, and Miruna Petrescu-Prahova. 2006. "Gendered Living Arrangements among Children With Disabilities." *Journal of Marriage and the Family* 68: 630–38.

Collins, Patricia Hill. 2005. *Black Sexual Politics: African Americans, Gender, and the New Racism*. New York: Routledge.

———. 1990. Black Feminist Thought: Knowledge, Consciousness, and the Politics of Empowerment. New York: Routledge.

Committee on Minority Representation in Special Education. 2002. *Minority Students in Special and Gifted Education*. Edited by M. Suzanne Donovan and Christopher T. Cross. Washington, DC: National Academy Press.

Connell, R. W. 1995. *Masculinities*. Berkeley: University of California Press.

Conrad, Peter. 2005. "The Shifting Engines of Medicalization." *Journal of Health and Social Behavior* 46: 3–14.

———. 1976. Identifying Hyperactive Children: The Medicalization of Deviant Behavior. Lexington, MA: D. C. Heath.

Conrad, Peter, and Deborah Potter. 2000. "From Hyperactive Children to ADHD Adults." *Social Problems* 47 (4): 559–83.

Cosh, Colby. 2007. "Broken Homes, Unfocused Minds." *National Post* (Canada). June 8.

Cotter, David, Paula England, and Joan Hermsen. 2010. "Briefing Paper: Moms and Jobs: Trends in Mothers' Employment and Which Mothers Stay Home." In *Families as They Really Are*, edited by Barbara Risman, 416–24. New York: Norton.

Crystal, Stephen, Mark Olfson, Cecilia Huang, Harold Pincus, and Tobias Gerhard. 2009. "Broadened Use of Atypical Antipsychotics." *Health Affairs* 28: 770–81.

Cullen, Kevin. 2010. "Standing Up for Phoebe." *Boston Globe*. March 30.

Davis, Lennard, ed. 2012. *The Disability Studies Reader*. 4th ed. New York: Routledge.

DeGrandpre, Richard. 2000. *Ritalin Nation*. New York: Norton.

DeParle, Jason. 2012. "Two Classes, Divided by 'I Do': Marriage for Richer; Single Motherhood for Poorer." *New York Times*. July 15.

DeVault, Marjorie. 1991. *Feeding the Family*. Chicago: University of Chicago Press.

Diller, Lawrence. 1998. *Running on Ritalin*. New York: Bantam.

Donzelot, Jacques. (1977) 1997. *The Policing of Families*. Baltimore: Johns Hopkins University Press.

dosReis, Susan, Matthew P. Mychailyszyn, MaryAnne Myers, and Anne W. Riley. 2007. "Coming to Terms with ADHD: How Urban African-American Families Come to Seek Care for Their Children." *Psychiatric Services* 58 (5): 636–41.

dosReis, Susan, Julie Magno Zito, Daniel J. Safer, Karen L. Soeken, John W. Mitchell Jr., and Leslie C. Ellwood. 2003. "Parental Perceptions and Satisfaction with Stimulant Medication for Attention-Deficit Hyperactivity Disorder." *Journal of Developmental and Behavioral Pediatrics* 24 (3): 155–62.

Doucet, Andrea. 2006. *Do Men Mother?* Toronto: University of Toronto Press.

Dumit, Joseph. 2004. *Picturing Personhood: Brain Scans and Biomedical Identity.* Princeton: Princeton University Press.

Eberstadt, Mary. 2004. *Home-Alone America: The Hidden Toll of Day Care, Behavioral Drugs, and Other Parent Substitutes.* New York: Sentinel.

———. 1999. "Why Ritalin Rules." *Policy Review* 94: 24–44.

Eckholm, Erik. 2012. "Minnesota School District Reaches Agreement on Preventing Gay Bullying." *New York Times.* March 7.

Ellison, Katherine. 2010. "Seeking an Objective Test for Attention Disorder." *New York Times.* June 1.

Elson, Jean. 2004. *Am I Still a Woman? Hysterectomy and Gender Identity.* Philadelphia: Temple University Press.

Engel, Susan, and Marlene Sandstrom. 2010. "There's Only One Way to Stop a Bully." *New York Times.* July 23.

Federation for Children with Special Needs. 2003. Basic Rights Training. Boston. http://fcsn.org/. Accessed March 30, 2004.

Ferguson, Ann Arnett. 2000. *Bad Boys: Public Schools in the Making of Black Masculinity.* Ann Arbor: University of Michigan Press.

Fildes, Valerie. 1986. *Breasts, Bottles, and Babies: A History of Infant Feeding.* Edinburgh: Edinburgh University Press.

Fine, Cordelia. 2010. *Delusions of Gender.* New York: Norton.

Fitzgerald, Terence. 2009. *White Prescriptions: The Dangerous Social Potential for Ritalin and Other Psychotropic Drugs to Harm Black Males.* Boulder, CO: Paradigm.

Fremstad, Shawn, and Rebecca Vallas. 2012. "Supplemental Security Income for Children with Disabilities." *Social Security Brief* 40 (November): 1–15.

Freud, Sigmund. (1930) 1961. *Civilization and Its Discontents.* New York: Norton.

Friedman, Richard. 2003. "What You Do Know Can't Hurt You." *New York Times.* August 12.

Fukuyama, Francis. 2002. *Our Posthuman Future: Consequences of the Biotechnology Revolution.* New York: Farrar, Straus and Giroux.

Fumento, Michael. 2003. "Trick Question: A Liberal 'Hoax' Turns Out to Be True." *New Republic* 228 (4): 18–21.

Furedi, Frank. 2008. *Paranoid Parenting.* 2nd ed. London: Continuum Press.

Garland-Thomson, Rosemarie. 2005. "Feminist Disability Studies." *Signs: Journal of Women in Culture and Society* 30 (2): 1557–87.

———. 2002. "Integrating Disability, Transforming Feminist Theory." *NWSA Journal* 14 (3): 1–32.

Gerstel, Naomi, and Natalia Sarkisian. 2006. "Marriage: The Good, the Bad, and the Greedy." *Contexts* 5 (4): 16–21.

Giddens, Anthony. 1991. *Modernity and Self-Identity: Self and Society in the Late Modern Age*. Cambridge, UK: Polity Press.

Goffman, Erving. (1963) 1986. *Stigma: Notes on the Management of Spoiled Identity*. New York: Touchstone.

Goldberg, Carey. 2007. "Bipolar Labels for Children Stir Concern." *Boston Globe*. February 15.

Goode, Erica. 2003. "British Warning on Antidepressant Use for Youth." *New York Times*. December 11.

Goode, Erica, and Jack Healy. 2013. "Focus on Mental Health Laws to Curb Violence Is Unfair, Some Say." *New York Times*. February 1.

Gorenstein, Dan. 2013. "How Much Is the DSM-5 Worth?" *Marketplace*. May 17. Accessed July 16, 2013. http://www.marketplace.org/topics/business/health-care/how-much-dsm-5-worth.

Gornick, Janet, and Marcia Meyers. 2005. *Families That Work*. New York: Russell Sage.

Gray, David E. 2003. "Gender and Coping: The Parents of Children with High-Functioning Autism." *Social Science & Medicine* 56: 631–42.

Gray, David E., and William J. Holden. 1992. "Psycho-Social Well-Being among the Parents of Children with Autism." *Australia and New Zealand Journal of Developmental Disabilities* 18 (2): 83–93.

Greenhouse, Linda. 2005. "Burden of Proof Now on Parents in School Cases." *New York Times*. November 15.

Griffith, Allison, and Dorothy Smith. 2005. *Mothering for Schooling*. New York: RoutledgeFalmer.

Guevara, J., P. Lozano, T. Wickizer, L. Mell, and H. Gephart. 2002. "Psychotropic Medication Use in a Population of Children Who Have Attention-Deficit/Hyperactivity Disorder." *Pediatrics* 109 (5): 733–39.

Hallowell, Edward. 2006. *Crazy Busy*. New York: Ballantine.

Hallowell, Edward M., and John J. Ratey. 1995. *Driven to Distraction*. New York: Simon and Schuster.

Hansen, Karen V. 2005. *Not-So-Nuclear Families: Class, Gender, and Networks of Care*. New Brunswick: Rutgers University Press.

Harmon, Amy. 2012. "The Autism Wars." Sunday Review, *New York Times*. April 8.

———. 2004. "How About Not 'Curing' Us, Some Autistics Are Pleading." *New York Times*. December 20.

Harmon, Kristen. 2013. "Growing Up to Become Hearing: Dreams of Passing in Oral Deaf Education." In *Disability and Passing: Blurring the Lines of Identity*, edited by Jeffrey Brune and Daniel Wilson, 167–98. Philadelphia: Temple University Press.

Harris, Gardiner. 2011. "Talk Doesn't Pay, So Psychiatry Turns Instead to Drug Therapy." *New York Times*. March 6.

———. 2006. "Proof Is Scant on Psychiatric Drug Mix for Young." *New York Times*. November 23.

———. 2004. "Pfizer to Pay $430 Million over Promoting Drug to Doctors." *New York Times*. May 14.

———. 2003. "Britain Says Use of Paxil by Children Is Dangerous." *New York Times.* June 11.

Harris, Gardiner, and Alex Berenson. 2009. "Settlement Called Near on Zyprexa." *New York Times.* January 14.

Harry, Beth, and Janette Klingner. 2006. *Why Are So Many Minority Students in Special Education? Understanding Race and Disability in Schools.* New York: Teachers College Press.

Harry, Beth, Janette Klingner, and Elizabeth Cramer. 2007. *Case Studies of Minority Student Placement in Special Education.* With the assistance of Keith M. Sturges and Robert F. Moore. New York: Teachers College Press.

Hart, Nicky. 2006. "Making the Grade: The Gender Gap, ADHD, and the Medicalization of Boyhood." With the assistance of Noah Grand and Kevin Riley. In *Medicalized Masculinities,* edited by Dana Rosenfeld and Christopher A. Faircloth, 132–64. Philadelphia: Temple University Press.

Hays, Sharon. 2003. *Flat Broke with Children.* New York: Oxford University Press.

———. 1996. *The Cultural Contradictions of Motherhood.* New Haven: Yale University Press.

Head, John F. 2007. "Why, Even Today, Many Blacks Are Wary about American Medicine." Review of *Medical Apartheid: The Dark History of Medical Experimentation on Black Americans from Colonial Times to the Present,* by Harriet A. Washington. *The Crisis* 114 (1): 48–49.

Hehir, Thomas. 2012. *Effective Inclusive Schools.* With Lauren Katzman. New York: Jossey-Bass.

Heimer, Carol, and Lisa Staffen. 1998. *For the Sake of the Children.* Chicago: University of Chicago Press.

———. 1995. "Interdependence and Reintegrative Social Control: Labeling and Reforming 'Inappropriate' Parents in Neonatal Intensive Care Units." *American Sociological Review* 60: 635–54.

Hickel, K. Walter. 2001. "Medicine, Bureaucracy, and Social Welfare: The Politics of Disability Compensation for American Veterans of World War I." In *The New Disability History,* edited by Paul K. Longmore and Lauri Umansky, 236–67. New York: NYU Press.

Hochschild, Arlie. 2009. "Crossroads: The State of Family, Class, and Culture." Sunday Book Review, *New York Times.* October 16.

———. 1997. *The Time Bind: When Work Becomes Home and Home Becomes Work.* New York: Henry Holt.

———. 1989. *The Second Shift.* With the assistance of Ann Machung. New York: Penguin.

Hogan, Dennis. 2012. *Family Consequences of Children's Disabilities.* New York: Russell Sage Foundation.

Hogan, Dennis, Carrie Shandra, and Michael Msall. 2007. "Family Developmental Risk Factors among Adolescents with Disabilities and Children of Parents with Disabilities." *Journal of Adolescence* 30 (6): 1001–19.

Holden, Stephen. 2011. "Even a Things-to-Do List Seems to Be Multitasking: Review of *I Don't Know How She Does It*." *New York Times*. September 15.

Home, Alice. 2002. "Challenging Hidden Oppression, Mothers Caring for Children with Disabilities." *Critical Social Work* 2 (2): 88–103.

Hondagneu-Sotelo, Pierrette. 2001. *Doméstica*. Berkeley: University of California Press.

Howell, Joseph. 1973. *Hard Living on Clay Street*. Garden City, NY: Anchor Press.

Huffington, Arianna. 1997. "Peppermint Prozac." *U.S. News & World Report*. August 18.

Jabr, Ferris. 2011. "Faulty Testosterone Cycle May Explain Male Autism Bias." *New Scientist*. February 17. Accessed May 30, 2013. http://www.newscientist.com/article/dn20143-faulty-testosterone-cycle-may-explain-male-autism-bias.html#. UjBvDxYjirA.

Jacobs, Jerry, and Kathleen Gerson. 2004. *The Time Divide*. Cambridge: Harvard University Press.

James, William H. 2008. "Further Evidence That Some Male-Based Neurodevelopmental Disorders Are Associated with High Intrauterine Testosterone Concentrations." *Developmental Medicine and Child Neurology* 50 (1): 15–18.

Jones, Kathleen W. 1998. "'Mother Made Me Do It': Mother-Blaming and the Women of Child Guidance." In *"Bad" Mothers: The Politics of Blame in Twentieth-Century America*, edited by Molly Ladd-Taylor and Lauri Umansky, 99–124. New York: NYU Press.

Jones, Nikki. 2010. *Between Good and Ghetto*. New Brunswick: Rutgers University Press.

Jordan-Young, Rebecca. 2010. *Brain Storm: The Flaws in the Science of Sex Differences*. Cambridge: Harvard University Press.

Jutel, Annemarie. 2009. "Sociology and Diagnosis: A Preliminary Review." *Sociology of Health & Illness* 31 (2): 278–99.

Kahn, Jennifer. 2013. "Reading, Writing, and . . . Emotional Intelligence." *New York Times Magazine*. September 15: 44–49.

Karp, David. 2001. *The Burden of Sympathy: How Families Cope with Mental Illness*. New York: Oxford University Press.

Katz, Jackson. 2011. "Advertising and the Construction of Violent White Masculinity: From BMWs to Bud Light." In *Gender, Race, and Class in Media: A Critical Reader*, 2nd ed., edited by G. Dines and J. Humez, 261–69. Thousand Oaks, CA: Sage.

Kimmel, Michael. 2008. *Guyland: The Perilous World Where Boys Become Men*. New York: Harper.

Kimmel, Michael, and Matthew Mahler. 2003. "Adolescent Masculinity, Homophobia, and Violence." *American Behavioral Scientist* 46 (10): 1439–58.

King, Marissa, and Peter Bearman. 2011. "Socioeconomic Status and the Increased Prevalence of Autism in California." *American Sociological Review* 76 (2): 320–46.

Klaus, Alisa. 1993. "Depopulation and Race Suicide: Maternalism and Pronatalist Ideologies in France and the United States." In *Mothers of a New World: Maternalist Politics and the Origins of Welfare States*, edited by Seth Koven and Sonya Michel, 188–212. New York: Routledge.

Koerner, Brendan. 1999. "Leo Sternbach, the Father of Mother's Little Helpers." *U.S. News & World Report*. December 27.

Koplewicz, Harold. 1997. *It's Nobody's Fault: New Hope and Help for Difficult Children and Their Parents*. New York: Three Rivers Press.

Kowalczyk, Liz. 2004. "Pfizer Unit Agrees to $430M in Fines." *Boston Globe*. May 14.

Kramer, Peter. 1993. *Listening to Prozac*. New York: Penguin.

Kristof, Nicholas. 2012. "Born to Not Get Bullied." *New York Times*. March 1.

Kureishi, Hanif. 2012. "The Art of Distraction." Sunday Review, *New York Times*. February 19.

Ladd-Taylor, Molly, and Lauri Umansky, eds. 1998. *"Bad" Mothers: The Politics of Blame in Twentieth-Century America*. New York: NYU Press.

Lareau, Annette. 2003. *Unequal Childhoods: Class, Race, and Family Life*. Berkeley: University of California Press.

———. 2000a. Home Advantage: Social Class and Parental Intervention in Elementary Education. 2nd ed. Lanham, MD: Rowman & Littlefield.

———. 2000b. "My Wife Can Tell Me Who I Know: Methodological and Conceptual Problems in Studying Fathers." Qualitative Sociology 23 (4): 407–33.

Lareau, Annette, and Erin McNamara Horvat. 1999. "Moments of Social Inclusion and Exclusion: Race, Class, and Cultural Capital in Family-School Relationships." *Sociology of Education* 71 (1): 37–53.

Lavoie, Denise. 2007. "Girl's Overdose Raises Questions about Psychiatric Meds for Kids." *Sentinel & Enterprise* (Fitchburg, MA). March 26.

Lee, David C., and Amit Gupta. 2010. "Lithium Toxicity." *Medscape Reference*. Accessed November 13, 2012. http://emedicine.medscape.com/article/815523-overview.

Legerski, Elizabeth Miklya, and Marie Cornwall. 2010. "Working-Class Job Loss, Gender, and the Negotiation of Household Labor." *Gender & Society* 24 (4): 447–74.

Leiter, Valerie. 2012. *Their Time Has Come: Youth with Disabilities on the Cusp of Adulthood*. New Brunswick: Rutgers University Press.

Leiter, Valerie, Marty Krauss, Betsy Anderson, and Nora Wells. 2004. "The Consequences of Caring." *Journal of Family Issues* 25 (3): 379–403.

Leiter, Valerie, and Patricia Rieker. 2012. "Mind the Gap: Gender Differences in Child Special Health Care Needs." *Journal of Maternal Child Health* 16: 1072–80.

Leonhardt, David. 2011. "Men, Unemployment, and Disability." Economix, *New York Times*. April 8.

Leslie, Laurel K., Jill Weckerly, John Landsverk, Richard L. Hough, Michael S. Hurlburt, and Patricia A. Wood. 2003. "Racial/Ethnic Differences in the Use of Psychotropic Medication in High-Risk Children and Adolescents." *Journal of the American Academy of Child and Adolescent Psychiatry* 42 (12): 1433–42.

Lewin, Tamar. 2012. "Black Students Face More Discipline, Data Suggests." *New York Times*. March 6.

"Lithium Toxicity." 2010. *MedlinePlus Medical Encyclopedia*. U.S. National Library of Medicine, National Institutes of Health. Accessed November 13, 2012. http://www.nlm.nih.gov/medlineplus/ency/article/002667.htm.

———. 2008. *MedTV*. Accessed November 13, 2012. http://bipolar-disorder.emedtv. com/lithium/lithium-toxicity.html.

Litt, Jacquelyn. 2004. "Women's Carework in Low-Income Households." *Gender & Society* 18 (5): 625–44.

———. 2000. *Medicalized Motherhood: Perspectives from the Lives of African-American and Jewish Women*. New Brunswick: Rutgers University Press.

Liu, Ka-Yuet, Marissa King, and Peter Bearman. 2010. "Social Influence and the Autism Epidemic." *American Journal of Sociology* 115: 1387–1434.

"Living with Autism." 2008. Easter Seals, conducted by Harris Interactive with Autism Society of America. Accessed February 22, 2010. http://www.actforautism.org/.

Loe, Meika, and Leigh Cuttino. 2008. "Grappling with the Medicated Self: The Case of ADHD College Students." *Symbolic Interaction* 31 (3): 303–23.

Losen, Daniel J., and Gary Orfield, eds. 2002. *Racial Inequity in Special Education*. Cambridge, MA: Harvard Education Press.

Losen, Daniel, and Russell Skiba. 2010. *Suspended Education: Urban Middle Schools in Crisis*. Montgomery, AL: Southern Poverty Law Center.

Lowrey, Annie. 2013. "When Problems Start Getting Real" *New York Times Magazine*. March 31: 12–13.

Lowrey, Annie, and Robert Pear. 2012. "Doctor Shortage Likely to Worsen with Health Law." *New York Times*. July 29.

Lubiano, Wahneema. 1992. "Black Ladies, Welfare Queens, and State Minstrels." In *Race-ing Justice, En-gendering Power*, edited by Toni Morrison, 323–63. New York: Pantheon.

Malacrida, Claudia. 2003. *Cold Comfort: Mothers, Professionals, and Attention Deficit Disorder*. Toronto: University of Toronto Press.

———. 2002. "Alternative Therapies and Attention Deficit Disorder: Discourses of Maternal Responsibility and Risk." *Gender & Society* 16 (3): 366–85.

MAPPS (Massachusetts Association of 766 Approved Private Schools). 2002. Directory of Member Schools, Wakefield, MA. Last modified 2008. http://www.spedschools.com/.

Marcus, Jon. 2011. "The Test Ahead." *Boston Globe Magazine*. October 9: 16–19, 26–29.

Markens, Susan. 1996. "The Problematic of 'Experience.'" *Gender & Society* 10: 42–58.

Martin, Emily. 1994. *Flexible Bodies*. Boston: Beacon.

Martin, Jack K., Bernice A. Pescosolido, Sigrun Olafsdottir, and Jane McLeod. 2007. "The Construction of Fear: Americans' Preferences for Social Distance from Children and Adolescents with Mental Health Problems." *Journal of Health and Social Behavior* 48: 50–67.

Mayes, Rick, Catherine Bagwell, and Jennifer Erkulwater. 2009. *Medicating Children: ADHD and Pediatric Mental Health*. Cambridge: Harvard University Press.

McCorkel, Jill. 2004. "Criminally Dependent? Gender, Punishment, and the Rhetoric of Welfare Reform." *Social Politics* 11 (3): 386–410.

McDowell, Linda. 1997. *Capital Culture*. Oxford: Blackwell.

McKeever, Patricia, and Karen-Lee Miller. 2004. "Mothering Children Who Have Disabilities." *Social Science & Medicine* 59 (6): 1177–91.

McLanahan, Sara. 2004. "Diverging Destinies: How Children Are Faring under the Second Demographic Transition." *Demography* 41: 607–27.

McLeod, Jane D., Bernice Pescosolido, David T. Takeuchi, and Terry Falkenberg White. 2004. "Public Attitudes toward the Use of Psychiatric Medications for Children." *Journal of Health and Social Behavior* 45: 53–67.

McPherson, Miller, Lynn Smith-Lovin, and Matthew Brashears. 2006. "Social Isolation in America." *American Sociological Review* 71 (3): 353–75.

Medina, John. 2010. *Brain Rules for Baby: How to Raise a Smart and Happy Child from Zero to Five.* New York: Pear Press.

Messner, Michael. 2000. "Barbie Girls versus Sea Monsters." *Gender & Society* 14: 765–84.

———. 1992. *Power at Play.* Boston: Beacon.

Metzl, Jonathan. 2003. *Prozac on the Couch: Prescribing Gender in the Era of Wonder Drugs.* Durham: Duke University Press.

Mink, Gwendolyn. 1995. *The Wages of Motherhood: Inequality in the Welfare State, 1917–1942.* Ithaca: Cornell University Press.

Mishel, Lawrence, Jared Bernstein, and Sylvia Allegretto. 2007. *The State of Working America, 2006–2007.* Washington, DC: Economic Policy Institute.

Morgan, Paul, Jeremy Staff, Marianne Hillemeier, George Farkas, and Steven Maczuga. 2013. "Racial and Ethnic Disparities in ADHD Diagnosis from Kindergarten to Eighth Grade." *Pediatrics* 132 (1): 85–93.

Mukherjee, Siddhartha. 2012. "Post-Prozac Nation." *New York Times Magazine.* April 22: 48–54.

Mullard, Asher. 2009. "What Is the Link between Autism and Testosterone?" *Nature.* January 1. Accessed May 30, 2013. http://www.nature.com/news/2009/090113/full/news.2009.21.html.

"Munchausen Syndrome by Proxy." 2010. *MedlinePlus Medical Encyclopedia.* U.S. National Library of Medicine, National Institutes of Health. Accessed June 9, 2013. http://www.nlm.nih.gov/medlineplus/ency/article/001555.htm.

Murkoff, Heidi Eisenberg, Arlene Eisenberg, and Sandee Hathaway. 2008. *What to Expect the First Year.* NY: Workman.

Murphy, Shelley. 2008. "Doctor Is Sued in Death of Girl, 4." *Boston Globe.* April 4.

Murray, Stuart. 2008. *Representing Autism.* Liverpool: Liverpool University Press.

Nadesan, Majia Holmer. 2005. *Constructing Autism.* New York: Routledge.

Nedelsky, Jennifer. 1999. "Dilemmas of Passion, Privilege, and Isolation: Reflections on Mothering in a White, Middle-Class Nuclear Family." In *Mother Troubles,* edited by J. Hanigsberg and S. Ruddick, 304–34. Boston: Beacon.

Nelson, Margaret K. 2010. *Parenting Out of Control.* New York: NYU Press.

NIH (National Institutes of Health). 2011. "What Is Dyslexia?" National Institute of Neurological Disorders and Stroke, National Institutes of Health. September 30. Accessed July 25, 2012. http://www.ninds.nih.gov/disorders/dyslexia/dyslexia.htm.

NIMH (National Institute of Mental Health). 2012. "Atypical Antipsychotic More Effective Than Older Drugs in Treating Childhood Mania, but Side Effects Can Be

Serious." *Science Update*. January 11. Accessed November 13, 2012. http://www.nimh.
nih.gov/news/science-news/2012/atypical-antipsychotic-more-effective-than-older-
drugs-in-treating-childhood-mania-but-side-effects-can-be-serious.shtml.

Nordal, Katherine. 2010. "Where Has All the Psychotherapy Gone?" *Monitor on Psychology* 41 (10): 17.

Oakley, Ann. (1974) 2005. "The Invisible Woman: Sexism in Sociology." In *The Ann
Oakley Reader*, edited by Ann Oakley, 189–205. Bristol, UK: Policy Press.

Omi, Michael, and Howard Winant. 1994. *Racial Formation in the United States*. New
York: Routledge.

Ong-Dean, Colin. 2009. *Distinguishing Disability: Parents, Privilege, and Special Education*. Chicago: University of Chicago Press.

Osher, David, Darren Woodruff, and Anthony E. Sims. 2002. "Schools Make a Difference: The Overrepresentation of African American Youth in Special Education and
the Juvenile Justice System." In *Racial Inequity in Special Education*, edited by Daniel J. Losen and Gary Orfield, 93–116. Cambridge, MA: Harvard Education Press.

Osteen, Mark. 2008. *Autism and Representation*. New York: Routledge.

Oswald, Donald P., Martha J. Coutinho, and Al M. Best. 2002. "Community and
School Predictors of Overrepresentation of Minority Children in Special Educa-
tion." In *Racial Inequity in Special Education*, edited by Daniel J. Losen and Gary
Orfield, 1–14. Cambridge, MA: Harvard Education Press.

Padden, Carol, and Tom Humphries. 2009. *Inside Deaf Culture*. Cambridge: Harvard
University Press.

Parish, Susan, and James Perrin. 2011. "Cutting SSI Would Only Hurt Children." Opinion, *USA Today*. October 26.

Park, Sarah. 2003. "Recalculating Needs." *Boston Globe*. June 20.

Parker-Pope, Tara. 2008. "Weighing Nondrug Options for ADHD." *New York Times*.
June 17.

Pascoe, C. J. 2007. *Dude, You're a Fag*. Berkeley: University of California Press.

"Pavlov's Dog." 2012. Nobel Media AB. Accessed March 16, 2012. http://www.nobel-
prize.org/educational/medicine/pavlov/.

Pear, Robert. 2012. "Next Health Law Battle: Insurance Exchanges." *New York Times*.
July 8.

Pearson, Allison. 2002. *I Don't Know How She Does It*. New York: Anchor.

Pearson, Catherine. 2013. "DSM-5 Changes: What Parents Need to Know about the
First Major Revision in Nearly 20 Years." HuffPost Parents, *Huffington Post*. May 20.
Accessed July 16, 2013. http://www.huffingtonpost.com/2013/05/20/dsm5-changes-
what-parents-need-to-know_n_3294413.html.

Perry, Brea, Bernice Pescosolido, Jack Martin, Jane McLeod, and Peter S. Jensen. 2007.
"Comparison of Public Attributions, Attitudes, and Stigma in Regard to Depression
among Children and Adults." *Psychiatric Services* 58 (5): 632–35.

Pescosolido, B., B. L. Perry, J. K. Martin, and J. McLeod. 2007a. "Stigmatizing Attitudes
and Beliefs about Treatment and Psychiatric Medications for Children with Mental
Illness." *Psychiatric Services* 58: 613–18.

Pescosolido, Bernice, Danielle Fettes, Jack Martin, John Monahan, and Jane McLeod. 2007b. "Perceived Dangerousness of Children with Mental Health Problems and Support for Coerced Treatment." *Psychiatric Services* 58 (5): 619–25.

Picoult, Jodi. 2010. *House Rules.* New York: Atria Books.

Pitts-Taylor, Victoria. 2010. "The Plastic Brain: Neoliberalism and the Neuronal Self." *Health* 14 (6): 635–52.

Pollack, William. 1998. *Real Boys: Rescuing Our Sons from the Myth of Boyhood.* New York: Random House.

Pollitt, Katha. 2012. "The New York Times Misses the Mark on Inequality, Marriage." *The Nation.* July 17. http://www.thenation.com/blog/168932/new-york-times-misses-mark-inequality-marriage#axzz2eafdkXcU. Accessed August 4, 2012.

Pope, Harrison, Katherine Phillips, and Roberto Olivardio. 2000. *The Adonis Complex.* New York: Simon & Schuster.

Porter, Eduardo. 2012. "Disability Insurance Causes Pain." *New York Times.* April 25.

Poteat, V., and D. Espelage. 2007. "Predicting Psychosocial Consequences of Homophobic Victimization in Middle School Students." *Journal of Early Adolescence* 27: 175–91.

Pratt, Laura A., Debra J. Brody, and Qiuping Gu. 2011. "Antidepressant Use in Persons Aged 12 and Over: United States, 2005–2008." *NCHS Data Brief,* no. 76. Hyattsville, MD: National Center for Health Statistics, Centers for Disease Control.

Rafalovich, Adam. 2005. "Exploring Clinician Uncertainty in the Diagnosis and Treatment of Attention Deficit Hyperactivity Disorder." *Sociology of Health & Illness* 27 (3): 305–23.

———. 2001. "The Conceptual History of Attention Deficit Hyperactivity Disorder." *Deviant Behavior* 22: 93–115.

Rascoe, Burton. (1938) 1998. "On a Hickory Limb." In *"Bad" Mothers: The Politics of Blame in Twentieth-Century America,* edited by Molly Ladd-Taylor and Lauri Umansky, 266–67. New York: NYU Press.

Ratey, John J. 2002. *A User's Guide to the Brain.* New York: Vintage.

Reich, Jennifer. 2005. *Fixing Families.* New York: Routledge.

Reinert, Sue. 2007. "DSS to Murder-Suspect Parents: Give Up Children." *Patriot Ledger* (Quincy, MA). May 17.

Requarth, Tim. 2013. "Bringing a Virtual Brain to Life." *New York Times.* March 19.

Rich, Motoko. 2011. "Moving from Disability Benefits to Jobs." Economix, *New York Times.* April 7.

Riesman, David. (1948) 1989. *The Lonely Crowd.* With the assistance of Nathan Glazer and Reuel Denney. New Haven: Yale University Press.

Riessman, Catherine Kohler. 1983. "Women and Medicalization." *Social Policy* 14: 3–18.

Rimer, Sara. 2004. "Unruly Students Facing Arrest, Not Detention." *New York Times.* January 4.

Roberts, Dorothy. 2011. *Fatal Invention: How Science, Politics, and Big Business Recreate Race in the Twenty-First Century.* New York: New Press.

———. 2002. *Shattered Bonds.* New York: Basic.

———. 1997. *Killing the Black Body*. New York: Pantheon.

Rose, Elizabeth. 1998. "Taking on a Mother's Job: Day Care in the 1920s and 1930s." In *"Bad" Mothers: The Politics of Blame in Twentieth-Century America*, edited by Molly Ladd-Taylor and Lauri Umansky, 67–98. New York: NYU Press.

Rose, Nikolas. 2007. *The Politics of Life Itself*. Princeton: Princeton University Press.

Rosenberg, Charles. 2006. "Contested Boundaries: Psychiatry, Disease, and Diagnosis." *Perspectives in Biology and Medicine* 49 (3): 407–24.

———. 2002. "The Tyranny of Diagnosis." *Milbank Quarterly* 80 (2): 232–60.

Rosin, Hanna. 2012. *The End of Men*. New York: Riverhead.

———. 2010. "The End of Men." *The Atlantic*. July/August. http://www.theatlantic.com/magazine/archive/2010/07/the-end-of-men/308135/. Accessed March 23, 2011.

Rutter, Virginia. 2009. "Divorce in Research vs. Divorce in Media." *Sociology Compass* 3–4: 707–20.

Safer, Daniel, and Michael Malever. 2000. "Stimulant Treatment in Maryland Public Schools." *Pediatrics* 106 (3): 533–39.

Safer, Daniel, Julie Magno Zito, and Susan dosReis. 2003. "Concomitant Psychotropic Medication for Youths." *American Journal of Psychiatry* 160 (3): 438–49.

Saguy, Abigail. 2013. *What's Wrong with Fat?* New York: Oxford University Press.

Schaffner, Laurie. 2006. *Girls in Trouble with the Law*. New Brunswick: Rutgers University Press.

Scheff, Thomas. (1966) 1999. *Being Mentally Ill*. Piscataway, NJ: Transaction.

Schor, Juliet. 1999. *The Over-Worked American: The Unexpected Decline of Leisure*. New York: Basic.

Schwartz, Casey. 2012. "Generation Rx? Review of *Dosed: The Medication Generation Grows Up*." *Daily Beast*. April 15.

Schwarz, Alan. 2012a. "Risky Rise of the Good-Grade Pill." *New York Times*. June 9.

———. 2012b. "Attention Disorder or Not, Pills to Help in School." *New York Times*. October 9.

Scott, Ellen K. 2010. "'I Feel as If I Am the One Who Is Disabled': The Emotional Impact of Changed Employment Trajectories of Mothers Caring for Children with Disabilities." *Gender & Society* 24 (5): 672–96.

Sears, William, and Martha Sears. 2003. *The Baby Book: Everything You Need to Know about Your Baby from Birth to Age Two*. New York: Little, Brown.

Shah, N. R., J. B. Jones, J. Aperi, R. Shemtov, A. Karen, and J. Borenstein. 2008. "Selective Serotonin Reuptake Inhibitors for Premenstrual Syndrome and Premenstrual Dysphoric Disorder." *Obstetric Gynecology* 111 (5): 1175–82.

Shandra, Carrie, Carrie Spearin, and Dennis Hogan. 2008. "Parenting a Child with a Disability: An Examination of Resident and Nonresident Fathers." *Journal of Population Research* 25 (3): 357–77.

Shelov, Steven, and Tanya Remer Altman, eds. 2009. *Caring for Your Baby and Young Child: Birth to Age 5*. 5th ed. New York: Bantam.

Shelton, Deborah. 2012. "Autism Doctor Loses License in Illinois, Missouri." *Chicago Tribune*. November 5.

Siebers, Tobin. 2004. "Disability as Masquerade." *Literature and Medicine* 23 (1): 1–22.

Siegel, Bryna. 1997. "Parent Responses to the Diagnosis of Autism." In *Handbook of Autism and Pervasive Developmental Disorders*, 2nd ed., edited by D. Cohen and E. Volkmar, 745–66. New York: Wiley.

Siegel, Daniel, and Tina P. Bryson. 2011. *The Whole-Brain Child*. New York: Delacorte Press.

Siegel, Daniel, and Mary Hartzell. 2004. *Parenting from the Inside Out: How a Deeper Self-Understanding Can Help You Raise Children Who Thrive*. New York: Tarcher/Penguin.

Silverman, Ed. 2012. "J&J Sees Male Breasts and Quickly Settles Risperdal Suit." *Forbes.* September 11. http://www.forbes.com/sites/edsilverman/2012/09/11/jj-sees-male-breasts-and-quickly-settles-risperdal-suit/. Accessed August 5, 2013.

Singh, Ilina. 2013. "Brain Talk: Power and Negotiation in Children's Discourse about Self, Brain, and Behavior." *Sociology of Health and Illness* 35 (6): 813–27.

———. 2011. "A Disorder of Anger and Aggression: Children's Perspectives on Attention Deficit/Hyperactivity Disorder in the UK." *Social Science Medicine* 73 (6): 889–96.

———. 2005. "Will the 'Real Boy' Please Behave: Dosing Dilemmas for Parents of Boys with ADHD." *American Journal of Bioethics* 5 (3): 1–14.

———. 2004. "Doing Their Jobs: Mothering with Ritalin in a Culture of Mother-Blame." *Social Science & Medicine* 59: 1193–1205.

———. 2003. "'Boys Will Be Boys': Fathers' Perspectives on ADHD Symptoms, Diagnosis, and Drug Treatment." *Harvard Review of Psychiatry* 11 (6): 308–16.

Smardon, Regina. 2008. "Broken Brains and Broken Homes: The Meaning of Special Education in an Appalachian Community." *Anthropology & Education Quarterly* 39 (2): 161–80.

Smith, Marissa M. 2006. "Medicalizing Military Masculinity: Reconstructing the War Veteran in PTSD Therapy." In *Medicalized Masculinities*, edited by Dana Rosenfeld and Christopher A. Faircloth, 183–202. Philadelphia: Temple University Press.

Smith, Rosa. 2003. "Race, Poverty, and Special Education: Apprenticeships for Prison Work." *Poverty and Race* 12 (6): 1–4.

Smith, Tovia. 2012. "Schools Get Tough with Third-Grade: Read or Flunk." *All Things Considered*, March 5. Accessed April 24, 2014. http://www.npr.org/2012/03/05/147980299/tough-love-reading-laws-target-third-graders.

Smith, Vicki. 2001. *Crossing the Great Divide*. Ithaca: Cornell University Press.

———. 1990. *Managing in the Corporate Interest*. Berkeley: University of California Press.

Solomon, Andrew. 2008. "The Autism Rights Movement." *New York Times.* May 25.

Sousa, Amy. 2011. "From Refrigerator Mothers to Warrior Heroes." *Symbolic Interaction* 34 (2): 220–43.

Sowell, Thomas. 2001. "Drugging Children." TownHall.com. August 23. http://www.townhall.com/columnists/thomassowell/2001/08/23/drugging_children/page/full. Accessed June 10, 2014.

Spitzer, Denise, Anne Neufeld, Margaret Harrison, Karen Hughes, and Miriam Stewart. 2003. "Caregiving in Transnational Context." *Gender & Society* 17 (2): 267–86.

Sroufe, L. Alan. 2012. "Ritalin Gone Wrong." Sunday Review, *New York Times*. January 28.

Stacey, Clare. 2011. *The Caring Self: The Work Experiences of Home Care Aides.* Ithaca, NY: ILR Press.

Stacey, Judith. 1990. *Brave New Families.* New York: Basic.

Steinberg, Jacques. 2008. "Talk Radio Host Stands by His Remarks on Autism." *New York Times.* July 22.

Sterzing, Paul A., Paul Shapiro, Sarah Narendorf, Mary Wagner, and Benjamin Cooper. 2012. "Bullying Involvement and Autism Spectrum Disorders." *Archives of Pediatric & Adolescent Medicine* 166 (11): 1058–64.

Stone, Pamela. 2007. *Opting Out? Why Women Really Quit Careers and Head Home.* Berkeley: University of California Press.

Stone, Robin. 2004. "Mind over Matter: A Conversation about African American Mental Health." Interview with Annelle Primm and John Head. *The Crisis* 111 (6): 32–35.

Stracuzzi, Nena. 2005. "Parenting in the Age of Prozac." PhD diss., University of New Hampshire, Department of Sociology, Durham, NH.

Strohschein, Lisa. 2007. "Prevalence of Methylphenidate Use among Canadian Children Following Parental Divorce." *Canadian Medical Association Journal* 176 (12): 1711–14.

"Study Finds No Ritalin Link to Later Drug Abuse." 2003. *New York Times.* January 6.

Sunderland, Margot. 2006. *The Science of Parenting: How Today's Brain Research Can Help You Raise Happy, Emotionally Balanced Children.* New York: Penguin.

Swarns, Rachel J. 2012. "Testing Autism and Air Travel." *New York Times.* October 28.

Szasz, Thomas. 1974. *The Myth of Mental Illness.* New York: HarperCollins.

Tanner, Lindsey. 2012. "DSM-5: Psychiatrists OK Vast Changes to Diagnosis Manual." HuffPost Healthy Lives, *Huffington Post.* December 1. Accessed December 8, 2012. http://www.huffingtonpost.com/2012/12/01/dsm-5-psychiatrists-ok-va_n_2224507.html.

Tavernise, Sabrina. 2011. "Married Couples Are No Longer a Majority, Census Finds." *New York Times.* May 26.

Taylor, Verta. 1996. *Rock-a-by Baby.* New York: Routledge.

Thoits, Peggy. 1985. "Self-Labeling Processes in Mental Illness." *American Journal of Sociology* 91 (2): 221–49.

Thomas, Katie, and Michael Schmidt. 2012. "Drug Firm Guilty in Criminal Case." *New York Times.* July 3.

Thornton, Davi Johnson. 2011. *Brain Culture.* New Brunswick: Rutgers University Press.

Tone, Andrea. 2008. *The Age of Anxiety: A History of America's Turbulent Affair with Tranquilizers.* New York: Basic.

UCP (United Cerebral Palsy). 2008. *The State of Disability in America.* Life without Limits Project. Accessed December 31. 2010. http://ucp.org/.

"U.S. Approves Prozac for Treating Children." 2002. *New York Times*. January 4.

U.S. Census Bureau. 2012. *Profile America, Facts for Features, Mother's Day 2012: May 13, 2012*. CB12-FF.08. March 19. Washington, DC. 20233. Accessed December 2, 2012. http://www.census.gov/.

U.S. Department of Education. 2013. "Special Education Fiscal Year 2013 Budget Request." Office of Special Education Programs. Washington, DC. 20202–7100. Accessed July 1, 2013. http://www.ed.gov/.

U.S. Department of Health and Human Services, Health Resources and Services Administration, Maternal and Child Health Bureau. 2008. *The National Survey of Children with Special Health Care Needs Chartbook, 2005–2006*. Rockville, MD: U.S. Department of Health and Human Services.

Vallas, Rebecca. 2009. "The Disproportionality Problem: The Overrepresentation of Black Students in Special Education and Recommendations for Reform." *Virginia Journal of Social Policy & the Law* 17 (1): 181–208.

Ventura, Stephanie. 2009. "Changing Patterns of Nonmarital Childbearing in the United States." *NCHS Data Brief*, no. 18. Hyattsville, MD: National Center for Health Statistics, Centers for Disease Control.

Von Bergen, Jane. 2006. "Mastering ADHD on the Job." *Philadelphia Inquirer*. November 12.

Waldman, Ayelet. 2009. *Bad Mother*. New York: Doubleday.

Walkup, John, and Michael Labellarte. 2001. "Current Thinking: Complications of SSRI Treatment." *Journal of Child and Adolescent Psychopharmacology* 11 (1): 1–4.

Wall, Glenda. 2010. "Mothers' Experiences with Intensive Parenting and Brain Development Discourse." *Women's Studies International Forum* 33 (3): 253–63.

———. 2004. "Is Your Child's Brain Potential Maximized? Mothering in an Age of New Brain Research." *Atlantis* 28 (2): 41–50.

Walsh, Mary. 2008. "Judge to Unseal Documents on the Eli Lilly Drug Zyprexa." *New York Times*. September 6.

Wang, Wendy, Kim Parker, and Paul Taylor. 2013. "Breadwinner Moms." Pew Research, Social and Demographic Trends. May 29. Accessed July 28, 2013. http://pewsocialtrends.org/.

Warner, Judith. 2010. *We've Got Issues: Children and Parents in the Age of Medication*. New York: Riverhead.

———. 2005. *Perfect Madness: Motherhood in the Age of Anxiety*. New York: Riverhead.

Watters, Ethan. 2010. "The Americanization of Mental Illness." *New York Times Magazine*. January 10: 40–45.

Wen, Patricia. 2011a. "Some in Congress Look at Incentives in Disability Benefit." *Boston Globe*. January 18.

———. 2011b. "Disability Program, Concerns on Rise." *Boston Globe*. July 11.

———. 2011c. "Children's SSI Program Examined." *Boston Globe*. October 26.

———. 2010a. "Case Spotlights Disability System." *Boston Globe*. January 17.

———. 2010b. "Mother Convicted in Girl's Drug Death." *Boston Globe*. February 10.

———. 2010c. "A Legacy of Unintended Side Effects: Call It the Other Welfare." *Boston Globe*. December 12.

———. 2007. "Drugs Doses Called Threat, Treatment in Dead Girl's Case Alarms Doctors." *Boston Globe*. February 10.

Will, George. 1998. "Mothers Who Don't Know How." In *"Bad" Mothers: The Politics of Blame in Twentieth-Century America*, edited by Molly Ladd-Taylor and Lauri Umansky, 280–82. New York: NYU Press.

Williams-Searle, John. 2001. "Cold Charity: Manhood, Brotherhood, and the Transformation of Disability, 1870–1900." In *The New Disability History*, edited by Paul K. Longmore and Lauri Umansky, 157–86. New York: NYU Press.

Wilson, Duff. 2010. "Child's Ordeal Reveals Risks of Psychiatric Drugs in Young." *New York Times*. September 2.

Wilson, William Julius. 1998. "The New Social Inequality and Affirmative Opportunity." *WorkingUSA* 1 (6): 74–91.

Winters, Marcus, and Jay Greene. 2007. "Debunking a Special Education Myth." *Education Next* 7 (2). Accessed May 12, 2012. http://educationnext.org/debunking-a-special-education-myth/.

Wolf, Joan. 2011. *Is Breast Best? Taking on the Breastfeeding Experts and the New High Stakes of Motherhood*. New York: NYU Press.

Woolhouse, Megan. 2011. "World's Apart." *Boston Globe*. December 18.

Wyatt, Edward. 2004. "New Salvo Is Fired in Mommy Wars." *New York Times*. November 2.

Wymbs, B., W. E. Pelham Jr., B. S. G. Molina, E. M. Gnagy, T. K. Wilson, and J. B. Greenhouse. 2008. "Rate and Predictors of Divorce among Parents of Youths with ADHD." *Journal of Counseling and Clinical Psychology* 76 (5): 735–44.

Zito, Julie Magno, Daniel J. Safer, Lolkje T. W. de Jong-van den Berg, Katrin Janhsen, Joerg M. Fegert, James F. Gardner, Gerd Glaeske, and Satish C. Valluri. 2008. "A Three-Country Comparison of Psychotropic Medication Prevalence in Youth." *Child and Adolescent Psychiatry and Mental Health* 2 (26): 1753–2000.

Zito, Julie Magno, Daniel J. Safer, Susan dosReis, James F. Gardner, Lawrence Magder, Karen Soeken, Myde Boles, Frances Lynch, and Mark A. Riddle. 2003. "Psychotropic Practice Patterns for Youth." *Archives of Pediatric and Adolescent Medicine* 157 (1): 17–25.

Zito, Julie Magno, Daniel J. Safer, Susan dosReis, James F. Gardner, Karen Soeken, Myde Boles, and Frances Lynch. 2002. "Rising Prevalence of Antidepressants among U.S. Youths." *Pediatrics* 109 (5): 721–27.

Zuvekas, Samuel, and Benedetto Vitiello. 2012. "Stimulant Medication Use in Children: A 12-Year Perspective." *American Journal of Psychiatry* 169 (2): 160–66.

INDEX

ADD: ADD-ogenic culture, 25–26, 29, 238; attention deficit disorder, 1–2; diagnostic uncertainty in, 20–21, 216; gender disparity, 228; heritability,76; prevalence, 2, 6, 20; shamefulness, 124. *See also* ADHD

ADHD: adult use of medication, 130–31; attention deficit hyperactivity disorder, 6; causes, 147; diagnostic uncertainty in, 20–21, 216; gender disparate prevalence: boys versus girls, 23, 26; history, 10–11; mothers raising kids with, 15; prevalence, 20; only as initial diagnosis or starting point, 16, 21; shamefulness, 124; treatment, 31. *See also* ADD; Diagnoses; Invisible disabilities/disorders; Medications; Ritalin

Advocate: educational, 49–51, 55, 76, 122–23, 135, 147, 159, 199, 227, 245; Federation for Children with Special Needs, 49. *See also* Support, commodified

American Psychiatric Association: *Diagnostic and Statistical Manual of Mental Disorders* (DSM), 20, 69–70, 266n49

American Psychological Association: decrease in psychotherapy, 12

Asperger syndrome, 17, 27, 69–70, 149, 238, 266n45; shamefulness, 124–25

Autism, 6, 142; airplane travel with autistic children, 103; in cultural studies, 27; in disability studies, 19; extreme male brain hypothesis for, 27, 208, 279n63; gender disparate prevalence,

23; mothers causing, 5; prevalence, 20; violating gender binary, 27–28. *See also* Bettelheim, Bruno; Brain, gendered; Invisible disabilities/disorders

Bettelheim, Bruno: "refrigerator" mothers, 5, 167, 240

Big Pharma, 7, 15, 85, 127–28, 243, 249, 256, 258n14, 271n68–70; a New Economy industry, 242; in popular culture, 284n35. *See also* Medications; Prozac; Ritalin

Bipolar disorder, 69–71; medication, 128; prevalence among youth, 265n38

Bourdieu, Pierre, 94–96, 99, 152, 181–83, 257n3; Bourdieusian, 120. *See also* Capital

Brain: children's, 29–30; gendered, 24–25, 262n108; in mothers' accounts, 35–36, 63, 73–76, 83; heritable deficiencies racialized, 10, 210, 349, 252–53, 256; New Economy high-tech metaphors for, 2, 13, 53–54, 75; plasticity, 53, 242; in popular advice, 72–73. *See also* Autism; Em-brained; Eugenics; Neuroscience

Bullying. *See* Victimization

Bureaucracies: "bureaucratic gymnastics," 43; "bureaucratic hurdles," 153, 158; dense, 36, 38, 42, 55–56, 133, 145, 154, 174; and gatekeeping, 254; health insurance, 43–44, 263n8; lone bureaucratic rangers, 87–88

Capital: body capital, 95, 99–100, 132, 181–85, 207; cultural capital, 14, 32, 88, 94–96, 98–100, 103, 113, 118–19, 121–22, 132–33, 139, 144, 150, 174, 217–18, 230, 245–46, 249, 259n36; social capital, 94–96, 102, 120; transmission of, 92, 94–96, 98–100, 104, 107–8, 111–12, 114, 116, 133–34, 136, 183, 230, 245–46. *See also* Bourdieu, Pierre; Lareau, Annette

Caregiving; gendered, 8–9, 177, 179; inequities in, 80–83; kin provided, 158; shaped by larger social forces, 133

Care work, 29, 54, 79, 106, 133; national devaluation of, 152, 253–54; paid, 132, 242

Children: in danger versus dangerous children, 11; gendered ideals for, 23–24. *See also* Brain; Department of Social Services (DSS). *See also* Medicalization, of childhood

Children of color: heritable deficiency, 10, 258n25; raising, 210–36. *See also* Brain, heritable deficiencies racialized; Eugenics; Masculinity, Black; Masculinity, boys of color "adultified"; Racial disparities; Special-ed racial disparities

Chodorow, Nancy, 177–79, 201–2, 276n7

Civil Rights: advocates, 216; post–Civil Rights era, 218, 233; research, 227. *See also* NAACP

Class transmission. *See* Capital

Columbine High School shooting, 278n41; influence of, 191, 193, 196, 223

Complex ambivalence. *See* Medications, complex ambivalence toward

Conrad, Peter, 15, 259n40

Conservative: arguments about gender and invisible disability, 28, 133; authors, 177–78; similar to left-wing media, 13; similar to liberal voices, 28

Cultural differences argument, 212, 216, 231, 234–35. *See also* Special-ed racial disparities

Department of Social Services (DSS), 161, 165–75, 197–98, 203, 279n50

Diagnoses: Diagnostic uncertainty, 20, 58, 123–24, 201–3

Dialectic of biology and culture, 7, 27, 243, 250, 267n97

Disabilities: beyond the social model, 267n97; history of, as masculine, 24; race, class, and gender in, 24; services on college campuses, 247; the social-antidiscrimination model, 19. *See also*, Invisible disabilities/disorders; Visible (traditional) disabilities/disorders

Disability rights legislation, 5–6, 45, 47, 49, 270n52. *See also* Individual Education Plan (IEP)

Disability studies, 18–19, 68

Divorce. *See* Marriage

Dyslexia, 38, 53, 61, 124, 271n60

Educational system: accountability movement in, 30; competing authority with medical system, 38, 43–45, 53, 61–62; public investment in, 255–56. *See also* Bureaucracies; Individual Education Plan (IEP); Schools; Special-ed parent groups (PACs); Teachers

Em-brained, 5, 147, 241; disorders, 19, 125; differentiated from mental illness, 69–71. *See also* Brain; Invisible disabilities/disorders

Emotional disorders, 6. *See also* Invisible disabilities/disorders

Ethnoracial others. *See* Others

Eugenics: discourse, 10; movements and scientific racism, 210, 233; school sorting, 12, 249, 252

Families: changing family forms, 2,138, 140, 259n30; fatherless, 138, 166, 169, 174, 248; gendered norms within, 26; hard-living, 22, 139, 161–65, 261n81; 272n4; lack of public policy support

Linda M. Blum is Associate Professor of Sociology at Northeastern University. She is the author of *Between Feminism and Labor: The Significance of the Comparable Worth Movement* (1991) and *At the Breast: Ideologies of Breastfeeding and Motherhood in the Contemporary United States* (1999).

CPSIA information can be obtained at www.ICGtesting.com
Printed in the USA
BVOW02*1333220215

388716BV00001B/3/P